Ubiquitous Cardiology: Emerging Wireless Telemedical Applications

Piotr Augustyniak
AGH University of Science and Technology, Poland

Ryszard Tadeusiewicz
AGH University of Science and Technology, Poland

Medical Information Science Reference

MEDICAL INFORMATION SCIENCE REFERENCE

Hershey · New York

Director of Editorial Content: Kristin Klinger
Senior Managing Editor: Jamie Snavely
Managing Editor: Jeff Ash
Assistant Managing Editor: Carole Coulson
Typesetter: Amanda Appicello
Cover Design: Lisa Tosheff
Printed at: Yurchak Printing Inc.

Published in the United States of America by
Information Science Reference (an imprint of IGI Global)
701 E. Chocolate Avenue, Suite 200
Hershey PA 17033
Tel: 717-533-8845
Fax: 717-533-8661
E-mail: cust@igi-global.com
Web site: http://www.igi-global.com/reference

and in the United Kingdom by
Information Science Reference (an imprint of IGI Global)
3 Henrietta Street
Covent Garden
London WC2E 8LU
Tel: 44 20 7240 0856
Fax: 44 20 7379 0609
Web site: http://www.eurospanbookstore.com

Library of Congress Cataloging-in-Publication Data

Tadeusiewicz, Ryszard.
Ubiquitous cardiology : emerging wireless telemedical applications / by Ryszard Tadeusiewicz and Piotr Augustyniak. p. ; cm.
Includes bibliographical references and index.
Summary: "This book, intended for biomedical experts, introduces scenarios of development in the area of telemedicine in the near future, with applications extending beyond the medical aspects"--Provided by publisher.
ISBN 978-1-60566-080-6 (h/c)
1. Ambulatory electrocardiography. 2. Telecommunication in medicine. I. Augustyniak, Piotr, 1965- II. Title.
[DNLM: 1. Electrocardiography--instrumentation. 2. Electrocardiography--methods. 3. Cardiovascular Diseases--diagnosis. 4. Technology Assessment, Biomedical. 5. Telemedicine--methods. 6. Telemetry. WG 140 T121u 2009] RC683.5.A45T33 2009
616.1'207547--dc22

2008052454

British Cataloguing in Publication Data
A Cataloguing in Publication record for this book is available from the British Library.

Table of Contents

Detailed Table of Contents

This chapter summarizes new needs, new opportunities, new challenges, and new fields for development of innovative IT methods for permanent and ubiquitous cardiological monitoring. The main idea for new generation of telecardiological devices goes as follows: *Bad heart always under permanent qualified observation, and every ill patient never without help—irrespective of moment of time and place on Earth.* The method proposed in this book for accomplishing such a goal and realization of the presented idea is based on three elements:

- individual patients' heart signal acquisition kits;
- advanced wireless communication equipment; and
- intelligent cardiological data analysis centers, based on the semantic-oriented and CI (computational intelligence) powered Web solutions.

This section offers a makeshift evaluation of the amount of information collected by a distributed personal cardiological data acquisition system, multiplied by the

The interoperability of diagnostic equipment is presented as an important aspect of patient safety. Since many diagnostic techniques are based on trends and series analysis rather than on single measurement, the independence of data from the equipment- or manufacturer-specific technical issues is crucial. The international initiative Open ECG is mentioned as an example of efforts towards interoperability.

This section offers a brief overview of the scope and structure of the proposed ubiquitous cardiology system. Included are specifications for the client terminal, the connection, and the software of the remote reader, along with considerations regarding the supervising center and central services.

The cardiac surveillance system for ubiquitous cardiology assumes the optimization of ECG signal interpretation justified on both medical and technical backgrounds. Consequently, in response to the changes in these aspects, the management software is supposed to continuously revise the interpretation task assignment between the remote PED and the central server. This section offers important criteria for this optimization, along with limitations and advantages of the proposed ubiquitous cardiology system.

One of the principal concepts introduced in the authors' research is the notion of optimal patient description. This and other scientific research areas needed for the proposed system to succeed are offered in this section.

The investigation of the local spectrum of the ECG signal is a common 'technical' approach to the temporal datastream variability. Several methods, including Short Term Fourier Transform and wavelets, were used to estimate the local spectrum of the ECG. The literature review and original authors' research results are presented in this section, along with highlights of their advantages and drawbacks.

The output-oriented approach of the ECG datastream assessment is based on the diagnostic parameters. The parameters set is weighted according to importance, and the resulting measure is used to correlate the diagnostic result deviation with the frequency and occurrence time of local bandwidth reduction. The main advantage of such an approach is the modulation of transmission channel requirements driven by diagnostic parameters derived automatically.

The perceptual approach to the informative contents of the ECG signal assumes the analysis of observer gaze points during the manual inspection of the trace. The examined study yielded several general rules on how the cardiology expert perceives the electrocardiogram and revealed important steps in human reasoning. The results of this research are applied to estimate the ECG signal features from medical findings and measurements of the waveforms.

The ECG signal contains some cardiac-independent components and represents the heart activity with limited reliability. The processing is based on many heuristics, expected signal features, and general knowledge, and implies an additional uncer-

The remote interpretation as a subscriber service needs two areas of data security to be considered, as outlined in this section. First is patient privacy and consistency of raw data, and the returned report. Second is the server security and immunity to the erroneous signal, network violation acts, or attempts to unauthorized access.

The prototype Internet service for diagnosis based on T wave dispersion was set up and afforded the authors an opportunity to meet several technical constraints for this idea. This section presents the small-scale network experimental results.

This section presents technical limitations of remote wearable recorders. These come mainly from high expectations of mobility and manifest themselves by short autonomy time, low computational power, limited resources, and the physical size.

Interpretation software is usually designed in the static mode and fulfills average diagnostic requirements in the average patient. The aim of personalization of interpretation software is to provide accurate information of the highest relevance depending on the variable status of the patient. A secondary benefit is uniformization of devices at the design and manufacturing stage, and customization by the software when in use according to patient-specific features.

This section describes further reprogrammability of the remote device lying in replacement of diagnostic procedures via wireless connection. The supervising center manages the remote device resources and puts to work the most suitable diagnostic procedures to derive an expected diagnosis. The interpretation chain

The common rule that a patient's examination frequency depends on his or her status has no analogy in automated diagnostics. This section proposes a medically justified modulation of reporting frequency implemented in a client-server cooperation model. The supervising center analyzes the incoming messages and other conditions, and issues the desired reporting interval back to the remote device. As a result of the authors' tests and simulations, this method may reduce wireless channel use and increase remote autonomy up to three times.

This section describes the common approach to the ECG interpretation, assuming the parameters are updated each time the input data are available. The heartbeat detector runs for each acquired sample, and arrhythmias are checked immediately after a positive detection of a heartbeat. This approach keeps the diagnostic parameters up to date at the cost of heavy computations. Slowly changing parameters are significantly oversampled, and consecutive values show high redundancy.

As mentioned in Chapter X, each diagnostic parameter has a specific update interval. Non-uniform reporting assumes the parameters are calculated and reported only by the end of validity of previous values. In this approach the computation costs are much lower without significant influence to the diagnostic quality, as long as the parameter-specific update frequency (or validity period) is set correctly. Besides the economy, this approach provides an advantage of modulating the update frequency of the patient status.

This section presents the concept of a packet-content manager. This procedure collects all requests concerning diagnostic parameter update and computation, supervises the propagation of validity attribute backwards through the processing chain, and provides an exceptional pathway for all abnormality alerts emerging in the processing chain. In the result, all parameters are reported as rarely as possible without breaking the Shannon rule—that the sampling frequency may be individually modulated in wide range depending on the patient's status, and computation costs are reduced providing longer autonomy.

Doctors are often considered conservative, but they are slowly moving towards the acceptance of the ubiquitous cardiology system because it has many advantages—some from the doctor's point of view. These advantages are discussed in this section.

The most important part of the ubiquitous cardiology system is the Central Station, equipped with a main computer, intelligent software, advanced communication devices, as well as a team of best cardiologists who can deal with any problem. From the patient's point of view, the system under consideration can be identified with the personal device described in this book—the PED. Acceptance and good assessment for the whole system depends on the PED's features, which are discussed in this section.

One aspect of novelty in the ubiquitous cardiology system is the evolution of the role of the human expert. He or she is no longer bored by the multitude of regular cases that affect his or her acuity to the emergency. All physiological records and most common pathologies are serviced automatically, leaving to a human expert only the unusual cases. The section addresses how doctors get a filtered set of difficult patients, and how they are required to consider them more carefully with a significantly higher level of expertise.

It is evident that once the ubiquitous cardiology system is born, it will become the target of attacks by traditional hospitals. In every hospital, every cardiological

Foreword

It is an honour to have been invited to write some words of introduction to this unique book. The authors and the publisher initially, somewhat graciously, suggested that this Foreword could be of sizeable length but the writer is of the view that you, the prospective reader, would rather move on to the meat of the text than spend a great deal of time reading this introductory commentary!

The authors have taken, as the basis of their book, a Personal Event Detector, or PED, which is a device for cardiac monitoring. In the first instance, this could be applied to individuals with certain forms of heart disease who are at higher risk of a cardiac event and who stand to benefit from this technique. Given the concept of sudden cardiac death in hitherto apparently healthy individuals, there might even be a case for suggesting that the whole population over a certain age should be continuously monitored, although this is really futuristic.

The authors have cleverly built the various sections of the book around various aspects of how a PED can be developed and utilised. This then allows a wide ranging review of the concept from the obvious generation of an electrocardiographic signal, through recording, analysis and interpretation to the point where an automated warning of an unusual finding can be transmitted to a central clinic where appropriate action can be initiated. The more sociological aspects of the concept are considered, including how such a technique could be funded through to the consequences of having a global system for cardiac surveillance.

Within each section of the book, the reader will find a review of relevant techniques and references to important publications and guidelines in the area under discussion.

The authors themselves suggest that the book should be of interest to researchers and manufacturers working in the field of cardiovascular monitoring, physicians/cardiologists with an interest in telemedicine, administrators interested in the future development of home care technology and finally, students of biomedical engineering. While there is the occasional section dealing with some of the more mathematical aspects of signal processing, the book is highly readable for the non mathematician. Thus, the text is very clearly within reach of a wide spectrum of readers.

The authors take an interesting look back at their childhood of the 60s at which time they looked ahead to the 21st century with many thoughts of "spacemen" and impressive communications throughout the universe. While some of these concepts might have been considered speculative at that time, they are nowadays reality. Similarly, there might be a degree of scepticism at the present time about the concept of Personal Event Detectors and the thought of many individuals being monitored centrally, with concern over false alarms and how a central monitoring station could handle multiple events occurring within a relatively short space of time. However, it might be as well to take the long view and think how the population of 2050 will be treated medically. The PED could be built today but nanotechnology enhances the prospects for development of extremely small, cheap PEDs capable of all of the functions discussed in this book. This writer does, however, wonder how increasing numbers of elderly individuals, with consequent increase in requirements for monitoring, could be handled in a realistic way. However, a lot can happen in 40 years and perhaps even the much talked about Polypill will reduce the problem of premature death from coronary heart disease though on the other hand, it might simply postpone such events without obviating the need for monitoring.

The information provided in this book will enable the reader to draw his or her own conclusions about the techniques involved in event monitoring and reach a personal conclusion as to its merits.

I would congratulate the authors on their novel approach to producing this text and on bringing together a wealth of information in the field. I am delighted to recommend this book to those potential readers previously listed – not to mention medical administrators and politicians who ultimately might be called upon to consider whether or not to provide the funding to support the concept.

Peter W. Macfarlane,
Professor of Electrocardiology,
University of Glasgow,
Glasgow, Summer 2008.

Preface

When I recall my first memories of kindergarten, I remember the drawing competition about Poland and the world in the year 2000. Because the date seemed so far away, the expectation of substantial change was evident. To be honest, some people were wearing antennas on their heads, but almost all our sketches were about space conquest and not about human life.

Now this magic date is behind us, and we—the children of the '60s—were right in having predicted the communication era for the year 2000; but we are not children anymore. Now, as engineers, we are responsible for the communication era. It manifests itself by the numerous applications of communication technology that exist, first in military and then in civilian life. Digital television and voice telecommunication, the Internet, global positioning systems, and global reference of time are the most common examples. We, the consumers of the early 21st century, are witnesses of the communication era.

Once more we—the children of the '60s—were right…unfortunately. In the communication era there is much attention on entertainment, on commerce and publicity, but still there is very little concern about human life. Who are we? The civilization that cares more about the primitive shows and worldwide games than about our health? Are we really responsible or are we still in our childhood?

Fortunately, the communication era already made its first marks in healthcare as well. We are witness to the triumphal spread of the idea of telemedicine all around the world. The use of modern technology for medical applications is a domain of fascination for both young engineers and young doctors; moreover it conquests little by little the buildings of old hospitals and the minds of traditionally educated physicians. Each year, computers and digital information-based solutions are more present in healthcare institutions and become more usable to doctors, who no longer must provide health using their own hands. Getting familiar with a computer considered as a diagnostic or surgical tool of the 21st century is not easy for doctors. In fact it is difficult from the technological point of view, because the service and maintenance of modern electronic and computer-powered medical devices demands education in information technologies. But more difficult is the adaptation of the traditional medical point of view and traditional habits of physicians to the new role of distribution between doctors, patient, and technical devices. We, the engineers, really appreciate the effort of medics, as we share their sense of responsibility. It is surely not the business of entertainment anymore.

Computers are also present in our homes. Surprisingly they are similar machines based on the von Neuman scheme, as used 30 years ago in military or civil calculation centers. In a common belief they are associated with serious things only, like scientific research, economical forecasting, and development of new technologies. In the '60s of the last century, everybody could imagine a spaceship with computers on board, but nobody could imagine a refrigerator with a computer build in. Nevertheless at the beginning of 21st century, advanced electronic devices and computers became general-purpose equipment of everyday use. The owner of a computer is currently not necessarily a scientist or a business analyst. Computers are very common as entertainment centers, home information resources, and communication tools. A simple reason for this comes from the fact that computers became available and acceptable during the past two decades. The secret of availability has its explanation in mass production and low price. What other smart device can be so cheap at the same time? Mass production achieved success thanks to the deep software customization of personal computers. And thanks to proper computer software development, this general-purpose device is a typewriter for a literate, an encyclopedia for an adolescent, a sampler for a music composer, a home studio for a digital videographer or photographer, and finally a newspaper or a means of communication for a bored housewife.

Acceptability is historically linked to ease of operation. Console-based operating systems are now reserved for professional computer systems administrators, while a significant majority of users prefer graphical interfaces designed with respect to human performance. Engineers adopt their design for merit correctness and technical effectiveness, but usability is a second important prerequisite.

This book is about medical devices, not about computers—though to tell the truth, almost every modern medical device today includes a build-in computer.

Nevertheless, the authors' wish is to follow the example of computers, which come from temple-like computational centers to the kitchen. Computers, originally used for very serious problems only (like designing new rockets or calculating bank accounts) and now available to help children with their homework and to help home cooks collect recipes, smoothed the way for home care devices.

With the progress of medical education in societies, people need medical devices designed with regard to patient performance—the devices must be cheap and commonly available. Today, cardiology monitors are symbols of restricted-to-professional intensive care units and their use is commonly associated with serious, even life-threatening situations. In the future, we believe a small cardiological recorder may be worn as a watch, but instead of speeding up our heart, it will make it safe. The authors' intention is that the new generation electrocardiographic device, described in this book under the name of PED (patient electronic device), will provide essential information and warnings about the most crucial cardiovascular system of our organism and will be commonly accepted in every house, even for personal use. The PED is intended to be used as an individual patient's heart signal acquisition kit integrated with a communication device, which can automatically call an emergency service in case of patient heart failure. Therefore it must be as cheap and as easy to operate as the mobile phones of today. The user in pain does not have to be concerned with the details of the recorder's operation, but instead must be provided with fast and reliable help.

THE CHALLENGE

The ubiquitous cardiology system is expected to be with a patient continuously and simulate the presence of his or her doctor, even during a trip far away from home. Fulfilling this task requires the personal recorder PED to be mobile and integrated as a part of a network. This seems difficult, but the example of mobile phones shows that it is possible. However, the medical knowledge embedded as ECG interpretation software demands much more computational power than voice processing performed by handsets. This limits the autonomous (performed by the PED itself) applications of personal cardio-monitors. With the use of wireless communication, the performance of the PED can be supported at any time with the data analysis performed by the SuSe (supervising server)—a large and powerful computer in the Central Station, which is a kernel element of the whole system's architecture. In most difficult cases, the distant care of the patient can be provided by the doctors employed at the Central Station as consultants. In the case of emergency, the appropriate service can be called automatically for direct help to the patient.

Another limitation for the ubiquitous cardiology system is the availability of the wireless connection. The data transmission is highly dependant on atmospheric or terrain conditions, and in remote areas the link quality may be very weak. In such cases the device must rely on the embedded intelligence, and therefore simple ECG recorders transmitting the unprocessed ECG over a digital link are not applicable.

Doctors are our natural choice as colleagues, as we work on the frontier between medicine and technology. Inspired by the relations between the doctors we took on the challenge to design and partly prototype a system intended to resemble the cardiologist or the cardiologists' group behavior much more than contemporary systems do. We believe that these relations, established through the history of medicine, are optimal and worth investigating and implementing into an automatic network-based surveillance system.

These investigations are addressed in this book. As a consequence of our early results, we designed and prototyped a limited-scale surveillance system that demonstrates the technical feasibility of a global scale cardiac surveillance network. The advantage of the prototype is the use of emerging but already matured technologies. We strongly hope that our findings will inspire other engineers to search for more human-oriented designs and also convince medical scientists to accept a new approach to diagnostic data considering reliability, uncertainty, and risk management issues.

PURPOSE OF THE BOOK

The authors of this book are scientists and engineers with some medical background working in biomedical engineering. Therefore we hope to find a common language with four groups of prospective readers:

- technology researchers and manufacturers working in the area of medical applications;
- medical doctors, in particular cardiologists involved in telemedicine;
- managers of caregiving institutions seeking future development of home care systems; and
- students of biomedical engineering, in particular those interested in electronic systems, telecommunication solutions in biomedicine, and dedicated information systems.

The book may be useful for experts aiming to predict the scenarios of development in the area of telemedicine in the near future, with applications extending beyond the medical aspects, intended for everyday personal use. Medical devices are currently considered high-tech, requiring highly qualified operators. Such opinion assumes the equipment is restricted to use in hospitals or doctors' offices, hindering the widespread use of artificial intelligence and telemedicine in home care. Though the devices are not reserved for outpatient use—or for use with impaired and elderly patients—these do seem to be quite a significant target group and therefore constitute a promising market. But our aim is to stimulate growth of common interest in general personal health, which would open up a nationwide market for personal health monitors responding to both needs: owner curiosity and personal safety. Healthy people could also be a target market for dedicated medical products in the future, as they are for entertainment products today.

In our opinion this book should stimulate some medical research and normalization in the field of diagnostics. Several drawbacks of methods currently in use are pointed out thanks to our metrological aspects. The conformance of the software and expert-derived diagnosis is judged from the results, instead of the similarity of data processing. This approach needs huge databases of human-annotated examples to provide the reasonable reliability of the software. For some rare diseases, the collection of a sufficient number of samples is difficult, making progress very expensive. The second issue is the absence in medical data of attributes commonly used in metrology to assess the data reliability in the value (e.g., amplitude) and time domains. We therefore seek to investigate the variability of the diagnostic parameters over time, and consequently to set the validity period for each parameter type. This would be the analogy of a Shannon theorem in medical measurements.

This book may also be useful for engineers as inspiration for their research on non-uniform systems. In electrical engineering and metrology, the assumption of data uniformity is a kind of sacrifice and thus is very rarely challenged. This can be partially explained, but not justified by the reason of commodity, since the theory of uniform data processing was established a century ago, and its counterpart concerning non-uniform data involves some modern mathematics. Our application shows that the non-uniform approach better simulates human behavior and due to the flexibility is much more suitable for adaptive systems. We are certain that this remark holds far beyond the cardiology for other automatic systems that are expected to replace and mimic human organs.

After introductory chapters presenting some known issues, we turn to more complicated matters. Therefore our primary reader is expected to be the technical and medical scientist or the advanced student. The authors hope, however, that this will not narrow the audience and that the future-oriented reader will also find this book interesting.

ORGANIZATION OF THE BOOK

The book is organized into two sections. Section I (Chapters II, III, and IV) presents the current state of the art in selected domains connected to telemedicine and computerized cardiology. Section II (Chapters VI, VII, VIII, IX, X, and XI) presents original achievements of the authors: the investigation of data uniformity and priority, the design and prototyping of system elements, and the validation of results. The remaining chapters (I, V, and XII) play the role of braces, justifying the research, and explaining the results applicability and the social impact of the proposed solutions. A brief description of each chapter follows.

Chapter I presents new needs, new opportunities, new challenges, and new fields for development of innovative IT methods for permanent and ubiquitous cardiologic monitoring. The authors present the general idea of an ECG recording device that is mobile and safe, thanks to the use of soft computing featuring high adaptability to the patient and to diagnostic needs.

Chapter II introduces basic concepts of electrocardiography—the anatomy and physiology of the heart, highlighting electrophysiological phenomena. This chapter also reviews computer procedures used to interpret the signal, and it presents basic regulation and example requirements on testing the performance of medical devices and software.

Chapter III presents the cardiovascular system as complicated, vulnerable, and very important to the organism, and it introduces the cardiovascular disease as the primary cause of mortality in developed countries. (In some counties, it is secondary only to cancer). The current state of the art of long-term monitoring is presented, followed by a short review of contemporary computer networking and digital communication technologies.

Chapter IV reviews the current issues concerning databases as reservoirs of data storage, retrieval, and interchange systems. The specificity of medical applications of the databases is highlighted as a result of the multitude of data modalities and the role the databases play in current information technology-based societies.

Chapter V stresses the need for an alternative approach to home care, personalized healthcare, and prevention in cardiology, and defines main postulates for the intelligent distributed surveillance system. Such a system benefits from current communication technology, agile software engineering, control theory, and from the observation of interpersonal relations. Three main aspects of novelty highlighted are:

- the experimental derivation of cardiologists' knowledge,
- the use of dynamic re-programmability, and
- the definition of additional data attributes setting their medical relevance.

The authors reveal differences in data handling between technical and medical measurements, and point out some areas for medical research concerning data quality and uncertainty.

Chapter VI presents investigations and results concerning the distribution of medical information in the ECG signal. Following a common belief in the medical relevance aspect, certain signal parts are more informative than others. We propose several methodological variants for quantitative measurement of the local signal relevance. The chapter ends with a proposal of application of the scan-path analysis for objective assessment of personal interpretation skills.

Chapter VII addresses various aspects of improvements in a typical ECG processing chain. Particular procedures designed for the computation of specified diagnostic results are usually developed as a result of long research projects and are rarely disclosed as a source code. Without challenging well-established methods, we tried to optimize the data flow and minimize the propagation of computational errors.

Chapter VII presents the idea of medical information interchange networks providing the signal and possibly image interpretation services. The proposal of distributed interpretation challenges the current definition of telemedicine because the software, instead of the human, is supposed to be the main agent in the network. The prototype of QT dispersion analysis service is presented as an example, with all the related technical issues.

Chapter IX presents new solutions for dynamic task distribution in a mobile client-server cooperation. The authors present the prototype PDA-based ECG-oriented recorder supporting the agile interpretation software and the adaptive reporting format. The optimization of the patient description is an issue of particular concern, since it drives the interpretive software adaptation. The chapter also provides results for detailed analysis of technical conditions of task relocating, as well as for the analysis of erroneous decisions and their consequences.

Chapter X discusses various forms of adaptive ECG reporting, which is a consequence of the modulated software functionality and variable status of the patient. The authors postulate a new approach to the diagnostic parameters time series and consequently investigate the validity time for main components of the ECG diagnostic report. The concept of non-uniform reporting is presented with the concern of regularization of the reports.

Chapter XI presents the concept of "on request" ECG interpretation. This idea assumes the data recipient calls for new measurement results at the end of current data validity. The request is propagated backwards to the front-end procedures, but considerable calculation and transmission savings are made on the metadata of long validity. This concept defines several unexploited concepts for further research, but is the closest to human reasoning when a doctor is giving the care to his or her patient.

Chapter XII concludes and presents principles of the Emerging Wireless Telemedical Applications used for ubiquitous cardiology in home care, risk assessment, and cardiovascular prevention. The authors consider issues of acceptance, availability, and social impact of the system and network, simulating the continuous presence of medics with the patient in motion.

Acknowledgment

This book presents results of our everyday scientific work for years; therefore, the authors would like to acknowledge the help of the AGH University of Science and Technology in Krakow, Poland, which financially supported the scientific research described in this book under the grant number 11.11.120.612. Countless people in the University helped us working as contractor researchers, colleagues, students or administrative emploees. It is very fascinating in the university (probably in any university in the World), that everybody can contribute by asking a pertinent question.

From outside of the University, we greatly appreciate the help of Professor Paul Rubel from INSA/INSERM-ERM-107, Lyon, France. He reviewed and constructively corrected the chapter concerning the CSE Database and initiative. Moreover, being three times a visitor to INSERM, Piotr Augustyniak experienced unforgettable hospitality and an atmosphere of collective work in an international team. We also wish to acknowledge the help of Andrzej Wrzesniowski PhD, president of Aspel SA., Poland's biggest manufacturer of the ECG equipment. Disregarding the risk of benefit for his own enterprise, he allowed implementing and testing of some of our unusual ideas in industrial conditions. Thanks to this experience, we were close to cardiologists, patients, industrial programming and science at the same time.

Special thanks also go to the publishing team at IGI Global, whose contributions throughout the whole process from inception of the initial idea to final publication have been invaluable. In particular to Julia Mosemann and Jessica Thompson who both supervised the project for two years motivating us, the authors, to concentrate and work hardly instead of putting our fingers to many things else. Our particular thanks goes, however, to Julia for her perfect solution concerning linguistic correction when our means were out.

Thanks to Maria Boyer, first for accepting the invitation for helping the book in its critical point and second, for not permitting our book to appear to the eyes of readers as it was first proposed. Let us keep confidential how much work and knowledge was required to organize our ideas to a readable English message.

Special thanks go to Peter Macfarlane, Professor of Electrocardiology and the President of Computers in Cardiology Inc. for his review of a semi-final draft of the manuscript and for many helpful suggestions for enhancing the book's content. His contribution to this book is much greater than the foreword, the reader may notice.

The authors thank the International Electrotechnical Commission (IEC) for permission to reproduce information from its International Standard 60601-2-51 ed.1.0 (2003). All such extracts are copyright of IEC, Geneva, Switzerland. All rights reserved. Further information on the IEC is available from www.iec.ch. IEC has no responsibility for the placement and context in which the extracts and contents are reproduced by the author, nor is IEC in any way responsible for the other content or accuracy therein.

In closing, we wish to thank our families for their patience and care continued even if sometimes we returned home still speaking a language of signal processing.

Piotr Augustyniak,
Ryszard Tadeusiewicz,
Krakow, Poland
November 2008

Chapter I
Introduction

This chapter summarizes new needs, new opportunities, new challenges, and new fields for development of innovative IT methods for permanent and ubiquitous cardiological monitoring. The main idea for new generation of telecardiological devices goes as follows: *Bad heart always under permanent qualified observation, and every ill patient never without help—irrespective of moment of time and place on Earth.* The method proposed in this book for accomplishing such a goal and realization of the presented idea is based on three elements:

- individual patients' heart signal acquisition kits;
- advanced wireless communication equipment; and
- intelligent cardiological data analysis centers, based on the semantic-oriented and CI (computational intelligence) powered Web solutions.

This chapter provides a makeshift evaluation of the amount of information collected by the distributed ECG data acquisition system multiplied by the expected number of patients. The results show that the total amount of data circulating in the system can be very large. The most important question is how to manage such huge information streams when the total number of physicians (especially professional cardiologists) employed in the system must be limited. The proposition of a multilayer system architecture will be described, in which two lower layers can interpret the common everyday records in a fully automatic way, and the middle layer, powered by artificial intelligence and based on a large amount of medical knowledge stored in the cooperating expert system, can solve many problems of an average level of diagnostic difficulty. The most difficult problems must still employ human experts.

INTRODUCTION

In this book we describe a biotechnological system, discovered, designed, and developed by the staff of the Biocybernetic Laboratory at the AGH University of Science and Technology, Krakow, Poland. The system under consideration can help many people suffering from heart diseases. Using our system, the patient can be mobile and be safe at the same time. Let us describe the problem and propose our solution.

Until now the patient with a serious heart problem had to be under the continuous control of diagnostic equipment and under the supervision of medical personnel. It was not necessary to engage medical care experts on a full-time basis, but at least one qualified nurse had to be concerned about the results of heart parameter recordings (provided by electronic sensors and monitors) in order to make decisions in the case of emergency. With serious cardiac problems, such a model must be continuously applied according to the intensive care regime expecting a sudden event. Therefore, patients with serious heart problems, even those who were feeling well, are hospitalized and subject to permanent observation.

But there are many other patients suffering from cardiac diseases of moderate severity. Such a patient can return home, can work, can walk—but his or her heart must also be observed all the time. Even if the probability of a crisis is very small, its occurrence can be very dangerous. Therefore, these patients must be observed all the time, although this observation not need be overly intensive.

Permanent observation is easy in patients' homes (by family members) and in stable workplaces (by coworkers). But when an ill person must travel, the problem becomes more complicated. Nowadays, people travel often for business and leisure. Modern businessmen, journalists, scientists, engineers, moviemakers, and many other professionals sometimes are called "contemporary nomads," because traveling makes up a large part of their lives. If this form of activity concerns the person with a cardiac disease, mobile surveillance systems have the opportunity to play their role.

It is evident that during a journey and when staying in new places with new people around, the ill person can be exposed to several dangers. His or her heart can fail at any moment without any alerting symptoms, but in an alien environment nobody will notice and a sick person can die.

In such difficult situations the only solution that can be provided is through modern technology. Therefore, we formulated the project based on this phrasing:

Your heart is with you always and everywhere.

Take the monitoring device always and everywhere with your heart, expecting a failure!

We planned to design a system in which *every heart at risk will always be under permanent qualified observation, and every ill patient will never be without help—irrespective of time and place.* This goal was very ambitious, and we had to formulate and solve many problems of scientific, technological, and also medical natures before we could reach it.

After six years of research and development, described in detail in papers listed in the bibliography at the end of this book, we have a working prototype of such a system. Describing its structure, principles, and functions is main purpose of this book.

At the beginning we can stress that although the total system is large and complicated, the basic principles can be explained clearly in a few words. The first assumption is:

Every patient can carry a small and cheap electronic device called the PED. Depending on the preferred technology, it can be a personal handheld computer, a cellular phone, a business organizer, and so forth. The PED contains its own software, which can continuously interpret the patient's heart activity, recorded with the use of wearable sensors, and help the bearer in case of emergency in various ways:

- The PED can serve the patient by giving him or her appropriate advice (e.g., "stop working" or "don't hurry") in the case of small heart problems reported by part of the system. Sometimes it can be enough to help the patient in the simplest situations. Consulting with the doctor's prescription registered in its memory, the PED can recommend to the patient an increase or decrease in the dosage of a particular drug and also tell him or her to take some specific pill exactly at a specified moment.
- When the problem with a patient's heart is complicated, the PED uses automatic wireless consultation mode with a large reference computer in the Central Station. Such a large and well-equipped computer, called the SuSe (supervising server), is in fact the kernel of the whole system under consideration. The

SuSe is part of the Central Station, where best decisions or best advice can be elaborated in almost unrestricted environment in the case of more complex situations. An important part of the Central Station are the well-educated doctors with long and good experience in cardiology who work as the "last line of defense."

- The highest expertise of doctors should be used only in rare circumstances. In typical situations, even if the PED reports rather complicated cardiological problems, the central computer finds an appropriate solution in an automatic way. This is very important, because if thousands of patients are connected via their own PEDs to one Central Station, the effectiveness of the doctors giving 'handmade' diagnoses and 'individually prepared prescriptions for treatment' can be dramatically insufficient. Automatic finding of adequate diagnosis and proper therapy will be faster and much more reasonable. The proposed solution is feasible because the SuSe is more powerful than the PED. Its power, expressed by computational speed and total processing performance, allows the use of more complicated algorithms based on artificial intelligence for solving patient problems. Moreover, the SuSe records a history of every patient, therefore his or her up-to-date situation can be considered and automatically evaluated with reference to the archival results. The SuSe can also solve many practical problems using the content of large medical databases, which can be efficiently searched and explored by means of fast disk devices. Taking into account a large cardiology database with many samples of symptoms recorded for the particular patient and other persons, as well as information about the best treatment examples (proven by the results of therapy), the SuSe can be very efficient. Analogy-based automatic reasoning can be very helpful in automatic solving of the problems reported by the PED of a particular patient. It can work in ways similar to some computer programs for chess players (like *Deep Blue*), which are based not only on artificial intelligence backgrounds, but mainly on a 'brutal force' approach, which uses a large database of millions of chess games. Similar to the chess program selecting the best move on the basis of past experiences, a similar approach can be applied for the selection of the best treatment and therapy for a particular patient on the basis of thousands of similar examples taken from caregiver databases.
- Artificial intelligence-based cardiological data analysis, as well as searching in medical databases, can be insufficient for extremely complicated situations. Therefore, it is very important to implement into the SuSe test procedure and criteria for recognition the situations when the automatic system must 'give up' and ask the human doctor for help. Initiated by the SuSe, consultations with qualified medical doctors (employed in the Central Station) should be very rare,

but must be taken into account when automatic analysis of the patient status fails. Even for a powerful computer in the Central Station system, finding a proper solution using automatic procedures or database searches cannot be guaranteed.

- All activities listed above are based on a remote analysis of the cardiological data collected and processed by the PED and the SuSe, and takes into account providing a remote therapy based on helpful advice and instant procedures. In some cases it is not enough. Such situations can be detected by the PED itself if the state of a patient becomes critical. Otherwise, this decision can be made by the central computer when the exact analysis of the patient's state, performed in the SuSe, shows that the situation is dangerous. Intervention can also be taken by the doctor, used as the last resort. In all these cases, the automatic wireless alerting of an appropriate medical emergency service is performed, using the data about the patient's current and previous medical situation, and taking into account his or her precise location (the PED can have this information both from the cellular phone network and from the GPS system). The decision made by the system can take into account automatically calculated distances from the rescue station and the current patient position, as well as the specific competences and/or specific equipment possessed by the particular emergency service teams, because sometimes the nearest does not mean the best.

From the properties defined above for the PED, we see a fundamental element of the design—missing from many personal electronic devices dedicated to patient use—is the central system, powered by a large computer named the SuSe. This equipment offers effective communication for the permanent exchange of information between all personal devices of all patients registered in the system. An added element is the employment of highly qualified specialists (cardiologists) who can help if the technological equipment fails.

Additional features of the described system include:

- Patient devices are equipped with a set of sensors, which can simultaneously observe the heart activity of a patient. In experimental devices used in the research phase of the system design, the contact between the PED and patient's body is based on a set of traditional electrodes located on the patient's chest using typical medical technology and connected to the PED by means of a system of wires. In the final version, the system must be equipped with a more comfortable method of data collection. Wearable sensors with dedicated preprocessing units (for conditioning and compression of signals) are planned in the final release. They use short distance wireless communication devices (e.g., Bluetooth) for sending data between the sensors and the PED processor.

- When the PED cannot solve the problem and contacts the SuSe for help in signal interpretation, as a response two streams of information are pushed from the SuSe to the PED. The first is devoted to solving the present problem. The patient needs advice and/or other types of help, and the SuSe must force the PED to carry out all the necessary activities. The second stream of information is the software modification for the PED processor. If the problem was too hard for the PED and it must ask the SuSe for help, it suggests that the present software located in the PED is not optimal: or the previous version of the PED software was out of date, or the status of the patient has become more complicated, or even a new cooperating SuSe is now selected and provides a new algorithm not available before. Nevertheless, of the cause and reason, the result is the same: the PED needs new software and the SuSe can send it.
- When the SuSe cannot solve the problem on the basis of algorithms and examples retrieved from the database, a doctor from the Central Station staff is asked for assistance. The result of the query in the form of a whole interpretation procedure performed by the doctor is stored in the SuSe system's central memory for further reuse in similar situations. This means that the system under consideration can be classified as the learning one.
- The personal computer of every particular patient can also learn on the basis of current events happening with the patient heart. If some activity was successful in a particular situation in the past, the same activity should be performed in circumstances classified as similar to the previous one. An additional form of PED learning is connected with the forced software modifications described above.

HOW CAN WE MANAGE THE FLOOD OF TELE-CARDIOLOGICAL DATA?

Every human heart is a source of a large amount of information. The datastream produced by the PED sensors can be estimated on the basis of digital ECG record volumes. For example, the records from the Massachusetts Institute of Technology-Beth Israel Hospital (MIT-BIH) database are sampled at 360 samples/second. For many purposes the sampling rate must be higher; for simple calculations let us consider 500 samples/second. Every sample is coded without compression in two bytes, and for full information about the total electrical activity of the heart, an eight-channel recording is necessary. It results in the datastream volume of 8 kilobytes/second per patient.

The system under consideration will be useful and properly defined both from the social and economic point of view, if it can serve for at least 10,000 and preferably 100,000 patients. This means approximately 100 to 1,000 megabytes/second of total source information capacity. Such an amount of data is no problem from a communications perspective, because contemporary wideband wireless telecommunication channels have enough efficiency. Moreover, most of the PEDs operated by patients can use different channels, therefore the occurrence of the "bottleneck effect" in this part of the system is not probable.

Although from the point of view of the SuSe, where all datastreams from all patients meet and must be analyzed simultaneously, such a large stream of data can cause several problems. Even if the central computer is a mainframe and is of supercomputer class (which is not a good solution because such large computers are very expensive), such a stream of information cannot be processed and analyzed in real time. This can lead to delays in answering, which are not acceptable in telecardiological applications. Therefore, the distributed processing of patients' signal analysis seems to be the only reasonable solution.

According to our assumptions, most of the recorded signals should be interpreted directly in the PED systems. This can also be performed in real time if processors mounted in the PEDs are small and cheap, because the front edge processing of the raw ECG data will be performed separately for every patient. If the result of this preliminary processing shows that the patient's heart works properly or if it detects a problem, that software located in the PED can solve the problem—the communication between the PED and the SuSe will be limited to a short message, meaning 'all right'.

Only when a serious and difficult problem is encountered on the level of preliminary analysis performed by the PED processor does the datastream of the information exchanged between the PED and the SuSe increase. First, the PED is sending a short alert signal to the central computer. The central computer rearranges the time schedule of continuous processing of all data from all the PEDs and reserves a larger quantity of its time for the processing and analyzing of a raw ECG signal coming from the alerting PED. Next, detailed information about the heart failure is sent from the PED to the SuSe and is the basis for advanced analysis at the Central Station. During this 'emergency action' all signals from the other PEDs are only occasionally processed (mainly only archived for complete documentation) unless the SuSe solves the signaled problem.

For illustrative purposes, the scheme sketched above is simplified. In practice during the processing of one 'emergency alert', another 'emergency signal' may happen. Therefore, a central computer must have an advanced scheduling system with priority services and apply a fast and accurate input filter, in order to select the most important (e.g., most dangerous) input signals from all the information sent by the PEDs. Especially the emergency rescue actions must be performed in a fast and accurate way. Therefore, the realization of the proposed system is closely connected with the solutions of problems, including artificial intelligence software, new methods of automatic signal processing, data analysis, valuable information extraction, and—last but not least—automatic decision making.

The necessary efficiency of the whole system is also a problem worth considering. Particular attention must be paid to very restrictive reduction of datastreams on every level of the system, but also by algorithms used in the system (especially by the SuSe) which must be optimized according to time efficiency.

With system growth, the number of patients can increase very quickly. A prototype single-kernel network can be managed by the most powerful computer in the Central Station and by means of software optimization. Nevertheless, when the system becomes very large, the two-layer structure (which includes only the PED layer and SuSe layer) cannot be efficient enough. Therefore, the next version of the system must be designed with the PED layer, the multiple-kernel layer of many SuSe subsystems (located for example according to the regional organization of the system, depending on an average number of patients predicted in particular regions), and one main control module. This supervisory layer is not involved in ECG interpretation, but is only responsible for the coordination of the work of the whole system, load-balance between local SuSe subsystems, and central distribution of the data (e.g., if a patient moves from one location to another, his or her historical data must be transferred from one SuSe subsystem to another). The twice-distributed organization of the system (one is distributed on the PED level and one is distributed between the local SuSe subsystems) can be very difficult for control and optimization, but only such complicated systems can be effective on a worldwide scale and face the permanently increasing needs of the patients.

HOW ABOUT MONEY?

At the end of this chapter we try to present some calculations, estimating how a described system, dedicated to the intensive and ubiquitous monitoring of cardiac-related parameters of many people simultaneously, can be applied in practice from an economic point of view. As described in previous sections, the system is rather complicated and its elements seem to be expensive. In fact, such modern and advanced technology can be cheaper than one may expect.

Let us cost the particular elements. Personal electronic devices must contain at least three subsystems: an ECG signal acquisition and processing subsystem, a cardiac data analysis subsystem, and a wireless communication subsystem. The two latter modules can be based on solutions already widely used in personal organizers, wireless connected palmtops, and also larger cell phones. This means that such elements, produced for mass application, although complicated in structure and equipped with very advanced technological elements, can be inexpensive because of the "scale effect."

The first part of the PED, closely connected with cardiological measurements only, cannot be produced on a very large scale, so it may be more expensive. Reduction of production costs can be achieved by using typical elements already used in other areas of biomedical technology applications—for example in hospital or telemedical systems. Moreover, it is possible that the whole cost or at least most of it will by paid by GSM, UMTS, LTE, or even the next generation of digital communication providers. They usually support such gadgets as built-in cameras. The application of smart-ECG modules is clearly increasing the providers' interest at the minimum risk level. The practical implementations of the ubiquitous cardiology system will increase the demand for wireless telecommunication and in the future will be a large source of income for all wireless communication providers.

After a short introductory period, new electronic (digital) heart signal recorders used in PEDs, as well as advanced wireless communication technologies used in whole systems, will become very popular and therefore inexpensive. At the beginning of the system implementation, typical ECG acquisition modules can be used, which are rather inexpensive. If the system becomes more popular, a dedicated wearable cardiological data acquisition system must be designed, because the maintenance of typical medical signal acquisition elements can be too complicated for many patients. The prototypes of wearable cardiological sensors (featuring communication with the data collection system via Body Area Network) are now too expensive. But if such technology becomes preferred by patients as especially easy to use, and if it becomes more popular, the prices will come down quickly. Therefore, we estimate the total cost of a PED (paid by the patient) as reasonably low.

Also the central part of the system, based on multilayer Web-based advances in computer architecture, can be very cheap when counting cost *per capita,* because of a huge number of users. Even if the central computer (the SuSe) is a large mainframe (or a supercomputer) equipped with a very fast disk storage system, powerful communication devices, and an advanced doctor alerting subsystem, we must take into account that such a singular system will be used by thousands of patients over many years. Counting one patient for one period (let say, one month) of the remote cardiological monitoring, the cost can be respectively low.

Summarizing all the facts and anticipations mentioned above, we can formulate this thesis:

Ubiquitous cardiology is a new opportunity in the wireless world, which can be properly designed from a technological point of view, successfully applied from the medical point of view, profitably used by many patients, and—last but not least—not very expensive.

In the chapters that follow, we attempt to explain step by step how the ubiquitous cardiology system is organized, how it works, and how to solve many scientific, technological, medical, psychological, and sociological problems connected with its implementation.

Let's start!

Chapter II
Background 1: ECG Interpretation:
Fundamentals of Automatic Analysis Procedures

This chapter briefly introduces the basic concepts of electrocardiography—the anatomy and physiology of the heart, highlighting the electrophysiological phenomena. This technical overview recalls facts concerning the heart action, only as far as it creates the background necessary for future technical considerations. Therefore, the origin of the signal and the principles of medical interest in electrical heart action representation are put forward. Particular attention is paid to physiological limitations of the signal variability, since this concept is a key for assessment of the limited signal predictability and expected local bandwidth. These terms, not yet common in the everyday ECG description, are a background to the auto-adaptive telemonitoring system proposed as a scientific challenge in Chapters VII to XI.

This chapter is organized as follows. It begins with principles of human ECG interpretation and fundamental algorithms for automated ECG interpretation. Examples of commonly used heartbeat detectors are discussed in the context of real-time and off-line processing. Basic concepts of clustering of QRS complexes follow, in the context of rhythm classification. The wave measurements technique, being the most complex procedure in the processing chain, decides the overall performance of the ECG interpretation and therefore is also considered in detail, using original research results of the authors.

Another interesting subject is a review of selected specialized procedures dedicated to arrhythmias detection, heart rate variability analysis, and ischemiae symptoms extraction. This part of the book is also based on the original research performed by the authors and gives the reader an idea of precision and reliability expected from the basic diagnostic parameters. These parameters are used for investigating the heartbeat sequences in aspects of alteration of active stimulus generator, rhythm stability, and control performed by the balance of sympathetic and parasympathetic nervous systems. Due to the dynamic nature of investigations in the area of cardiology itself, it is hardly possible to give an accurate and well-balanced description of diagnostic parameters currently in use. The actual choice of diagnostic methods applied depends on the latest medical communications, available tools, and in particular on the patient status. This last dependence is widely exploited in the proposed auto-adaptive system, which we expect to behave like a doctor much more than any other currently available solution.

At the end of this chapter we present tools and methodology used for the performance assessment of automatic ECG interpretation procedures. The databases with reference signals and annotations are discussed in the context of statistical methods used to validate software performance. The chapter is concludes with references of international standards (IEC) and conformance tests used to validate the requirements for safety and accuracy of commercial ECG interpreting software.

ORIGINS AND FUNDAMENTALS OF THE ELECTRICAL CARDIAC ACTIVITY

The Electrocardiogram as a Representation of the Heart Function

This chapter does not pretend to be a source of medical knowledge in cardiology, but to give some insight about ECG generation and recording, and its main characteristics, and highlight the clinically meaningful information that can be extracted from the ECG.

The electrocardiogram is the paper or digital record of the cardiac electrical activity. In most cases it is taken at the body's surface via a noninvasive and painless procedure, not implying discomfort to the patient and extremely cheap compared with other methods to assess heart function. The intracardiac recordings and other modalities are reserved for use in specialized cases and will not be discussed in this book.

The electrocardiogram has been extensively used in clinical medicine for more than 80 years, and is now a primary diagnostic tool for many cardiac and other diseases (Fisch, 2000; Van Mieghem, Sabbe, & Knockaert, 2004).

It is recorded as a temporal representation of the electrical field resulting from the electrical activity of the heart muscle issue at the cell level. By using several electrodes placed on the skin, it is possible to access several simultaneous aspects of spatial phenomena, known as electrocardiographic leads.

Due to their electrical nature, some congenital heart abnormalities and thickness or damage in the heart muscle are just two examples of the many diseases that may be detected and diagnosed prior to or during heart attacks (myocardial infarction). Cardiologists may also notice evidence of acutely impaired blood flow in the heart.

Abnormal electrical activity of the heart is detected as an unusual representation of particular elements of the heart cycle in time or amplitude. Such variations of externally measurable electrical parameters are caused by too fast/slow or irregular rhythms and abnormal generation or conduction of the cardiac electrical impulses. Specified changes in some of these parameters may represent life-threatening conditions, therefore the evaluation of the cardiac rhythms is a problem of major importance.

As far as the importance of the cardiac diagnosis being recognized, the systematic diagnosis concerned the considerable percentage of populations, and new disease-oriented modalities of the ECG were implemented into clinical practice. The use of automatic analysis systems was found essential in two ways:

- interpretation efficiency, namely in cases of very long records and for automatic preselection of events and suspicious signal segments for further analysis performed by a cardiologist; and
- standardization of the interpretation process which was systematized in the global scale in order to avoid the inter and intra observer variability.

The electrocardiogram of today is interpreted manually (or better said, visually) only in rare cases in which the software fails to give the right solution due to unusual disease, unstable recording conditions, or inconsistent results. The interpretation software is currently implemented as firmware in a wide range of stand-alone bedside ECG recorders and as general-purpose operation system-based interpretive workstations in the cardiologists' offices. The second implementation benefits from the large computational capacity usually available on personal workstations and gives the cardiologists an opportunity for interaction.

The Origin of the Electrocardiogram

The heart is the principal organ in the vascular system which is propelling the blood and consequently assuring the transportation of substances throughout the body.

The heart has two upper chambers (atria) collecting the blood at each beat and sending it to the lower chambers (ventricles) that pump the blood to the vessels of the circulatory system. The chambers on the right side feed the pulmonary circulation with venous blood to be oxygenated and the left side receives the arterial blood from the lungs and pumps it to all other parts of the body (Wagner & Marriott, 1994).

Living cells present a negative electrical potential at relaxation state (~90mV) and are quickly depolarized by the electrical stimulus. This voltage variation acts over compressible and electrically excitable proteins inside those cells, producing mechanical contraction of the heart muscle. The spreading of the electrical wavefront causes the contraction in muscular cells, which results in changes in chamber volume.

In order to pump the blood effectively, the mechanical phenomena of muscular contraction and distraction is repeated, perpetually initiated by the electrical activation and recovery of the myocardial cells that constitute the cardiac muscle. A specialized system provides initiation and synchronization of different muscular areas in order to allow correct timing between atrial and ventricular contractions as well as simultaneous contraction of muscle fibers filling each heart chamber. The wall of the heart consists of three different structures: an internal membrane (endocardium), a middle muscular layer (myocardium), and an external serous membrane (pericardium).

In physiological cases, a heartbeat is electrically initialized by a group of cells located in the upper part of the right atrium, known as sinoatrial node (SA), having the ability of a spontaneous discharge.

The resulting wavefront is spread through the atrial paths and stimulates contraction of both atria, forcing the blood into the ventricles. The electrical impulse is conducted, with an approximate speed of ca. 4m/s through the atrioventricular pathways (Bachmann, Wenckebach, and Thorel bundles) being physiologically the only structure capable of transmitting electrical impulses from atria to ventricles. In the atrioventricular node, the wavefront is delayed about 120 ms due to significantly lower electrical conductivity (ca. 0,05m/s). Within this time, the content of atria (ca. 400 ml of blood) is moved to the ventricles through the atrioventricular valves. The large size of ventricles is compensated by the existence of specialized conducting pathways (Purkinje fibers) that accelerate the propagation of the electrical wavefront, allowing the efficient pumping of the blood throughout the whole body (Wagner & Marriott, 1994; Malmivuo & Plonsey, 1995). After the depolarization the cells are not immediately able to receive or transmit a new electrical stimuli unless the relaxation potential is not rebuilt up to –65 mV. In consequence the stimulation wavefront dies down after achieving the latter cell of the heart muscle tissue. This mechanism prevents the spontaneous action of the heart muscle parts without the control of the sinoatrial node. The refractory period (approximately 200 ms) represents the biologically possible minimum interval between two heartbeats (Iyer et al., 2006; Rolls et al., 2006).

The ECG signal corresponds to the different action potential (AP) curves, representing the electrical activity over time in each heart region accumulating at the body surface. As described above, the propagation of the electrical wavefront is appropriate for several heart regions that are stimulated at different stages of the cardiac cycle, producing AP curves with corresponding characteristics. Each heartbeat is typically represented by the sequence of five principal waves known as P, Q, R, S, and T, as illustrated later in Figure 2.3, corresponding to different cardiac phases (Garibyan & Lilly, 2006):

- The atrial activation (depolarization) produces a small amplitude smooth wave denoted as the P wave, marking the beginning of a new beat.
- The ventricular activation results in a group of three sharp waves known as the QRS complex, composed of an initial small wave Q (depolarization on the wall between the ventricles), followed by a dominant bigger wave with opposite polarity R (depolarization on the left ventricle external wall), and a small wave appearing in the end finishing the ventricular activation S (depolarization of upper part of ventricles).

Figure 2.1. Fundamentals of anatomy of the heart conductive system

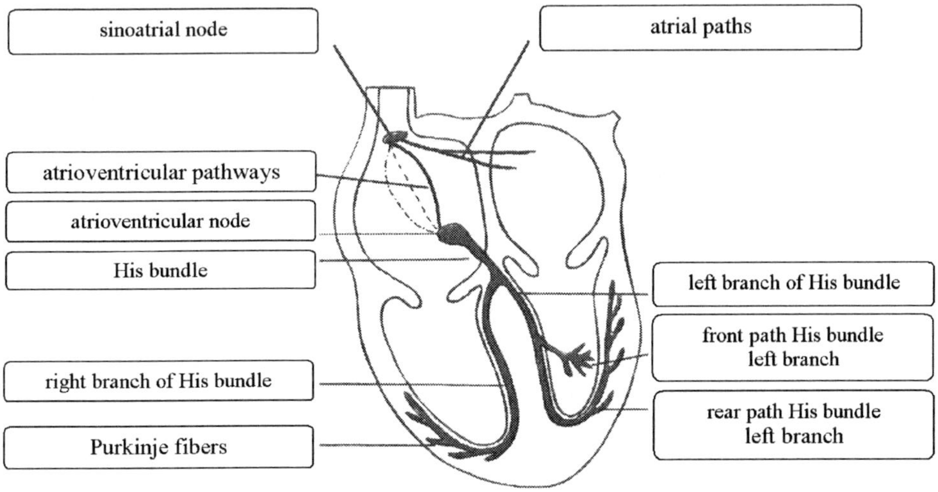

- The ventricular repolarization (recovery) is represented by a smooth T wave of variable morphology, sometimes followed by an extra small U wave of unknown origin.

Due to the standardized positions of recording electrodes, the polarity of the waves reflects the spatio-temporal projection of the electrical field vector to the segment determined in the space by the heart center and the electrode position (unipolar derivatives: Goldberger, Wilson) or two electrode positions (bipolar derivatives: Einthoven, Frank). The P wave can be positive, negative, or biphasic (with two subsequent peaks of opposite polarity). In the QRS complex, the first negative wave is named the Q wave, the first positive wave is referred to as the R wave, the second negative deflection as the S wave, and the second positive deflection as R' (CSE Working Party, 1985). The dominant wave is positive in physiological case in all Einthoven derivatives, and for that reason this group of waves is known as the QRS complex, regardless of actual content.

The T wave can show any of the morphologies—positive, negative, bimodal, biphasic—or even be only an upwards or downwards deflection (corresponding to a baseline-level change). Opposite of the P wave, which is not present in cases of ventricular-originated heartbeats, the T wave is always present after the QRS complex, however in some leads it may hardly be visible. The recovery of the atria is not noticeable in the ECG as a separate event, because of simultaneous occurrence with the dominant QRS complex (Garibyan & Lilly, 2006).

Lead Systems

According to the dipole hypothesis, the electrical activity of the heart can be approximated by a time-variant electrical dipole, called the electrical heart vector (EHV). Thus, the voltage measured at a given lead is merely the projection of the EHV into the unitary vector defined by the lead axis (Malmivuo & Plonsey, 1995).

This is a theoretical basis for using an orthogonal 3-lead system, allowing the recording of vectocardiogram (VCG) as a canonical representation of EHV given by a three-dimensional record. Although the electrical activity has some non-dipolar components, this approximation is widely used as spatial representation of the ECG. According to the dipole hypothesis, any hypothetical lead can be synthesized by an adequate projection of the VCG. This allows synthesizing the signals of one lead system from the recordings made with a different lead system (Dower, 1984; Levkov, 1987). The corrected Frank system is the most used orthogonal system. It is based on three orthogonal body axes defined from the observer point of view as right-to-left (lead X), head-to-foot (lead Y), and front-to-back (lead Z).

The lead set most widely used in clinical practice is a standard 12-lead system (Wagner & Marriott, 1994; Malmivuo & Plonsey, 1995). Despite its redundancy, it reflects the history of electrocardiography and is widely supported for the convenience and habits of experts. Although all leads acquire the signal being a projection of the same electrical phenomena, the waves morphology (shape) and amplitude depend on the lead position with reference to the heart position. For the same reason, different aspects result in various durations on the electrical phenomena reported from each lead viewpoint. Thus, depending on the spatial orientation, a wave can raise up or fall down in one lead before another, and even not be visible at all. In the 12-lead system, the leads span two orthogonal planes:

- The frontal plane, the vertical plane corresponding to the thorax of a standing individual, contains the three limb bipolar leads (named I, II, and III after Einthoven) and three augmented unipolar leads (named aVL, aVR, and aVF after Goldberger).
- The transversal plane, the horizontal plane that crosses the thorax orthogonally to the frontal plane, contains the six precordial unipolar leads (named V1, V2, V3, V4, V5, and V6 after Wilson).

Taking as origin the heart location on the thorax, each lead is defined by a vector that gives the direction along which electric potentials are measured. Symmetric vectors (with reverse polarity) correspond to symmetric ECG signals. Different lead

Figure 2.2. Electrode placement for the standard 12-lead electrocardiogram

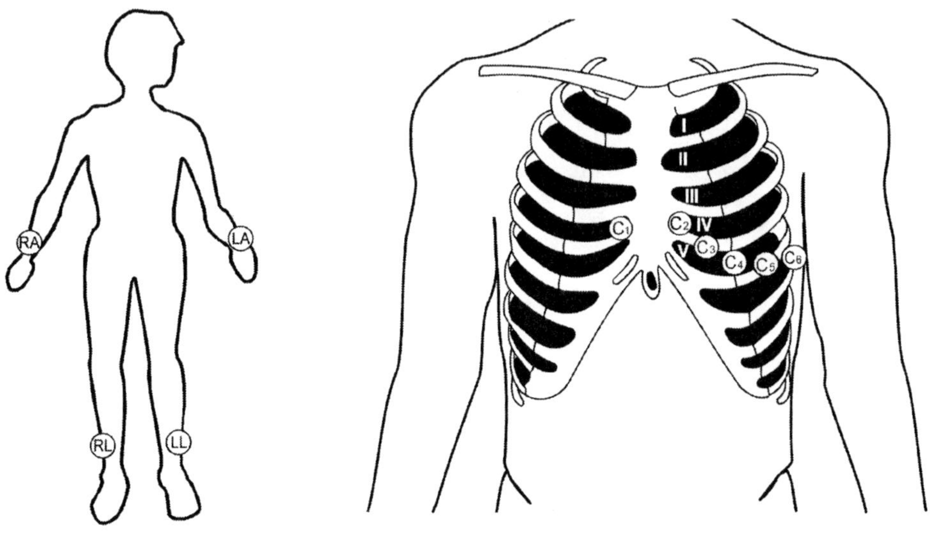

systems have been proposed and used for clinical and investigation purposes—from orthogonal 3-lead systems to the extremely redundant body surface mapping using as many as 80 or 120 leads. The relations between the leads of the standard system are used to recover all limb leads from any two of them basing on a Kirhoff law. This helps avoid the transmission and storage of redundant signals. Another linear transformation was defined by Dower (1984) and Levkov (1987) to derive the Frank orthogonal system (VCG) from the 12-lead system and vice versa. In terms of the lead axis, the Frank leads correspond respectively to leads I, aVF, and -V2, but the X, Y, and Z leads are constructed taking into consideration the distortions caused by the boundary and internal inhomogeneities of the body (Malmivuo & Plonsey, 1995).

The Clinical Use of ECG Modalities

Contemporary ECG usage is no longer a single technology, but developed different modalities. Depending on the patient condition and diagnostic hypothesis, the recording can be done in several different ways (Malik & Camm, 2004; Sörnmo & Laguna, 2005):

rest ECG	12-leads short time recording of simultaneous ECG leads on a lying down position	is commonly used to diagnose permanent conditions
exercise stress test	12-leads ECG + blood pressure rest phase (5 min.) followed by exercise protocol defining the applied workload during the stress phase and recovery phase (up to 15 min.)	aims to study the heart's ability to cope with increased need of oxygen resulting from the normative physical work
Holter monitoring	ambulatory 3- or 12-lead ECG, using a portable recorder; typically 24-hour records are obtained, covering all sorts of daily routine activities, including sleep, awake, moderate exercise such as walking, etc.	to analyze situations of transient symptoms, long-term regulatory mechanisms, pacemaker functions, drug influence, etc.

Except for the subject's heart condition, the ECG signal also reflects other body conditions such as electrolyte abnormalities (Van Mieghem et al., 2004). Also, the heart as a part of the cardiovascular system is closely related to respiration. Both systems are under the control of the autonomic nervous system (ANS), which relays the involuntary coordination and control of the basic body functions. ANS is responsible for the organism global response to external stimuli and for adapting the body functions to the needs inherent to different activities (such as sleep, digestion, exercise, etc.). It has two components with antagonistic functions: the sympathetic system, which rules the functions' activation, and the parasympathetic system, which rules relaxation states. The correct working of the physiological functions and the survival of the individual depends on the balance between these two subsystems (Franchini & Cowley, 2004). Using ECG recording, specific tests can be performed with the particular goal of testing the ANS condition.

As the electrodes are placed on the body surface, the recorded ECG reflects the conductivity of tissues crossed from heart to skin. The different structures in the thorax causes anisotropic propagation of the electrical field, producing changes in

Figure 2.3. Correspondence of cardiac cycle components and their representation in the ECG

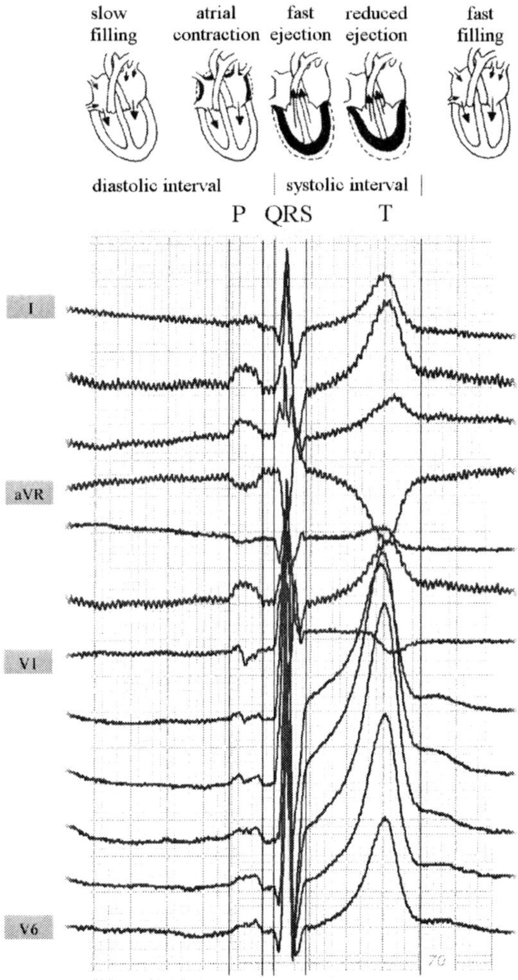

the signal that need to be taken into consideration for its interpretation (Gulrajani, 1998). Also, the ECG is likely to be affected by extracardiac electrical fields, either of biological origin (other muscular activity) or external (electric power interference) and events such as electrodes' contact liability, which can produce artifacts or signal loss. Clinical ECG commonly presents high levels of noise and interferences, in particular for life-recorded signals, making its visual study difficult and subjective. Automatic systems avoid inter and intra observer variability, can easily deal with large amounts of data, and much of the processing can be done in real time. Thus automatic systems are currently referred to as an indispensable tool for today's electrocardiography.

Temporal relations (durations) of the heart's electrical phenomena and their variations over time are parameters of primary clinical relevance. Since these phenomena correspond to subsequent ECG waves (fig. 2.3), their durations can be measured as time intervals between adequate fiducial points on the ECG, such as peaks (maximum or minimum of a waveform), onsets (departure from the baseline level), and ends (return to the baseline).

Except for detailed description of the heart muscle behavior during each beat, low variations of cycle-based parameters are also considered as clinically very important, because they reflect heart regulatory processes. Such sequences of interval measures, indexed to the heartbeat, are known as cardiovascular series. The RR interval series (tachogram) and the QT series are particularly important. The RR series is currently used as a heart rate signal and expresses the cardiac rhythm.

Physiologically the beats are generated by the SA node under the ANS influence. The abnormal heartbeats can be initiated by other cells instead of the SA node (ectopic focus) or be produced by pathogenous conduction of the electric wavefront. If the heart rate or the coordination between atrial and ventricular contractions is

Table 2.1. Fundamental heart intervals

interval name	interval measure	related physiological event
RR interval	time interval between consecutive R waves	ventricular cycle duration
PP interval	time interval between consecutive P waves	atrial cycle duration
PQ interval	time between the onset of the P wave and the onset of the QRS complex	atrio-ventricular delay
QT Interval	time between the onset of the QRS complex and the end of the T wave	total duration of the ventricular depolarization and repolarization

severely affected, the efficiency of pumping can be at risk, and potentially fatal situations can occur. Abnormal QT interval length and beat-to-beat variations are associated with several pathological conditions and increase risk factor. These series differ significantly in terms of mean value and variability level.

Pursuit of Depolarization Effects

Although the physiological cardiac cycle initiates with the atrial activation, the RR interval is commonly used as the cardiac cycle duration (Task Force of the ESC/ASPE, 1996) instead of the interval between the consecutive P waves. The RR interval is easier to measure due to the dominance of QRS over the smooth shape of the P wave. The heart rate (HR) is defined as 60/RR and expressed in beats per minute (bpm). The heart rate reported or displayed for diagnostic purposes is usually the average value of seven consecutive RR intervals. Excluding two shorter and one longer intervals from the averaging increases the HR report stability in the presence of missing or extra detections. The instantaneous HR and its beat-to-beat variations (HR variability, or HRV) have been studied for many years, particularly in the framework of investigation of the ANS balance.

The rate of normal sinus rhythm (NSR), triggered at rest by the sinoatrial node in humans, lies between 60 and 100 bpm (Zaret et al., 1999; Rolls et al., 2006). The rhythm variations are modulated by the autonomous nervous system (ANS) according to the expected need of oxygen from the organs. In periods of stable HR, there are small beat-to-beat variations that result from the balance between the sympathetic system and the parasympathetic system. For this reason any pharmacologic agent that acts over ANS functions also influences the heart rate (Rolls et al., 2006). Lower rhythms (sinus bradycardia, below 60 bpm), resulting from the prevalence of a parasympathetic system, occur in states of deep relaxation or in athletes with enlarged stroke volume. Higher rhythms (sinus tachycardia, above 100 bpm) are caused by the dominance of a sympathetic system and appear during physical effort or mental stress.

Physiologically, the sinoatrial node SA is the structure with the highest discharge rate, and the generated stimulus propagated through the heart discharges other structures of the conductive system including those showing the pacemaking ability. If the normal pacemaker is decelerated, an ectopic pacemaker is not externally discharged within its own automaticity period and can take over producing an escape beat. Another pathology lies in shortening the discharge time in automatic cells not belonging to the SA node. The discharge appears earlier than the ANS-modulated stimulus would be generated and propagates through the heart conductive system discharging muscle fibers and the sinoatrial node. Such a premature beat, called ectopic beat, can occur frequently in healthy subjects without any serious consequence (Rolls et al., 2006). However, the prevalence of ectopic beats makes the ANS inefficient and also seriously affects the pumping efficiency because of lack of coordination of the contraction and relaxation of the cardiac chambers. If the SA node is permanently malfunctioning, an artificial pacemaker needs to be implanted to ensure a correct heartbeat (Batsford, 1999).

Uncoordinated discharge, except for premature beats, may also lead to very serious rhythm abnormalities, as ventricular tachycardia (rapid heartbeat initiated within the ventricles) or even ventricular fibrillation that usually evolves in death in a few minutes, unless not interrupted by an external electric discharge (McPherson & Rosenfeld, 1999).

The electric conduction can also be altered as a result of reduced conductivity of the tissue (blocked area) that delays (partial block) or inhibits (total block) the stimulus propagation. Damaged areas result frequently from a myocardial infarction (heart attack). The implantation of an artificial pacemaker can be necessary to substitute the damaged pathway and restore the coordination of ventricular contraction. Delayed conduction may also result in an asynchronous refractory period of adjacent cells. As a result some recovering cells receive the delayed impulse as if it were a new beat. In this case the electric impulse can even be spread backwards (reentry phenomena) causing dangerous arrhythmias (McPherson & Rosenfeld, 1999).

Investigation of Ventricular Repolarization

Pathological electric conduction cannot only change the cardiac rhythm, but it also affects the duration of each cardiac phase. In particular, ventricular repolarization alterations have been reported in situations of increased risk by Extramiana et al. (1999a), Lass, Kaik, Karai, & Vainu (2001), Pellerin et al. (2001), Valensi et al. (2002), Cuomo et al. (2004), Milliez et al. (2005), among others.

Therefore, despite averaging the ventricular electrical activity of the whole heartbeat, the QT interval is currently considered an index of the ventricular repolarization (VR) time. Variations of this interval have high predictive value for stratifying the risk of malignant ventricular pro-arrhythmicity or even sudden death (Gaita et al., 2003; Yap & Camm, 2003).

The QT interval measure relies on the correct location of both QRS onset and T wave end. The technical problem of precise measurement of T wave boundaries is caused by its smoothness and shape varying through the channels. Consequently, the same stands for many other indexes for VR characterization that also require the location of T wave boundaries, including T wave area and symmetry.

Some approaches use alternative VR measures relying on Tapex (wave peak) instead of T wave end location. The use of the RTapex interval to assess VR is based on the assumption that the cardiac cycle length dependence of VR is concentrated on the early portion of the QT interval (Stramba-Badiale, Locati, Martinelli, Courvillet, & Schwartz, 1997). However, in spite of being easier to measure, RTapex presents even shorter length than QT interval, which additionally reduces the variability range and ignores fluctuations in VR that mainly affect the last part of the T wave. Thus:

- The interval T apex to T end was reported as independent of HR and QT (Merri et al., 1989; Benhorin et al., 1990).
- The interval from T peak to T end represents transmural dispersion of repolarization and therefore may be considered as an index for arrhythmic risk (Yan & Antzelevitch, 1998).

Electrocardiogram and Respiration

The pulmonary respiration cycle consists of inspiration and expiration performed alternately and is controlled partly by the ANS and partly voluntary as long as the subject is awaken. The mean respiratory frequency is taken as the inverse of the mean respiratory cycle duration and usually lays slightly above the 0.15 Hz (Yasuma & Hayano, 2004). The respiration is closely related with the ECG, and several methods were proposed to derive the respiratory curve from the electrocardiogram (Moody, Mark, Zoccola, & Mantero, 1986; Bailón, Sörnmo, & Laguna, 2006a, 2006b). The common points of these two signals (fig. 2.4) are:

- Lung expansion and contraction during the respiratory cycle change the heart position and consequently the electrical axis within the chest, resulting also in scaling and rotation on the ECG. Thus respiratory activity has several effects over the ECG signal recorded at the body surface, namely in the wave's morphology.
- The ANS controls and coordinates many other body functions besides the heart rate, in a way to make the body work properly. Thus the HRV and variations of respiratory frequency have a common source, and respiration induces changes in cardiac cycle length. This modulation of respiration over HRV in known as respiratory sinus arrhythmia (Yasuma & Hayano, 2004). During inspiration the HR increases and during expiration it decreases.
- Volume of the air in lungs varying during the respiratory cycle also changes the electrical properties of the lung tissue. During inspiration the resistance increases and the amplitude of the electrocardiogram is lower.

A detailed study of these electrocardiogram-derived respiration signals shows that heart position-based methods are sensitive to the voluntary breath pauses,

Figure 2.4 Respiration-modulated electrocardiogram

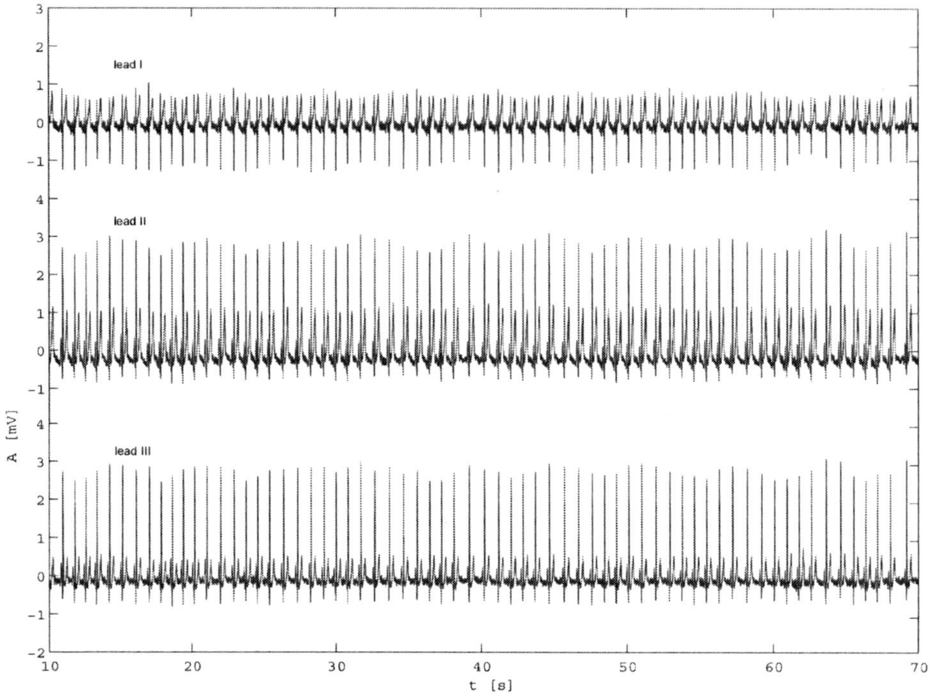

while heart rate-based methods are sensitive only for apnea induced by ANS defects. Regarding ECG-based telemonitoring, a very important conclusion is the possibility of a reliable assessment of respiration without the use of any additional equipment or sensors.

BASIC AUTOMATED INTERPRETATION PROCEDURES: HEARTBEAT DETECTION, RHYTHM CLASSIFICATION, AND WAVE MEASUREMENTS

General Considerations

In contemporary clinical practice, physicians overread and correct computerized ECG interpretive reports. If similar waveforms are analyzed subsequently, the computer software makes the same diagnostic error over and over. Although it is desirable for an ECG interpretation system to "learn" from its mistakes, there is no current commercial system that improves its performance by analyzing its errors.

The modem microprocessor-based interpretive machines include eight ECG amplifiers in order to simultaneously sample and store eight leads—I, II, and V1-V6 (see fig. 2.2). Then they synthesize the four redundant leads—III, aVR, aVL, and aVF. These machines include enough memory to store all the leads for a 10-second interval at a clinical sampling rate of 500 samples per second (sps).

The approach for computerized interpretation of the ECG used in modern commercial instrumentation is based on decision logic (Pordy et al., 1968; Macfarlane, Lorimer, & Lowrie, 1971). A computer program mimics the human expert's decision process using a rule-based expert system. The decision logic approach is based on a set of rules operating on the measurement matrix derived from the ECG. The rules are assembled in a computer program as a large set of logical IF-THEN statements. The rules are usually developed based on the knowledge from human experts. The pathway through the set of IF-THEN statements ultimately leads to one or more interpretive statements that are printed in the final report. Unfortunately, it is well known that a group of cardiologists typically interpret the same set of ECGs with less than 80% agreement. In fact, if the same ECGs are presented to one cardiologist at different times, the physician typically has less than 80% agreement with his or her previous readings. Thus, a decision logic program is only as good as the physician or group of physicians who participate in developing the knowledge base.

One advantage of the decision logic approach is that its results and the decision process can easily be followed by a human expert. However, since its decision rules are elicited indirectly from human experts rather than from the data, it is likely that such a system will never be improved enough to outperform human experts. Unlike human experts, the rule-based classifier is unable to make use of the waveforms directly. Thus, its capability is further limited to looking at numbers that, being extracted from the waveforms, may include some measurement error. Also, with such an approach, it is very difficult to make minor adjustments to one or a few rules in order to customize the software to a particular group of patients. Even slightly changing one rule may lead to modification of many different pathways through the logic statements (Hamilton & Tompkins, 1986; Kohler, Hennig, & Orglmeister, 2002).

In early years an alternative approach considered the ECG interpretation as a pattern classification problem and applied a multivariate statistical pattern recognition method to solve it (Klingeman & Pipberger, 1967). For the multivariate statistical pattern recognition approach to ECG interpretation, each decision is made directly from the data; hence this approach is largely free from human influence. Decisions are based on the numbers in the ECG measurement matrix being within certain statistical ranges calculated from the known probabilities of these numbers for a large set of patients. Since this technique is dependent directly on the data and not on the knowledge of human experts, it is theoretically possible to develop an interpretive system that could perform better than the best physician.

However, unlike the decision logic approach, which can produce an explanation of how the decision is reached, there is no logic to follow in this approach, so it is not possible to present to a human expert how the algorithm made its interpretation. This is the major reason that this technique has not been adopted in commercial instrumentation.

ECG interpretation chainThe ECG interpretation usually starts with feature extraction, which has two parts:

- waveform recognition to identify the waves in the ECG including the P and T waves and the QRS complex, and
- measurement to quantify a set of amplitudes and time durations that is to be used as background for the interpretation process.

The first step in waveform recognition aims at identifying all the heartbeats in the *raw signal* using a QRS detection algorithm. Next, the similar beats in each channel are time-aligned and an average (or median) beat is calculated for each of the 12 or for selected leads. These 12 representative beats are analyzed to identify additional waves within the heart cycle and other features of the ECG. The set of *measurement results* (metadata or semantic description) is then assembled into a matrix. These values are analyzed by subsequent processes (e.g., feature extraction) and result in a set of numbers called the *diagnostic parameters*. These parameters are fed to a decision logic or statistical process that completes the interpretation process while assigning predefined natural *language tokens* belonging to a closed standardized dictionary to describe the patient condition. The roadmap of the standard ECG processing is presented in Figure 2.5.

Heartbeat Detection Algorithm

Various techniques used to implement a QRS detector include linear digital filters, nonlinear transformations, decision processes, and template matching (Thakor, 1978; Thakor, Webster, & Tompkins, 1980, 1983, 1984b; Ahlstrom & Tompkins, 1981; Fumo & Tompkins, 1982; Pan & Tompkins, 1985). Typically, two or more of these techniques are combined together in a detector algorithm. It is necessary to extract the signal of interest, the QRS complex, from other noise sources such as the P and T waves (Friesen et al., 1990). Besides the QRS, the ECG waveform contains other waves, 60-Hz noise from powerline interference, EMG from muscles, motion artifacts from electrodes and skin interface, and possibly interferences from other sources (e.g., electro-surgery equipment in the operating room).

Figure 2.5. The roadmap of standard ECG processing

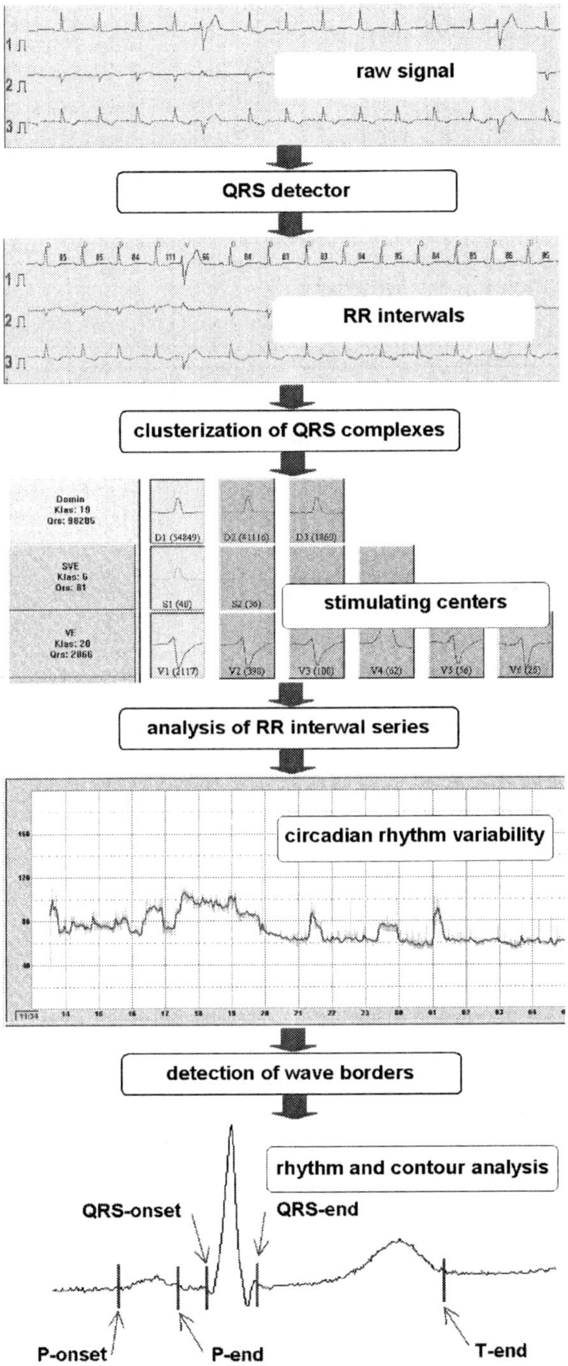

Bandpass Filters Technique

From the power spectrum analysis of various signal components in the ECG signal, an effective filter can be designed to select the QRS complex from the ECG. Another study examined the spectral plots of the ECG and the QRS complex from 3875 beats (Thakor et al., 1984a). The result revealed that the maximum signal-to-noise ratio (SNR) value is obtained for a bandpass filter with a center frequency of 17 Hz and a factor Q (slope stepness) of 3.

Differentiation

Differentiation is included in many QRS detection algorithms. Since it acts as a high-pass filter, the derivative amplifies higher frequencies characteristic of the QRS complex while attenuating the lower frequencies of the P and T waves.

An algorithm based on first and second derivatives originally developed by Balda, Diller, Deardorff, Doue, and Hsieh (1977) was modified for use in the high-speed analysis of recorded ECGs by Ahlstrom and Tompkins (1983). Friesen et al. (1990) subsequently implemented this algorithm as part of a study to compare noise sensitivity among certain types of QRS detection algorithms.

The absolute values of the first and second derivative are calculated from the ECG signal. These two data buffers, $y_0(nT)$ and $y_1(nT)$, are scaled and then summed. The data buffer $y_1(nT)$ is now scanned until a certain threshold is met or exceeded $y_2(T)>1.0$. Once this condition is met, the next eight points are compared to the threshold. If six or more of these eight points meet or exceed the threshold, then the segment is suspected to be part of the QRS complex. In addition to detecting the QRS complex, this algorithm has the advantage that it produces a pulse that is proportional in width to the complex. However, particular sensitivity to higher-frequency noise is an important disadvantage of this algorithm.

Template Matching

The most common approach in contemporary commercial ECG instrumentation is based on template matching. A model of the normal QRS complex, referred to as a template, is extracted from the ECG during a learning period for a particular patient. This template is compared with the subsequent incoming real-time ECG to look for a possible match, using a mathematical distance criterion. A signal close enough to the template represents a detected QRS complex. If the analyzed waveform does not match to the normal template but is a suspected abnormal QRS complex, it is treated as a separate template, and future suspected QRS complexes are compared with it. Although related to the human recognition process, the process requires significant computational power for matching the templates to the real-time signal.

The correlation coefficient is commonly used to quantify the degree of match between the shapes of two or more signals. A QRS detection technique designed by Dobbs, Schmitt, and Ozemek (1984) uses cross-correlation. This technique of correlating one signal with another requires that the two signals be aligned with one another. In this QRS detection technique, the template of the signal that we are trying to match stores a digitized form of the signal shape that we wish to detect. Since the template has to be correlated with the incoming signal, the signal should be aligned with the template. Dobbs et al. (1984) describe two ways of implementing this.

The first way of aligning the template and the incoming signal is by using the fiducial points on each signal. These fiducial points must be assigned to the signal by some *external process*. If the fiducial points on the template and the signal are aligned, then the correlation can be performed.

Another implementation involves continuous correlation between a segment of the incoming signal and the template. Whenever a new signal data point arrives, the oldest data point in time is discarded from the segment (a first-in-first-out data buffer). A correlation is performed between this signal segment and the template segment that has the same number of signal points. This technique does not require processing time to assign fiducial points to the signal. The template can be thought of as a window that moves over the incoming signal *one data point at a time.* Thus, alignment of the segment of the signal of interest must occur at least once as the window *moves through the signal.*

The value of the cross-correlation coefficient always falls between +1 and -1. A value of +1 indicates that the signal and the template match exactly. As mentioned earlier, the value of this coefficient determines how well the *shapes* of the two waveforms under consideration match. The magnitude of the actual signal samples does not matter. This shape matching, or recognizing process of QRS complexes, conforms with our natural approach to recognizing signals. The algorithm begins by saving a segment of the incoming ECG signal that corresponds to the QRS waveform. This segment or template is then compared with the incoming ECG signal. Each point in the incoming signal is subtracted from the corresponding point in the template. When the template is aligned with a QRS waveform in the signal, the subtraction results in a value very close to zero. This algorithm uses only as many subtraction operations as there are points in the template.

Semantic-Domain Template Matching

Fumo and Tompkins (1982) developed a QRS detector that is based on concepts from automata theory. The algorithm uses basic techniques that are common in many pattern recognition systems. The ECG signal is first reduced into a set of predefined tokens, which represent certain shapes of the ECG waveform. The sequence of tokens is the input to the finite state automaton, which is a state-transition diagram that can be implemented with IF-THEN control statements available in most programming languages. The sequence of tokens is fed into the automaton. For example, a sequence of tokens such as *zero, normup, normdown,* and *normup* would result in the automaton signaling a normal classification for the ECG.

The sequence of tokens must be derived from the ECG signal data. This is done by forming a sequence of the differences of the input data. Then the algorithm groups together those differences that have the same sign and also exceed a certain predetermined threshold level. The algorithm then sums the differences in each of the groups and associates with each group this sum and the number of differences that are in it.

This QRS detector has an initial learning phase where the program approximately determines the peak magnitude of a normal QRS complex. Then the algorithm detects a normal QRS complex each time there is a deflection in the waveform with a magnitude greater than half of the previously determined peak. The algorithm now teaches the finite state automaton the sequence of tokens that make up a normal QRS complex. The number and sum values (discussed in the preceding paragraph) for a normal QRS complex are now set to a certain range of their respective values in the QRS complex detected. The algorithm can now assign a waveform token to each of the groups formed previously based on the values of the number and the sum in each group of differences. For example, if a particular group of differences has a sum and number value in the ranges (determined in the learning phase) of a QRS upward or downward deflection, then a *normup* or *normdown* token is generated for that group of differences. If the number and sum values do not fall in this range, then a *noiseup* or *noisedown* token is generated. A *zero* token is generated if the sum for a group of differences is zero. Thus, the algorithm reduces the ECG signal data into a sequence of tokens, which can be fed to the finite state automata for QRS detection.

Thresholding

The set of thresholds that Pan and Tompkins (1985) used for this stage of the QRS detection algorithm were set such that signal peaks (i.e., valid QRS complexes) were detected. Signal peaks are defined as those of the QRS complex, while noise peaks are those of the T waves, muscle noise, and so forth. After the ECG signal has passed through the band-pass filter stages, its signal-to-noise ratio increases. This permits the use of thresholds that are just above the noise peak levels. Thus, the overall sensitivity of the detector improves. A peak is determined when the signal changes direction within a certain time interval. Thus, the signal peak is the peak that the algorithm has recognized as corresponding to the QRS complex—while noise peak is any peak that is not related to the signal of interest. New values of thresholds are calculated from previous ones and with regard to the amplitude of the detected peak. Consequently, the algorithm adapts to changes in the ECG signal from a particular person.

Whenever a new peak is detected, it must be categorized as a noise peak or a signal peak. If the peak level exceeds a threshold during the first analysis of the signal, then it is a QRS peak. If a search-back technique is used, then the signal peak should exceed a lower value of threshold to be classified as a QRS peak.

Search-Back Technique

To implement the search-back technique, this algorithm maintains two RR-interval averages. One average is that of the eight most recent heartbeats. The other average is that of the eight most recent beats that had *RR* intervals that fell within a certain range. Whenever the QRS waveform is not detected for a certain interval, then the highest peak between the established thresholds (mentioned in the previous section) within this time interval is considered as QRS and influences further threshold values. Since the research is considering twice a certain interval of the ECG, this technique is known as *search-back.*

TESTING

The performance of the heartbeat detection algorithm is usually tested on the 24-hour annotated MIT/BIH database, which is composed of half-hour recordings of ECGs of 48 ambulatory patients (MIT/BIH ECG Database Distribution, n.d.). This database, available on the CD-ROM and partly on the Internet, was developed by the Massachusetts Institute of Technology and the Beth Israel Hospital in Boston. The total error in analyzing about 116,000 beats is 0.68%, corresponding to an average error rate of 33 beats per hour. In fact, much of the error comes from four particular half-hour tape segments (i.e., two hours of data from the total database). Another available ECG database was developed by the American Heart Association (AHA, 1967).

Pattern Clustering

Several approaches are developed for the task of heartbeat classification or, better said, clustering. The procedure is typical for off-line long-term ECG analyzers like Holter systems. Traditional bedside recorders acquire a short strip of the signal and do not require patterns to represent the cardiac cycles. The stress testers are expected to deliver real-time information on every extra-sinus beat, therefore they instead use pattern recognition, like correlation or semantic description-based methods. The aim of the clustering is to reveal the number and contribution of extra-sinus stimulators. The clusters are assumed to contain physiologically similar but not electrically identical heartbeats. The interest of the procedure exists in representation of the group of beats by a reference pattern on which the most time-consuming processing is done. Such processing aims at deriving the origin of the stimulation, and the physical location of an ectopic physiological stimulator is just as important, as the stimulator contributes to the global rhythm. The existence of patterns limits the calculations to 200-300 beats instead of about 100,000 when a typical 24-hour record is interpreted.

Since the stimulus generation process and conduction pathways are reflected in the shape of the heartbeat in a multilead record, the most natural way to detect the irregular conduction is a multidimensional comparison in the amplitude domain. Even for 8-channel recordings, the correlation between channels is high, and thus the comparison dimensionality may be reduced to three channels selected as the most independent. The comparison is based on the difference in the amplitude domain referred to an empirical threshold or tolerance margin. The beats falling between the margin or differences below the threshold are accepted and considered as members of a given class. The threshold, as the crucial factor for the successful clustering, is set by the operator in interactive systems, as a compromise of total cluster number and the probability of merging two beats significantly differing in medical aspect. The advantage of amplitude-domain clustering is that the tolerance threshold expressed as a percentage of signal amplitude has a precise meaning in the operator imagination, which is not as easy in cases with a features domain. The drawback is the necessity of correct beat alignment before the beat shapes are compared. Some systems use tolerance margins extended at both ends of the pattern in order to neglect the differences distant from the pattern center.

Because clustering consists of a huge number of repetitive amplitude comparison operations, multi-pass clustering methods also use beat matching in the feature domain. Once a heartbeat is detected, its representation in a feature domain is computed. This needs additional computation time, but because the feature vector size is always significantly shorter than a three-dimensional amplitude representation, the comparison operation is reduced and does not last as long. This second option for the classification is used mainly in unsupervised systems, because the operator has no practical reference to the specific feature. Besides speeding up the process, its additional advantage is the possible choice of synchronization-invariant features for beat representation. In such a case no additional computation is necessary for the temporal alignment of compared beats. Example features are:

- the QRS area to periphery ratio,
- the count of samples where signal derivative exceeds a double value of average derivative, and
- the maximum signal derivative to average signal derivative ratio.

Real-time ECG interpreters usually employ single-pass clustering. Once the decision about membership is taken, it is always final. The incoming heartbeat is tested for membership to every existing cluster. A new cluster is set with the failure of the last test, until the maximum cluster number is reached. The testing order is optimized by two factors—last success and the cluster population—in order to achieve the positive test result as soon as possible which limits the test number and consequently the computation expenses. Clusters are represented by their kernels, which are usually the first incoming real heartbeat representations. In rare real-time systems, there is time to recalculate kernels with each new acceptance to the cluster.

Multi-pass clustering used in off-line systems—or in some high-speed, computer-based stepping real-time interpreters—use the single-pass clustering as the initial pass of the multi-pass process. After completing a clustering pass, the cluster kernels are recalculated as the average of the members' representation. Cluster memberships are stored but remain invisible for the next clustering pass. The clustering in the second and subsequent passes uses cluster kernels calculated previously, and creation of new classes is limited. At the end of those passes, the resulting memberships are compared with the previous pass results. The occurrence of identical results ends the multi-pass process. Multi-pass clustering is much more computation expensive, however the final result usually contains less errors. A limit for iteration count should be set, because according to the theoretical proof, the process may not be converging.

Wave Detection and Delimitation

Wave detection is a gateway to the contour analysis of the ECG, since it determines the regions of signal considered as belonging to a specified wave. Primary ECG diagnostic parameters are based on temporal dependencies between the waves, representing the conduction of stimulus through a specified tissue or contraction of muscle. There are three main waves in heart evolution. Their temporal order is P, QRS, and T, following the consequent action of a single isolated stimulus propagating through the heart. Nevertheless, the wave first recognized is usually the QRS complex, which is the most apparent component of the electrocardiogram and therefore may be easily recognized. The QRS complex represents the contraction of the ventricular muscle and starts with a sudden and broad depolarization front, but ends smoothly with depolarization of most distant cells in the muscle tissue. Consequently, in the electrical representation, the QRS complex in particular at the beginning is a rapid and energetic phenomena, which facilitates its detection. The point usually called QRS-onset is indicated by the software as an index of signal sample when the stochastic character of the baseline noise is no longer a dominant component of the signal. Because of the anatomy of the conductive branches, the extra-ventricular beats are significantly more rapid at the beginning than the ventricular escape beats. Because of better synchronicity of muscular contraction, the extra-ventricular QRS waves are usually also significantly shorter.

The QRS-end point is determined with much lower precision because of the smooth nature of the late depolarization phase and because of overlapping of the early repolarization manifesting itself by the S-T slope. The S-T section may not return to the baseline level, and the best background for the QRS-end detection is the return of the noise statistics to the values similar to those from before the QRS-onset. However, this method will not reach a true result if the final part of the QRS complex is affected by late ventricular potentials produced by isolated fibers with affected recovery latency.

The T wave represents the repolarization process, hence it is the electrical consequence of the QRS complex. Its existence is evident, however in some leads it may be hard for detection. The beginning of the T wave is extremely hard to determine, however this point is not very important in calculation of primary diagnostic parameters. For the assessment of the ST section, usually the QRS-end or maximum of QRS is taken as a reference, and the measurement points J, ST, and E are set in a fixed or HR-dependent position. On the contrary, the T-end has a widely recognized clinical significance. The first difficulty in T-end determination is the possible smoothness of the signal, however sometimes the T wave ends so abruptly that the T-end is confused with the QRS-onset. The second problem is that the T wave ends with different delays in particular leads, which is caused by various geometrical aspects on this rather linear process. The differences were even a background for a set of QT dispersion diagnostics, recently disputed for its inaccuracy and partly abandoned. The third problem that may emerge during the detection of a T-end is the existence of a local signal minimum before (in the sense of time) the actual T-end. For rapid heart rhythms, the software may confuse this residuum with a baseline between the T-end and P-onset of subsequent evolution. The end of a T wave is usually determined with the use of multi-channel correlation or by curve fitting to the terminal sector of the wave.

The P wave is detected as the last wave, because the processing often requires the removal of QRS and T waves of significantly higher energy. The existence of the P wave represents the atrial action; thus for the junctional beats the P wave is visible directly before the QRS, and for ventricular beats the P wave is absent. In the case of atrioventricular block, the QRS may be preceded by none, one, or several P waves. In the case of atrial fibrillation or flutter, a continuous perpetual atrial action appears as a seamless train of P waves. The two latter cases are very difficult for automatic wave detection, and therefore atrial fibrillation is usually detected before the P wave and a positive result inhibits P wave detection. The P wave may be negative, positive, or bipolar. The variation of forms creates additional difficulty for automatic border detection.

To illustrate computational complexity of the wave border detection, the easiest case of QRS-onset detection is presented, as developed in the Lyon interpretation program (Morlet, 1986):

1. In a 200 ms section before the heartbeat detection point, the 15 ms sliding window is searched which contains only samples of absolute value of signal derivative (speed) below a given threshold. If the window does not exist, the search is repeated for augmented threshold value.
2. The first reference point *QD* is assigned to the earliest of the samples from that window. It is assumed that *QD* is earlier than a true QRS-onset.
3. For samples later than *QD*, the value of signal second derivative (acceleration) is calculated and averaged over a 20 ms interval. The earliest point where the acceleration exceeds the value of 2 is considered as approximate QRS-onset *Q-SAPR* and as a starting point for more precise research.
4. The exact baseline level is determined as the average value of samples in the 20 ms section preceding the *Q-SAPR*.
5. In the 50ms bidirectional neighborhood of *Q-SAPR*, the surface function is calculated as a root of the sum of the squares for corresponding signal samples in every considered lead.
6. In the narrowed neighborhood, a second derivative of surface function *AS* is calculated from samples in 10 ms intervals. For points earlier than *QD*, the extremum values of *AS* are determined and their difference is used as an estimate of baseline noise level *BN*.
7. In the interval from *QD* to *Q-SAPR*+32 ms, the earliest sample is searched for which the value of *AS* exceeds the *BN*. If such a point is found, a directly preceding sample is considered as the QRS-onset. Otherwise, the *Q-SAPR* is considered as the QRS-onset and the software issues an inaccuracy warning.

Determination of Electrical Axes for Waves

The waves duration alone give a principal insight to the temporal aspects of stimulus conduction in the heart. The complementary spatial aspects are represented by the approximate electrical axes determined separately for each wave. The precise determination of axes is possible with a three-dimensional recording technology like vectocardiography. This technique defines heart axis as the direction in space determined by the product electrical vector in the moment it has the largest length. Similar definitions are accepted locally for the QRS axis, which is equal to the heart axis, and for computation of the axes within P and T waves.

Since 12-lead ECG systems do not assume the leads orthogonality, the wave axes may only be estimated. The computation is performed on limb lead signals because the frontal projection of a three-dimensional vector is the subject for assessment.

Although reflected by respiration, pregnancy, and other factors influencing the heart position within the human body, the QRS axis helps to estimate the correctness of stimulus conduction. If the conduction is affected by the local necrosis of a heart wall tissue or by the His bundle branch block, the heart axis has a permanently altered position referred to as a right or left axis deviation. In a physiological condition the frontal projection of the heart vector falls between the right horizontal line (0 degrees) and the downward vertical line (90 degrees). In case of downward-left orientation (more than 90 degrees), the right axis deviation is reported, and for the upward right position (less than 0 degrees), the left axis deviation is stated.

The P wave axis represents the distribution of the stimulus to the left ventricle and through atrioventricular pathways. These phenomena could be diagnosed with the P-axis, however due to the small amplitude of the P wave, the role of the P-axis is to determine the beat-to-beat stability of these phenomena. As far as the P-axis being found stable within a given margin, the early conduction phases are considered repetitive and controlled by the sinoatrial node. Together with the stability of PQ interval, the stability of the P-axis is essential for statement of normal sinus rhythm (NSR).

The T wave axis is rarely considered in everyday diagnostics except for the case of T wave alternans. The alternans manifests itself by the alternate shapes and polarity of the T wave and has a significant predictive value for early recognition of ventricular tachycardia.

SELECTED SPECIALIZED PROCEDURES: RESEARCH FOR ARRHYTHMIAS, HEART RATE VARIABILITY, AND ISCHEMIAE SYMPTOMS

This section presents selected aspects of advanced ECG interpretation procedures. The selection key was the current usage of diagnostic parameters issued by presented analysis techniques in telemedicine. Consequently, analysis domains included: the detection of atrial and ventricular arrhythmias, the analysis of heart rate variability in time and frequency domains, and the detection of ischemia symptoms based on the analysis of ST section.

The reader should be conscious that the analyses presented as examples in the next few pages are each widely described domains and therefore the presentation here is as concise as possible. Interested readers are encouraged to read more about the examples and relevant diagnostic techniques in the sources cited. Contour analysis, infarct detection, His bundle block detection, and hypertrophy are only a few examples of ECG analytical techniques relevant today, yet rarely represented in telemedicine and therefore not yet considered as parts of ubiquitous cardiology. The future will prove their application.

Arrhythmia Analysis

Ambulatory electrocardiographic monitoring is an important diagnostic tool in patients with supraventricular arrhythmias (Biblo & Waldo, 1986). The ambulatory ECG can also be used to assess therapeutic procedures. Most sustained supraventricular arrhythmias are diagnosed by recording a standard 12-lead ECG, either alone or with an appropriate rhythm strip. However, transient arrhythmias may cause symptoms that may not last long enough to be captured with a conventional ECG unless acquired at home. For those patients, the ambulatory ECG is critical for diagnosis. If the arrhythmic events are sufficiently frequent in a 24-hour period, or if the expectation is that the arrhythmia will occur in a 24-hour period, then the continuous 24-hour ambulatory ECG is most useful.

In patients whose symptoms include syncope or near syncope, the continuous ambulatory ECG is critical for diagnosis. It is also critical to diagnose events that may occur during sleep, or events that may be suspected but are associated with either no symptoms or such minimal symptoms that they do not elicit a response from the patient that would urge the use of an event monitor.

The continuous 24-hour ambulatory ECG is essential for the diagnosis of the sick sinus syndrome (Vera & Mason, 1981). Invasive electrophysiologic tests, such as sinus node overdrive suppression and sinoatrial conduction time assessment, may be completely normal in patients with marked sinus node dysfunction. Thus, the best diagnostic tool for this disorder is continuous ECG monitoring. Abnormalities of AV conduction can also be recognized using 24-hour ambulatory ECG monitoring. In addition, continuous ambulatory ECG monitoring is useful in the assessment of autonomic dysfunction.

The principal applications of ambulatory ECG monitoring of supraventricular arrhythmias currently include:

1. assessment of symptoms (frequent, preferably daily) possibly associated with a transient arrhythmia,
2. characterization of known or suspected supraventricular arrhythmias,
3. assessment of sinus node dysfunction,
4. correlation of the effects of the activities of daily living with supraventricular arrhythmias,
5. assessment of AV conduction, and
6. determination of the effectiveness of antiarrhythmic therapy (drug therapy, pacemaker therapy, ablative therapy, or surgical therapy).

Ambulatory ECG monitoring supplements the role of invasive electrophysiologic testing in characterizing some tachyarrhythmias, such as AV re-entrant tachycardia and AV nodal re-entrant tachycardia, and in characterizing some AV conduction abnormalities, such as aberrant ventricular conduction during a supraventricular arrhythmia.

Continuous 24-hour ambulatory ECG remains the most reliable tool for diagnosing *sinus node dysfunction*. Recordings must be quite long, as abnormalities that are diagnostic may be episodic. Sinus pauses or sinus bradycardia when associated with appropriate symptoms are usually representative of sinus node dysfunction. The correlations with symptoms is invaluable, though not always a requisite. Furthermore, it is important to emphasize that markers of apparent sinus node dysfunction may be normal under certain circumstances. For instance, in the well-trained athlete, sinus bradycardia and even sinus pauses greater than 3 seconds may reflect normal sinus node function (Swiryn, McDonough, & Hueter, 1984). Many of the markers of sinus node dysfunction that occur when a person is awake are not abnormal when he or she is asleep. Standards for abnormal sinus node function during sleep are not well established. Thus, abnormal findings that occur during the day almost always have more significance, especially when associated with symptoms.

Atrial fibrillation can be documented by many different methods. When the rhythm is sustained, a patient can present him or herself to a medical facility for a conventional 12-lead ECG examination. However, in some instances it is preferable to make the diagnosis using a 24-hour ambulatory ECG or an ECG event monitor. Clearly, the ambulatory ECG is useful when symptoms are episodic. In addition, asymptomatic episodes of atrial fibrillation are not uncommon. Furthermore, there are unique applications of the 24-hour ambulatory ECG in atrial fibrillation, particularly in understanding the relationship to autonomically mediated atrial fibrillation. The patterns of vagally mediated or adrenergically mediated paroxysmal atrial fibrillation should be identifiable on a 24-hour ambulatory ECG. Close attention to heart rate changes that occur in proximity to the onset of the arrhythmia is necessary. A mixed picture of vagal and adrenergic atrial fibrillation may be difficult to identify.

Atrioventricular re-entrant tachycardia is associated with the presence of one or more accessory AV connections. When antegrade conduction is possible over the accessory AV connection, a delta wave is present in the ECG during sinus rhythm as a result of ventricular pre-excitation. The most common form of ventricular pre-excitation is associated with Wolff-Parkinson-White syndrome (WPW). The presence of one or more accessory AV connections may be associated with a constellation of arrhythmias, the most common of which is atrioventricular re-entrant tachycardia (AVRT). In some patients, the accessory AV connection only conducts in one direction because of the presence of unidirectional block (antegrade or retrograde). Most commonly, the block is antegrade, and the presence of an accessory AV connection is not apparent from the ECG.

The ambulatory ECG is invaluable in diagnosing and directing therapy of arrhythmias present in patients with Wolff-Parkinson-White syndrome. For two reasons the arrhythmias associated with WPW and related syndromes are important to diagnose:

1. The identification of the presence of the arrhythmia serves to direct therapy made by radio frequency ablation of the accessory AV connection.
2. Patients with WPW are at significant risk to develop atrial fibrillation or atrial flutter, and critically, the accessory AV connection in some patients will be capable of conducting most or all the atrial impulses to the ventricles, resulting in very rapid, often life-threatening ventricular rates and rhythms, including ventricular fibrillation.

The ambulatory ECG is invaluable in assessing *abnormalities of AV conduction*, particularly when either minimally symptomatic or episodic. The correlation with symptoms remains essential to the appropriate consideration of permanent pacing. Occasionally, these abnormalities may be secondary to a treatable or reversible cause, most often drug therapy.

Screening for AV block is generally not indicated unless a patient has symptoms. However, in the presence of known disorders like sarcoidosis or calcified aortic stenosis, a screening Holter monitor is reasonable to exclude paroxysmal AV block.

Ventricular premature beats (VPBs) are ubiquitous and even short runs of ventricular tachycardia (VT) may by seen in asymptomatic people (Marcus, 1986). In normal, healthy subjects aged 10-30 years, the incidence of VT—defined as three or more consecutive VPBs—is in the range of 1-3%. The prevalence of frequent VPBs increases with age, as does the prevalence of ventricular couplets and VT. In a group of healthy elderly people aged 60-85 years, ventricular couplets were observed during 24-hour ambulatory ECG monitoring in 11% and ventricular tachycardia of 3-13 beats in 4%.

These data indicate that there is an appreciable prevalence of ventricular arrhythmias among an asymptomatic population, as well as in patients who have cardiac disease with impaired left ventricular function. When ambulatory ECG monitoring is used for diagnostic purposes to evaluate the cause of syncope or pre-syncope, there needs to be a correlation between the symptoms and the ventricular arrhythmias. Conversely, the lack of ventricular arrhythmias when pre-syncope or syncope occurs is particularly useful to exclude ventricular arrhythmias as an etiology of the symptoms.

The development and commercial availability of the ambulatory ECG recorder in the 1960s allowed studying the relationship between the frequency and complexity of ventricular arrhythmias after *myocardial infarction* and subsequent mortality. The yield of recording VPBs during six hours of ambulatory ECG monitoring was increased twelve-fold compared with that of a 36-second ECG (Moss, Schnitzler, Green, & DeCamilla, 1971). About 10 days after a myocardial infarction, only 15-25% of patients have 10 or more VPBs per hour (Moss, Bigger, & Odoroff, 1987). It was found that ventricular arrhythmias are a risk indicator for subsequent mortality, independent of the associated left ventricular dysfunction.

With the information that ventricular arrhythmias after a *myocardial infarction* are an independent risk factor, it was reasonable to assume that ventricular premature beats isolated or in runs could trigger VT or ventricular fibrillation, and that suppression of the ventricular ectopy would decrease the mortality in the first few years after hospital discharge.

Since VT and couplets, and possibly VPB frequency, *predict increased mortality* in heart failure, it would be expected that a decrease in ventricular ectopy would be associated with a decrease in mortality rate, particularly in sudden cardiac death. This hypothesis appears to be true in patients treated with ACE inhibitors, but not necessarily in patients treated with *antiarrhythmic drugs*. Several small trials of amiodarone in heart failure have shown that this unique drug does in fact effectively reduce ventricular ectopy, and most trials have reported a trend towards decreasing mortality.

Ambulatory ECG monitoring is now a well-accepted method to identify patients who are at higher risk of subsequent mortality among those who have recovered from an acute myocardial infarction. This information, combined with other data such as heart rate variability, signal-averaged late potentials, or other means of assessing autonomic tone such as carotid sinus sensitivity, may identify a sufficiently high-risk subgroup upon which to base the strategy to prevent sudden cardiac death. The use of ambulatory ECG monitoring to guide selection of antiarrhythmic drugs to prevent recurrent ventricular tachycardia or cardiac arrest remains controversial.

Figure 2.6. Examples of atrial and ventricular arrhythmias: (a) ventricular escape beat (VEB), (b) persistent supraventricular tachycardia (PSVT), (c) couplet, (d) irregular rhythm, (e) bigeminy, (f) pause, (g) salvo, (h) idiopatic ventricular rhythm (IVR), (i) ventricular tachycardia (VT, three traces)

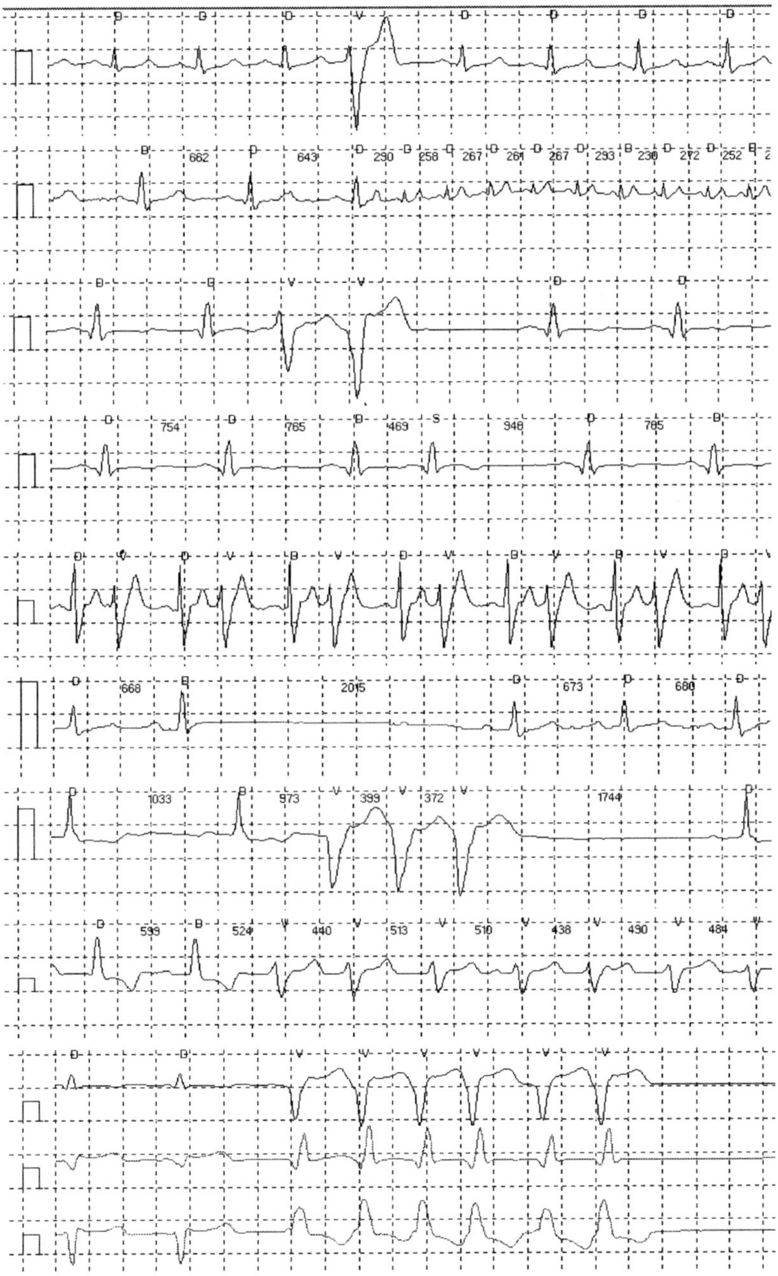

The Analysis of Heart Rate Variability

There are numerous ways of expressing the variability of heart rate and heart periods (Malik, 1995; Malik & Camm, 2004). The initial methods predominantly applied to the assessment of fetal rate variability were, for practical reasons, oriented to processing of short-term tachograms and periodograms, and involved rather simple arithmetic formulas in order to express the variability in quantitative terms.

As the measurement of heart rate variability was being applied to wider groups of laboratory investigations and clinical conditions, the need emerged for developing methods based on a more solid mathematical basis, and the so-called statistical methods appeared. These methods treat the sequence of RR intervals or of pairs of adjacent RR intervals as a set of unordered data and express its variability by conventional statistical approaches—for example, by applying the formula for calculating standard deviation.

Thanks to detailed physiological studies, the distinction of different components of heart rate variability was made with respect to individual regulatory mechanisms. This need led to the application of spectral methods to a series of RR intervals in which their original order was carefully recorded.

Statistical and spectral methods both require a high precision and a reliable quality of RR interval data, which is difficult to maintain when analyzing long-term ECGs recorded under conventional clinical conditions. This difficulty led to the introduction of the so-called "geometrical methods," which were developed in order to provide approximate assessment of heart rate variability even when applied to RR interval data containing low levels of errors and artifacts.

The physiologic and pathophysiologic mechanisms governing heart rate and its oscillations are not only complex, but also substantially irregular in their periodicity. There are in principle two broad categories of methods for heart rate variability measurement. The spectral methods treat the RR interval data as a time-ordered series, and the non-spectral methods process the sequence of RR intervals or their pairs without paying any attention to the original order and timing of individual intervals.

Substantial numbers of non-spectral methods (but not all of them) report the results of heart rate variability in units of time, for example, in milliseconds. For this reason, the whole group of non-spectral methods is frequently called 'time-domain methods'.

Statistical Methods

The task of expressing numerically the variability of a series of data is a standard requirement of *descriptive statistics*. Thus, having the data on the durations of individual RR intervals or on heart rate in consecutive segments of an ECG, the application of the formula for calculating standard deviation is an obvious choice, at least from a mathematical or statistical point of view. A solely mathematical approach such as the application of the standard deviation formula does not reflect any physiological or pathophysiological aspects of heart rate variations.

To provide meaningful results, similar quality and contents of data are required by the statistical methods. However, the automatic or semiautomatic way of obtaining data from electronically recorded ECGs, and especially long-term ECGs, is not sufficiently accurate in the case of a distorted signal. Thus before applying any statistical method to the data of RR interval durations of consecutive heart rates, visual checks and manual corrections of the automatic ECG analysis or other additional data preparation phases must ensure that all coupling intervals and compensatory pauses of premature cycles have been excluded and that, on the other hand, all sinus rhythm QRS complexes were correctly recognized and included into the datastream. In order to specify this character of intervals included in the analyzed datastream and to postulate that extra care has been given to the quality of the datastream, the term "normal-to-normal" intervals (or NN intervals) has been proposed and widely accepted.

In NN interval series obtained from short-term recordings, the formula of standard deviation can be applied either to durations of individual intervals or to the differences between the neighboring intervals. The first possibility leads to the so-called *SDNN* (Standard Deviation Normal-to-Normal) measure of heart rate variability (2.1).

$$SDNN = \frac{rr_i - \overline{rr}}{\overline{rr}} \qquad (2.1)$$

Because in practically all ECGs that are recorded for at least tens of seconds, the mean of differences between successive NN intervals is substantially different from zero only during individual phases of respiratory arrhythmia and during similarly fast adaptations of heart rate, the so-called *RMSSD* (Root Mean Square of Successive Differences, equation 2.2) measure is used instead of *SDNN*. To avoid a zero value, the mean of the differences is squared, averaged, and the square-root obtained.

$$RMSSD = \sqrt{\frac{\sum_{i=1}^{n}(rr_i - rr_{i-1})^2}{\sum_{i=1}^{n} rr_i^2}} \qquad (2.2)$$

When assessing heart rate variability in long-term recordings, the mean NN interval may be found for individual segments (in other words, the reciprocal of the heart rate may be calculated in each segment, usually five minutes) and statistical formulas applied to the resulting series of samples of the mean NN interval. Calculating standard deviation of five-minute means of NN intervals results in the so-called *SDANN* (Standard Deviation of Averaged NN intervals, equation 2.3) measure.

$$SDANN = \frac{\sum_{t0}^{t0+300s}\left(rr_i - \overline{rr}\right)}{\overline{rr}} \tag{2.3}$$

The five-minute duration of individual segments into which the long-term recording is subdivided has historical rather than physiological or valid practical justification. Indeed, the observations of more recent physiological studies might possibly be interpreted as suggesting that a division of long-term recording into much shorter segments might perhaps lead to more physiologically related measures of heart rate variability.

From a physiological point of view, the fastest changes of heart rate can be attributed to the changes in the parasympathetic tone and to fast-acting neurohumoral regulation. Indeed, release of acetylcholine from the vagal fibers is associated with marked prolongation of RR intervals that can create large differences between two consecutive cardiac cycles. Similarly, neurohumoral regulation is responsible for immediate increases in heart rate, such as those associated with sudden fright. In order to reveal these rapid changes being masked in SDNN or RMSSD by the extent of slower regulatory mechanisms and external stimuli, the relative count concept assumes the measurement of the immediate changes in heart rate separately from the more gradually acting regulations.

For a selected threshold *t* of RR interval prolongation or shortening, one can count the number of cases in which an NN interval is prolonged or shortened by more than *t* within one cardiac cycle; that is the number of NN intervals that are longer than NN' -*t* or longer than NN' +*t*, where NN' is the duration of the immediately preceding NN interval.

The performance of such a method naturally depends on the value of the threshold *t*. The method has been proposed and widely used with a threshold of 50 ms. The numerical values of NN+50, NN-50, and NN50 crucially depend on the length of the recording. For this reason, the concept of relative counts has been proposed. The value of heart rate variability measure pNN50 (and similarly pNN+50 and pNN-50) is defined as the relative numbers of NN intervals differing by more than 50 ms from the immediately preceding NN interval (equation 2.4); in other words *pNN50* equals NN50 divided by the number of NN intervals in the whole analyzed ECG.

$$p50NN = \frac{\sum_{i=1}^{N} rr : \left|rr_i - rr_{i-1}\right| > 50ms}{\sum_{i=1}^{N} rr} \cdot 100\% \tag{2.4}$$

Geometric Methods

As the name suggests, the geometric methods use the sequence of RR intervals to construct a geometric form and extract a heart rate variability measure from this form. The geometric forms used in different methods are based on the sample density histogram of NN interval durations, on the sample density histogram of differences between successive NN intervals, or on the so-called Lorenz plots or Poincare maps which plot the duration of each NN or RR interval against the duration of the immediately preceding NN or RR interval.

The way in which the heart rate variability measure is extracted from the geometric form varies from one method to another. In general, three approaches are used:

1. Measurements of the geometric form are taken (e.g., the baseline width or the height of a sample density histogram) and the measure is derived from these values.
2. The geometric pattern is approximated by a mathematically defined shape, and heart rate variability measures are derived from the parameters of this shape.
3. The general pattern of the geometric form can be classified into one of several predefined categories, and a heart rate variability measure or characteristic is derived from the selected category.

The most studied geometric methods include the sample density histogram of NN interval durations. All incorrect measurements of RR interval fall outside the major peak of the distribution histogram and can frequently be clearly identified.

The geometric methods processing the histogram reduce the effect of the incorrect NN intervals by concentrating on the major peak of the sample density curve. The so-called *HRV triangular index* is based on the idea that, if the major peak of the histogram were a triangle, its baseline width would be equal to its area divided by one-half of its height (Malik, Farrell, Cripps, & Camm, 1989). The HRV triangular index approximates the heart rate variability as the baseline width of the histogram by a simple fraction A/H. The height H of the histogram equals the number of RR intervals with modal duration, and the area A of the histogram equals the total number of RR intervals. The numerical value of the index must consider the sampling applied to construct the histogram that is the discrete scale used to measure the NN intervals.

The so-called triangular interpolation of NN interval histogram (the *TINN* method) is a modification of the HRV triangular index method, which is less dependent on the sampling frequency. Using the method of minimum-square-difference interpolation, the highest peak of the sample density histogram is approximated by a triangle, and heart rate variability is expressed as the length of the base of this triangle.

Both these methods are particularly suited when the NN interval histogram contains only one dominant peak. This is frequent in recordings obtained from subjects exposed to a stable environment without physical and mental excesses. Such an environment is often present during in-hospital recordings, while 24-hour recordings of normally active healthy individuals frequently register two distinct intervals maximum, corresponding to active day and resting night periods.

Simple visual judgment of heart rate variability in a long-term ECG is perhaps best facilitated by the *Lorenz plot*, which is a map of dots in Cartesian coordinates. Each pair of successive RR or NN intervals is plotted as a dot with coordinates [duration RR(i), duration RR(i+1)].

Coupling intervals and the compensatory pauses of atrial and ventricular premature beats or incorrectly measured RR intervals lead to easily visible outliers in the map of the plot. Thus, compared with the histograms of RR durations, Lorenz plots are even more appropriate to judge the quality of the RR intervals that were identified in a long-term electrocardiogram, although such a possibility is not frequently exploited in commercial Holter systems. Preserved physiologic RR interval variations lead to a wide-spreading Lorenz plot while a record with markedly reduced heart rate variability produces a compact pattern of the plot. Based on such a visual judgment, some studies have led to proposals for classification of patterns of Lorenz plots and distinguished shapes.

Frequency Domain Analysis of Heart Rate Variability

Frequency domain analysis of heart rate variability (HRV) includes a variety of applications of a noninvasive methodology that has been utilized in different experimental and clinical conditions to evaluate the autonomic control of cardiovascular function and to identify subgroups of patients with increased cardiac mortality (Lombardi, 2001).

The basic assumption underlying this technique is that every periodic signal, such as RR interval or systolic arterial pressure, may be decomposed into a series of oscillatory components with different frequency and amplitude. However, as the number of oscillatory components that can be detected is also dependent on the duration of the time series, different results are obtained when considering short-term (a few minutes) or long-term (24 hours) recordings.

Physiological interpretation of spectral components is the main advantage of frequency domain HRV analysis. For short-term recordings (5-10 min.), spectral analysis of HRV is characterized by three major components at different frequency ranges (tab. 2.2).

Spectral analysis of short-term recordings can be performed by either parametric or nonparametric models. The first of them utilizes simpler and faster algorithms (Fast Fourier Transform) available in most mathematical libraries, whereas the second (autoregressive modeling technique) allows an easier post processing of the spectrum with an automatic computation of the power and the center frequency of each detected component. The center frequency of LF and HF varies in relation to the respiratory rate and to additional factors that may affect autonomic modulation of sinus node.

The quantification of the major rhythmical oscillation present in the HRV signal could provide relevant information on the neural mechanisms responsible at sinus node level for beat-to-beat variations of the heart period. Thus, the respiration-related component was proposed as an index of vagal modulation of sinus node, although other neural and non-neural mechanisms are involved for this frequency. The LF component interpretation is more controversial, but its amplitude increases in almost all conditions characterized by the sympathetic activation. The interpretation of the VLF component is even more critical and used primarily in long-term recordings. The averaging process by filtering the components at higher frequencies emphasizes the energy distribution within the ULF and VLF ranges. The variations of RR interval in relation to the subject being asleep and being awake, to periodic physical activity, as well as to circadian neurohumoral activation, are also responsible for the predominance of these components in the analysis of long-term recordings.

Spectral analysis of HRV is usually performed on the time series of RR intervals recorded during controlled conditions or during 24-hour Holter monitoring. In the first case, it is possible to simultaneously record a respiratory signal and to obtain a noninvasive continuous evaluation of arterial pressure. By doing so, it is possible

Table 2.2 Frequency ranges of frequency domain heart rate variability

name	frequency range	physiological background
high-frequency (HF)	0.15-0.40 Hz	a measure of the physiological respiratory sinus arrhythmias
low-frequency (LF)	0.04-0.15 Hz	rhythmicity of systolic arterial pressure frequently observed in experimental conditions of sympathetic activation
very low-frequency (VLF)	0.0033-0.04 Hz	often not characterized by a discrete spectral peak but rather by a progressive decrease of power as the component frequency is closer to the border of LF range
ultra low-frequency (ULF)	below 0.0033Hz	

to analyze the effects of the respiratory pattern on the HRV signal, as well as to obtain indices of the coupling between the spontaneous fluctuations of heart period and systolic arterial pressure.

One must be even more careful in performing spectral analysis of time series derived from Holter recordings, because one of the critical requirements of spectral analysis is the stationary state of the data—a property of the time series often assessed by visual inspection in the absence of a general consensus on how to define and measure it.

Currently, there are several commercial instrumentation systems that offer the possibility of analyzing HRV in time and frequency domain. These show critical differences in sampling rate and processing of the data that may vary, not only in relation to the algorithm used (e.g., FFT vs. AR) but also to some more technical aspects such as windowing, de-trending, or re-sampling of the time series or choice of the model order utilized to estimate the spectral density. Another limitation is due to the fact that during a 24-hour Holter recording, it is impossible to control and take note of several factors such as extent of physical activity, effects of environmental factors, quality of sleep, or changes in respiratory patterns. In clinical practice, the results of spectral analysis of 24-hour Holter recordings are often disregarded, as the time domain parameters are much easier to understand, less time consuming, and more robust to interferences present in the ECG record.

HRV Methods Summary

Statistical methods, especially those based on the standard deviation formula, can be applied to any recording ranging from five-minute to 24- or 48-hour—or possibly even longer—ECGs. The results provided are stable and have suitable statistical properties. For processing of short-term recordings, the statistical measures are the method of choice in cases that are not suitable for processing by spectral methods. Thus, SDNN and/or RMSSD are also valuable for physiological studies when the tachogram of the recorded ECG is not stationary. Statistical methods are preferential for the analysis of short-term recordings that contain too many premature beats, the interpolation around which would affect the result of the more detailed spectral analysis. If the frequency methods are excluded for the above-mentioned or other reasons, the statistical methods are the only possibility for heart rate variability measurement. In long-term recordings, statistical methods should be used when the quality of the NN interval data is guaranteed. In such recordings, the SDNN measure characterizes the overall variability of heart rate while the RMSSD measure assesses the fast components. The SDANN measure using five-minute averages is believed to be a measure of the very slow components of heart rate variability. The major disadvantage of the statistical methods, especially when they are used for processing of long-term ECGs, is their sensitivity to the quality of NN interval data. The need for having high-fidelity NN data applies to all statistical methods.

The geometric methods are capable of providing a reasonable assessment of heart rate variability even when the quality of data does not permit the use of conventional statistical and spectral methods. Their results are only approximate and they are not as precise as the more exact statistical and spectral analyses. The approximate nature of the results of geometrical methods is their limitation. Another important limitation of the methods is a consequence of a substantial number of RR or NN intervals (at least 20 minutes) needed to construct a representative geometrical pattern. Naturally, the longer the recording, the better is the definition of the derived geometric pattern. Thus, it is optimal to apply geometric methods to 24-hour or even longer recordings.

The need to record a sufficient number of cardiac cycles excludes the geometric methods from being used in short-term recordings made under specific conditions. However, the accuracy and quality of recordings obtained during such studies in usually high and careful manual editing of short records can easily be performed. In principle, this removes the need to use geometric methods in physiological studies and makes the statistical and spectral methods more appropriate.

Thus the application of geometric methods should be restricted to clinical investigations and to cases in which obtaining an error-free sequence of RR intervals is impractical. Clinical studies that employed these methods demonstrated that the practical value of their assessment of global heart rate variability is not inferior to that of the statistical and spectral methods.

ST Segment Analyzer

The ST segment represents the period of the ECG just after depolarization, the QRS complex, and just before repolarization, the T wave (Badilini, Zareba, Titlebaum, & Moss, 1986). Changes in the ST segment of the ECG may indicate that there is a deficiency in the blood supply to the heart muscle. Thus, it is important to be able to make measurements of the ST segment (Weisner, Tompkins, & Tompkins, 1982a, 1982b).

The ST segment is the portion of the electrocardiogram that goes from the end of the QRS complex to the beginning of the T wave. This segment reflects the second phase of the transmembrane action potential (TAP) of ventricular myocardial cells. This phase may last well over 100 milliseconds and is characterized by a rather low membrane conductance to all ions. Since there is little change in TAP during this phase, the ST segment is usually isoelectric in normal subjects. Abnormalities of the ST segment are seen in several pathologic conditions, including myocardial ischemia, hypertension, and pericarditis (Armstrong & Morris, 1983; Cosby &

Herman, 1962; Hull, 1961). These abnormalities consist of displacements of the ST segment either above the isoelectric line (elevation) or below it (depression). During these situations the electrical equilibrium characteristic of the plateau phase is disturbed as ion currents are allowed to flow between the inside and outside of the cells (Nelson, Kou, & Annesley, 1989). Changes of the ST segment morphology can often be transient, as is the case with exercise-related myocardial ischemia. Consequently, the ambulatory recording is a useful tool for the monitoring and evaluation of transient episodes of pathological ST displacements.

Long-term ECG analysis of episodic ST segment displacement dates back to 1974 (Stern & Tzivoni, 1974). The ambulatory approach deals with the monitoring of ST segment displacements in a 24-hour timeframe (Biagini et al., 1982). Each value of deflection is generally obtained by averaging the measurements made for several adjacent beats (the epoch), so that one result may be associated with many cardiac complexes. The trend of ST segment displacements is then compared with that of the heart rate to evaluate physiological correlations. The need for a more complete understanding of the cause-and-effect mechanisms that trigger transient ischemia and regulate its relationship with ST segment deflections is apparent. In this regard, a beat-to-beat approach is preferable since it allows direct evaluation of the dynamicity of the ST segment and of its direct relationship with other beat-to-beat series.

The advancements achieved in modern technology, and in particular the advent of high-sampling-rate digital recordings, have dramatically improved the quality of ST segment analysis, and made practical a beat-to-beat approach to ST segment analysis. The ST segment can thus be treated as a discrete-time series for the well-known time series of RR intervals. A classical approach for biological signals is the analysis of variability, either in the time domain (by means of a standard deviation analysis) or in the frequency domain (study of signal variability at various frequencies).

The main technical issue involves the measurement of an appropriate ST level, including:

- the identification of reliable fiducial isoelectric points,
- the correction for baseline low-frequency drifts, and
- the selection of an opportune heart-rate adjusted ST segment.

Baseline Estimation and Removal

Any ECG measurement involving amplitude relies on a clear definition of so-called 'isoelectric line' (or baseline). The measurement of ST segment displacement consists of the assessment of amplitude shifts between the voltage levels of points in the ST segment and the physiologic zero of the ECG signal. The physiologic zero does not coincide with the electrical reference of the digitized ECG since the baseline may wander. In many studies found in the literature, the isoelectric level is estimated from the voltage level of a single point—the fiducial point—identified in the PR segment, which is the segment between the offset of the P wave and the onset of the subsequent QRS complex (Akselrod et al., 1987). The rationale for this choice stems from the physiologic interpretation of the ECG, according to which the PR segment is thought to be the most reliable isoelectric reference of the electrocardiographic complex. The exact position of the fiducial point within the PR segment is generally found using minimization techniques. Any deviation measurement is then conventionally performed by taking the difference between the voltage level of the ECG signal in correspondence with the ST points of interest and the voltage level of the point selected in the PR interval.

Low-frequency baseline wander usually lasts for a few seconds. Consequently, for a specific heartbeat the baseline information can be gathered in the period immediately preceding and following the appropriate fiducial points. One way to obtain better estimates of the baseline specifically for each single ST segment is through the interpolation made between consecutive fiducial points. Among the different types of interpolation, cubic spline—that is, third-order polynomials fitted between consecutive fiducial points (Pottala, Bailey, Horton, & Gradwohl, 1989)—seems to provide the best compromise between accuracy and computation time. With use of interpolation, the values of ST displacement of each beat are measured not with respect to the level of the preceding baseline but with respect to an estimated baseline that is synchronous with each individual ST segment. Cubic-spline interpolation as a baseline estimator has a serious advantage: not being a filter, it avoids the problem of phase distortion so critical in the analysis of ST segments (Tayler & Vincent, 1985). The reliability of the cubic-spline estimation of the ambulatory ECG baseline has been tested against the presence of white noise in the ECG and against variations in the segment length used to find the fiducial point. This study suggested the use of a segment of about 90 ms prior to the R wave peak, and the number of fiducial points taken as interpolation knots equals 6.

Beat-to-Beat Measurements

Ambulatory recording studies have not been consistent in defining the exact location on the ST segment to quantify the amount of deflection. Common practice is to use the end of the QRS complex as a reference point (the so-called J point) and to measure ST displacement at constant time intervals after the J point (typically 40, 60, and 80 ms). Mathematically, the J point is defined as the point following the QRS complex where a sensitive decrease of ECG slope is observed. On high-frequency

12-lead ECGs, identification of the J point is a simple task, as the sensitive decrease in ECG slope can easily be identified visually. This is more complicated in case of most ambulatory ECGs, where the J point is difficult to identify automatically, especially in records acquired at low sampling rates.

A better reference in ambulatory recordings may be found in the QRS peak (R wave peak). Indeed, various algorithms have been shown to detect this point accurately, among them parabolic interpolation and matched filtering. Choice of this point as opposed to the J point is further supported by the fact that the RJ interval is generally constant in subjects without particular conduction defects, the situation in which ST segment analysis is generally carried out. A second important factor usually not considered in conventional ST analysis is the effect of heart-rate dependency. The duration of the ST segment is a function of the repolarization duration. At a heart rate of 120 bpm (RR = 500 ms), the ST segment length is reduced to 28 ms, whereas at 40 bpm (RR = 1500 ms), the ST segment is enlarged to 49 ms.

Once a heart-rate-adjusted ST segment window has been defined, measurements of displacement can be taken in the two points ST1 and ST2 with respect to the previously estimated baseline. A global indicator of ST displacement could be identified in the average of all the possible displacements that can be measured within the ST window. The number of measurable displacements depends on the sampling rate and on the window length that shortens at faster heart rates.

Correction of Respiratory-Related Modulation

Before performing a beat-to-beat analysis of ST segment displacement variability, the correction must be performed for motion-related respiratory modulation. To explain the background of this modulation, one can consider the ECG signal as the projection on an ideal line connecting the surface leads of a time-varying electrical vector. The dynamic of this vector reflects the time variations of the electrical status of the heart during the contraction phenomena. It is the different timing of depolarization and repolarization through different zones of the heart muscle that allows the inscription of the characteristic ECG waves.

In addition to these variations strictly related to the cellular activity of the heart, other noncardiac effects can cause the direction of the dipole to be shifted, thus influencing the projections on the exploring leads. The most typical undesired effect is caused by chest movements during inhalation and exhalation, which induce a relative motion between the surface leads and the heart.

The measured ECG can be characterized by modulations synchronous with the respiratory activity. This modulation causes the amplitudes of the ECG characteristic waves to be cyclically increased and decreased synchronously with the respiratory activity. This is a background of a family of algorithms for calculation called electrocardiogram-derived respiratory signals (Moody et al., 1986). Variability of ST segment displacement time series is also seriously influenced by this modulation, which may hide other physiological components.

Clinical Impact of ST Segment Diagnosis

Clinical and laboratory observations suggest that asymptomatic ST segment depression on ambulatory Holter recordings may be an important indicator of silent myocardial ischemia reflecting advanced and potentially unstable coronary occlusive disease (Moss, 1986). These concerns are derived from the ST segment shifts that occur with acute coronary disease, with vasospastic coronary disease (Prinzmetal's variant angina), and with exercise testing. In 1969, Parker (Parker J.O., di Giorgi S., & West R.O, 1966) reported that anginal pain was a late event during pacing-induced ischemia in coronary patients with typical effort angina. ST depression accurately reflected the onset, presence, and disappearance of metabolically defined myocardial ischemia (lactate production). Clinical episodes of spontaneous myocardial ischemia reflect an imbalance of myocardial oxygen supply and demand. The overwhelming evidence indicates that the pathogenetic mechanism involved in spontaneous ischemia during daily life is similar to that responsible for exercise-induced ischemia—that is, increased myocardial oxygen demand in the setting of restricted coronary flow.

In 1974, Stern and Tzivoni (1974) reported the detection of silent ischemic heart disease with 24-hour Holter monitoring during everyday activities in 80 patients with angina pectoris and normal resting 12-lead electrocardiograms. Holter monitoring was interpreted as positive for ischemia if transient ST depression or elevation of at least 1 mm (100 μV) and/or major T wave inversion were detected for several beats. During the course of the next 20 years, many descriptive studies using the Holter technology for the detection of transient myocardial ischemia (ST segment shifts) were reported, with only a few prospective studies reporting on the prognostic significance of Holter-detected ST segment depression in stable coronary patients.

The criteria for defining an episode of transient myocardial ischemia on the Holter recording were derived from exercise-testing criteria and from clinical experience with the Holter technique. A conventional definition evolved, and most Holter investigators utilize the following criterion for 'ischemia': an episode of transient ST segment depression of s 1 mm (0.1 mV) at 80 ms after the J point from the baseline ST segment position, lasting for over one minute in consecutive beats. This conventional definition has never been validated as truly indicating myocardial ischemia.

At present, most Holter systems utilize 3-lead 24-hour ECG high-quality digital recordings. Most systems also provide a complete record of every complex in compressed time and voltage scales. The resolution of these 'full disclosure' records is insufficient to accurately detect morphologic ST segment shifts. No technique provides perfect discrimination between physiologic signals and noise or artifact. Transient ST segment depressions are, for the most part, due to myocardial ischemia, but physiologic events other than ischemia may produce similar ST segment shifts (postural changes, tachycardia, hypertension, sympathetic activity, hyperventilation, left ventricular dimension and pressure changes, alterations in intraventricular conduction, and drug-level fluctuations).

PERFORMANCE REQUIREMENTS AND TESTING OF AUTOMATED INTERPRETATION PROCEDURES

All the solutions of technical support for cardiology diagnoses must meet specified criteria of safety and reliability before they can be implemented for use with medical devices. Various aspects of quality requirements standardization are presented in the remainder of this chapter:

- the most general FDA regulations concerning safe medical device and the use of unapproved device;
- the IEC regulation concerning interpretive cardiograph performance; and
- the CSE recommendation on the precision of ECG waves delimitation, as well as testing database and methodology descriptions.

The safety regulations for medical devices are purposely mentioned in the initial chapter, just after medical introduction and highlights of current technical approaches to the automated signal interpretation. Our aim is to stress the high importance of quality and reliability, which is higher in medical applications (including the software) than in any other civil application of technology.

Quality assessment is the practical process of determining the value of a new or emerging technology in and of itself or against existing or competing technologies using safety, efficacy, effectiveness, outcome, risk management, strategic, financial, and competitive criteria (Bronzino, 2000). Technology assessment also considers ethics and law as well as health priorities and cost effectiveness compared to competing technologies. A "technology" is defined as devices, equipment, related software, drugs, biotechnologies, procedures, therapies, and systems used to diagnose or treat patients. Technology assessment is not the same as technology acquisition/procurement or technology planning. The latter two are processes for determining equipment vendors, soliciting bids, and systematically determining a hospital's technology-related needs based on strategic, financial, risk management, and clinical criteria. The informational needs differ greatly between technology assessment and the acquisition/procurement or planning processes. This section focuses on the resources applicable to technology assessment.

There are nearly 400 (private, academic, and governmental) organizations worldwide, providing technology assessment information, databases, or consulting services. Some are strictly information clearinghouses, some perform technology assessment, and some do both. For those that perform assessments, the quality of the information generated varies greatly from superficial studies to in-depth, well-referenced analytical reports.

Selected FDA Regulations

Responsibility for regulating medical devices falls to the Food and Drug Administration (FDA) under the Medical Device Amendment of 1976 (Bronzino, 2000). This statute requires approval from the FDA before new devices are marketed and imposes requirements for the clinical investigation of new medical devices on human subjects. Although the statute makes interstate commerce of an unapproved new medical device generally unlawful, it provides an Investigational Device Exemption (IDE) to allow interstate distribution of unapproved devices in order to conduct clinical research on human subjects. Clinical research involving a significant risk device (e.g., orthopedic implants, artificial hearts) cannot begin until an Institutional Review Board (IRB) has approved both the protocol and the informed consent form, and the FDA itself has given permission. This requirement to submit an IDE application to the FDA is waived in the case of clinical research where the risk posed is insignificant. In this case, the FDA requires only that approval from an IRB be obtained certifying that the device in question poses only insignificant risk. In deciding whether to approve a proposed clinical investigation of a new device, the IRB and the FDA must determine the following (Bronzino, Flannery, & Wade, 1990a, 1990b):

1. Risks to subjects are minimized.
2. Risks to subjects are reasonable in relation to the anticipated benefit and knowledge to be gained.
3. Subject selection is equitable.
4. Informed consent materials and procedures are adequate.
5. Provisions for monitoring the study and protecting patient information are acceptable.

The FDA allows unapproved medical devices to be used without an IDE in three types of situations: emergency use, treatment use, and feasibility studies.

FDA Unapproved Devices in Emergency Use

The FDA insists that emergencies are circumstances that reasonable foresight would not anticipate. Particularly important here is the nature of the patient's consent. Individuals facing death are especially vulnerable to exploitation and deserve greater measures for their protection than might otherwise be necessary:

"The FDA has authorized emergency use where an unapproved device offers the only alternative for saving the life of a dying patient, but an IDE has not yet been approved for the device or its use, or an IDE has been approved but the physician who wishes to use the device is not an investigator under the IDE." (Bronzino et al., 1990a, 1990b)

Because the purpose of emergency use of an unapproved device is to attempt to save a dying patient's life under circumstances where no other alternative is at hand, this sort of use constitutes practice rather than research. Its aim is primarily to benefit the patient rather than to provide new and generalizable information. The FDA requires that a physician who engages in emergency use of an unapproved device must "have substantial reason to believe that benefits will exist. This means that there should be a body of pre-clinical and animal tests allowing a prediction of the benefit to a human patient" (Bronzino et al., 1990a, 1990b).

A second requirement that the FDA imposes on emergency use of unapproved devices is the expectation that physicians "exercise reasonable foresight with respect to potential emergencies and make appropriate arrangements under the IDE procedures. Thus, a physician should not 'create' an emergency in order to circumvent IRB review and avoid requesting the sponsor's authorization of the unapproved use of a device" (Bronzino et al., 1990a, 1990b).

FDA Unapproved Devices in Treatment

The FDA has not approved treatment use of unapproved medical devices, but it is possible that a manufacturer could obtain such approval by establishing a specific protocol for this kind of use within the context of an IDE. The criteria for treatment use of unapproved medical devices are the following:

- The device is intended to treat a serious or life-threatening disease or condition.

- There is no comparable or satisfactory alternative product available to treat that condition.
- The device is under an IDE, or has received an IDE exemption, or all clinical trials have been completed and the device is awaiting approval.
- The sponsor is actively pursuing marketing approval of the investigational device.

The treatment use protocol would be submitted as part of the IDE, and would describe the intended use of the device, the rationale for use of the device, the available alternatives and why the investigational product is preferred, the criteria for patient selection, the measures to monitor the use of the device and to minimize risk, and technical information that is relevant to the safety and effectiveness of the device for the intended treatment purpose (Bronzino et al., 1990a, 1990b).

As with emergency use of unapproved devices, the patients involved in treatment use would be particularly vulnerable patients. Although they are not dying, they are facing serious medical conditions and are thereby likely to be less able to avoid exploitation than patients under less desperate circumstances. Consequently, it is especially important that patients be informed of the speculative nature of the intervention and of the possibility that treatment may result in little or no benefit to them.

The Safe Medical Devices Act

On November 28, 1991, the Safe Medical Devices Act of 1990 (Public Law 101-629) went into effect. This regulation requires a wide range of healthcare institutions, including hospitals, ambulatory-surgical facilities, nursing homes, and outpatient treatment facilities, to report information that "reasonably suggests" the likelihood that the death, serious injury, or serious illness of a patient at that facility has been caused or contributed to by a medical device. When a death is device related, a report must be made directly to the FDA *and* to the manufacturer of the device. When a serious illness or injury is device related, a report must be made to the manufacturer *or* to the FDA in cases where the manufacturer is not known. The new law extends this requirement to users of medical devices along with manufacturers and importers. This act represents a significant step forward in protecting patients exposed to medical devices.

IEC International Standard 60601-2-51

The International Standard 60601-2-51—first issued by the International Electrotechnical Commission, (IEC) in 2003 and entitled, "Medical Electrical

Equipment—Particular Requirements for Safety, Including Essential Performance, of Recording and Analyzing Single Channel and Multichannel Electrocardiogra phs"—specifies the testing range and conditions as well as the requirements for results provided by the automatic analysis embedded in the electrocardiographs or released as independent software packages.

Three chapters of the standard specify the principal aspects of measurements accuracy requirements (IEC 60601-2-51).

Requirements for Amplitude Measurements (50.101.2)

The manufacturer shall disclose in the *accompanying documents* in which way amplitude values for the P, QRS, ST, and T waves are determined. If an *analyzing electrocardiograph* provides measurements, their accuracy shall be tested.

Amplitude measurements given for P, Q, R, S, ST, and T shall not deviate from the reference values by more than ±25 μV for amplitudes 500 μV or by more than 5% for amplitudes >500 μV. The differences between the amplitude measurements and the reference values for leads I, II, V1, ..., V6 shall be determined for all provided P, Q, R, S, ST, and T waveforms.

If the calibration and analytical ECGs are fed into the system after digital-to-analogue conversion via the ELECTRODE cables, the tests shall be performed five times. If the *electrocardiograph* can be tested with digital input of calibration and analytical ECGs, the test needs to be performed only once. The differences between measurements and reference values shall be calculated either from the single test or from the mean values of the five tests. If there are obvious fiducial point (P-, QRS-onset/end, and T-end) errors, exclude the differences in the affected amplitude measurements. Exclusion of differences resulting from not more than two fiducial point errors shall be allowed. The difference for each remaining amplitude measurement shall not deviate from the reference value by more than ±25 μV for reference values d 500 μV, or by more than 5 % or ±40 μV (whichever is greater) for reference values >500 μV.

Requirements for Interval Measurements

The manufacturer shall disclose in the *accompanying documents* in which way the isoelectric segments within the QRS complex are treated: whether they are included in or excluded from the Q, R, or S waves. He shall specifically explain whether isoelectric parts (I wave) after global QRS-onset or before global QRS-end (K wave) are included in the duration measurement of the respective adjacent waveform. If the measurements are provided for the *ECG record*, their accuracy shall be according to 50.101.3.1-50.101.3.2 presented below.

Requirements for Absolute Interval and Wave Duration Measurements (50.101.3.1)

These measurements shall be derived from the global interval and the wave duration measurements on the sixteen calibration and analytical ECGs. Acceptable tolerances for the mean differences of global durations and intervals and Q-, R-, and S-duration measurements are given in Table 2.3.

The calibration and analytical ECGs shall be fed into the electrocardiograph under test; simultaneous acquisition of all *leads* is assumed.

For each of the global measurements (P-duration, PQ-interval, QRS-duration, and QT-interval), there will be 16 numbers representing difference in each signal. If there are obvious fiducial point (P-, QRS-onset/end, and T-end) errors, the differences in the affected global and individual *lead* intervals may be excluded from the statistics. Exclusion of differences resulting from not more than two fiducial point errors shall be allowed. From the remaining differences, the two largest deviations shall be removed from the mean (outliers) for each measurement. The means and standard deviations of the remaining differences are computed and shall not exceed the tolerances given in Table 2.3. For each of the individual *lead* measurements (Q-, R-, and S-durations), the differences for *leads* I, II, V1 ... V6 (if the wave is present) are computed for all the *calibration and analytical* ECGs belonging to the control set. Exclude differences resulting from fiducial point errors as described above. From the remaining differences the two largest deviations from the mean (outliers) are removed for each measurement. The means and standard deviations of the remaining differences are computed and shall not exceed the tolerances given in Table 2.3.

Requirements for Interval Measurements on Biological ECGs (50.101.3.2)

One hundred (100) real test ECGs shall be fed into the *electrocardiograph* (either digitally or after D/A-conversion) and analyzed by the system under test. Measurement results shall be analyzed according to the following rules.

If there are obvious fiducial point (P-, QRS-onset/end, and T-end) errors, the differences in the affected global intervals may be excluded. Exclusion of differences resulting from not more than four fiducial point errors shall be allowed. From the remaining differences, the four largest deviations may be removed from the mean (outliers) for each measurement. The means and standard deviations of the remaining differences are computed and shall not exceed the tolerances given in Table 2.4.

Table 2.3. Acceptable mean differences and standard deviations for global intervals and Q-, R-, and S-durations on calibration and analytical ECGs (all dimensions in milliseconds, Copyright © 2003 IEC Geneva, Switzerland.www.iec.ch, used with permission from IEC 60601-2-51)

Measurement	Acceptable Mean Difference	Acceptable Standard Deviation
P-duration	±10	8
PQ-interval	±10	8
QRS-duration	±6	5
QT-interval	±12	10
Q-duration	±6	5
R-duration	±6	5
S-duration	±6	5

Table 2.4. Acceptable mean differences and standard deviations for global durations and intervals for biological ECGs (dimensions in milliseconds, Copyright © 2003 IEC Geneva, Switzerland.www.iec.ch, used with permission from IEC 60601-2-51)

Global Measurement	Acceptable Mean Difference	Acceptable Standard Deviation
P-duration	±10	15
PQ-interval	±10	10
QRS-duration	±10	10
QT-interval	±25	30

CSE Recommendations on the Precision of ECG Waves Delimitation

Ten European centers, five North American and one Japanese (including commercial manufacturers) were involved in a Common Standards for Quantitative Electrocardiography project of analysis for the given set of 250 original and 310 artificial ECG records containing simultaneous ECG and VCG traces of 10 seconds duration (Morlet 1986, Willems 1987, Willems 1990). The records were processed by 10 interpretive systems designed for 12-lead ECG and 9 systems using spatial

Table 2.5. Composition of the CSE Multilead Database (datasets 3 and 4) © 2008 Prof. Paul RUBEL (On behalf of the CSE Working Party). Used with permission.

Electrocardiographic abnormality dataset:	Cases Nbr 3	4	Electrocardlographic abnormality	Cases Nbr 3	4
Normal	33	33	Ischemic ST-T changes	3	3
Incomplete right bundle branch block	5	6	Bigeminy	3	3
Complete right bundle branch block	9	9	Trigeminy	0	1
Left anterior fasclcular block	12	13	Multiple PVC's	9	7
Complete left bundle branch block	7	7	Multiple APC's	6	5
Acute myocardial infarction	2	2	Supraventricular Tachycardia	3	1
Anterior myocardial infarction	13	12	Aerial flutter	1	1
Postero-diafragmatic MI	12	13	Atrial fibrillation	9	9
Lateral or high-lateral MI	4	3	1st AV-block	3	1
Apical myocardial infarction	2	2	2nd AV-block	1	1
MI + IVCD (QRS > 120 msec)	6	6	3rd AV-block	1	0
Left ventricular hypertrophy	12	12	Wolf-Parkinson-White Syndrome	2	2
Right ventricular hypertrophy	3	3	Pacemaker	2	2
Pulmonary emphysema	3	3	Other*	2	1

*Abbreviations ; APC - atrial premature contraction, IVCD - intraventricular conduction defect; MI - myocardial infarction; PVC - premature ventricular contraction; *Reversed arm electrodes, dextrocardia, pericarditis*

vectocardiographic leads. For each fiducial point the outcome of the software was compared with the reference collected from several independent cardiologists. The median value for each class of interpretive systems was compared to the reference and considered as representative for the state of the art in automatic detection of fiducial points.

The comparison consisted in the calculation of the difference between the software outcome and the human expert annotation. The negative value of the difference means that the beginning or end of the wave has been estimated by the software too early, while the positive value of the difference indicates that the software estimated wave border is too late. The average value represents the systematic error and the standard deviation approaches the result variability (Figure 2.5).

Figure 2.7 Testing the example ECG interpretation software for the wave borders accuracy with use of CSE Multilead Database: absolute accuracy (left plots) and

Figure. 2.7 Testing the example ECG interpretation software for the wave borders accuracy with use of CSE Multilead Database: absolute accuracy (left plots) and accuracy ranking in relation to other ECG interpreting systems whose results are available in the Database (right plots).

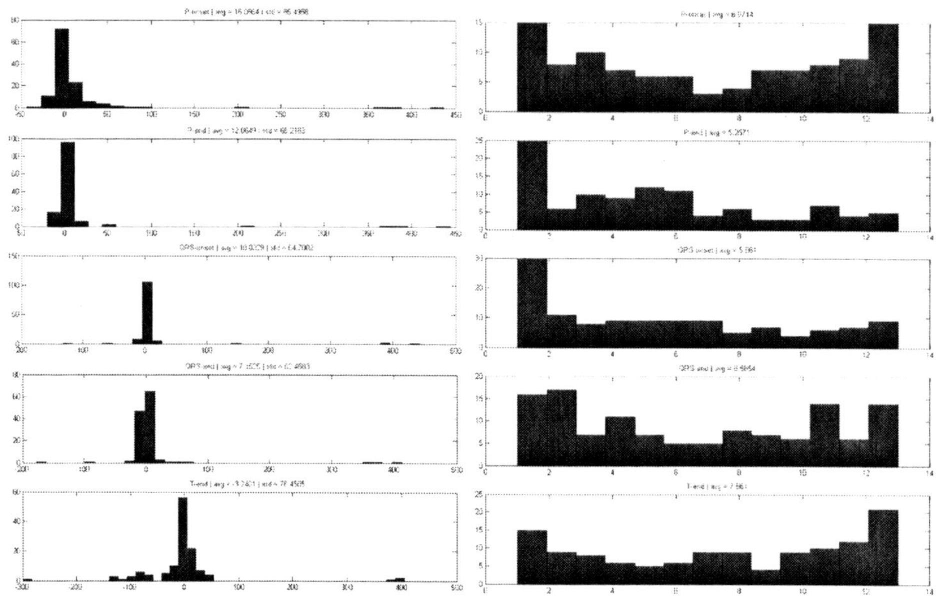

accuracy ranking in relation to other ECG interpreting systems whose results are available in the Database (right plots).

The result of a median software was very close to the references provided by the experts. In terms of statistical variability, each software system considered separately had a worse result than the median. Therefore, the CSE consortium recommends the use of the CSE database as a reference standard for evaluation of the fiducial point determinant software. The software under test should meet the following criteria (Morlet 1988):

- issue a result for QRS complex borders for at least 95% of input files for QRS, and respectively 90% for T wave and 85% for P wave after exclusion of the cases which do not show a P wave,
- issue a result best approximating the reference values (minimum systematic error),

- the standard deviation computed after excluding respectively 2% of the highest differences for onset and end of QRS and 3% for the onset of P and end of P and T shall be less than two standard deviations of the difference between the individual and final referee estimates (Willems 1985).

There are 3 CSE reference data bases on the CD-ROM (Willems 1990). Two have been developed for the testing and development of ECG measurement programs: the first for ECGs in which 3 leads have been recorded simultaneously in the standard sequence, i.e. leadgroup I, II, III; leadgroup aVR, aVL, aVF; leadgroup VI, V2, V3; leadgroup V4, V5, V6 and finally the Frank leads X, Y, Z. In the second data base all leads, i.e. the standard 12 leads plus the 3 Frank leads have been recorded simultaneously. The statistical contents of the CSE Multilead Database is presented in Table 2.5. The diagnostic interpretations of the ECG records of data sets 1-4 are only indicative of the complexity of the ECG records. A third CSE data base has been developed for the assessment of diagnostic ECG and VCG computer programs. This data base also comprises multilead recordings both of the standard ECG and the VCG. All cases have been sampled at 500 Hz. The goals of the CSE, the methods used for data collection and analysis, as well as many processing results have been published in (Willems 1990).

The 3-lead CSE measurement data base consists of 250 original and 310 so-called artificial ECG recordings. They have been divided into two equal sets, i.e. data set one and data set two. The multilead measurement data base is also composed of original and so-called artificial ECG recordings. This data base has been split into two equal sets i.e. data set three and data set four. The so-called artificial ECG data are made out of strings of identical selected beats up to fill a specified recording time.

The onsets and offsets of P, QRS and T of these beats have been analyzed by a group of cardiologists during an extensive iterative Delphi review process in the CSE project. The review was performed for all files in 3-Lead Database, while for the Multilead database, only around 21% of the cases have been analysed by the referees. In the Multilead Database, the truth has been obtained by taking the median of the values computed by 14 independent ECG/VCG programs. The results of this analysis have been released only for data sets one and three included in CD-ROM. Those of data sets two and four are kept secret in the CSE Coordinating Center for testing purposes.

The diagnostic data base (also called CSE data set 5) has been developed primarily for testing the performance of diagnostic ECG and VCG computer programs. For this data base only the digitized ECG data (1220 cases) have been released by the CSE Coordinating Center, without the clinically validated diagnoses. The clinical truth of the Diagnostic database is kept secret in the coordination center and

Table 2.6. Composition of the CSE Diagnostic Database (dataset 5) © 2008 Prof. Paul RUBEL (On behalf of the CSE Working Party). Used with permission.

Diagnostic category	Number of cases
Normal (NL)	382
Left ventricular Hypertrophy (LVH)	183
Right ventricular Hypertrophy (RVH)	55
Biventricular Hypertrophy (BVH)	53
Anterior myocardial Infarction (AMI)	170
Inferior Myocardial Infarction (IMI)	273
Anterior and Inferior Myocardial Infarction (MIX)	73
Hypertrophy and Myocardial Infarction (VH+MI)	31
Total	1220

will be used for the assessment of the interpretation programs results sent to the coordination center. Release of the 'true' clinical diagnoses of the cases has therefore by definition not been possible. The composition of CSE diagnostic library is provided in Table 2.4.

REFERENCES

AHA. (1967). *AHA ECG database.* Available from Emergency Care Research Institute, Plymouth Meeting, PA.

Ahlstrom, M. L., and Tompkins, W. J. (1981) An inexpensive microprocessor system for high speed QRS width detection. *Proceedings of the 1st Annual IEEE Compmedicine Conference* (pp. 81-83).

Akselrod, S., Norymberg, M., Peled, I. et al. (1987). Computerized analysis of ST segment changes in ambulatory electrocardiograms. *Medical and Biological Engineering and Computing, 25,* 513-519.

Armstrong, W. F., & Morris, S. N. (1983). The ST segment during ambulatory electrocardiographic monitoring. *Annals of Internal Medicine, 98,* 249-250.

Badilini, F., Zareba, W., Titlebaum, E. L., & Moss, A. J. (1986). Analysis of ST segment variability in Holter recordings. In A. Moss & A. Stern (Eds.), *Noninvasive electrocardiology—clinical aspects of Holter monitoring.* London: Saunders Co.

Bailón, R., Sörnmo, L., & Laguna, P. (2006a). ECG-derived respiratory frequency estimation. In G. D. Clifford, F. Azuaje, & P. E. McSharry (Eds.), *Advanced methods and tools for ECG data analysis* (pp. 215-244). Boston, Artech House.

Bailón, R., Sörnmo, L., & Laguna, P. (2006b). A robust method for ECG-based estimation of the respiratory frequency during stress testing. *IEEE Transactions on Biomedical Engineering, 53,* 1273-1285.

Balda, R. A., Diller, G., Deardorff, E., Doue, J., & Hsieh, P. (1977). The HP ECG analysis program. In J. H. van Bemmel & J. L. Willems (Eds.), *Trends in computer-processed electrocardiograms* (pp. 197-205). Amsterdam: North Holland.

Batsford. W. (1999). Pacemakers and antitachycardia devices. In: B.L. Zaret, M. Moser & L.S. Cohen (Eds.) *Yale University School of Medicine Heart Book*, pp. 331-338. Hearst Books. New York. Available online at http://www.med.yale.edu/library/heartbk/ (accessed in November 2008)

Biagini, A., Mazzei, M. Z., Carpeggiani, C. et al. (1982). Vasospastic ischemic mechanism of frequent asymptomatic transient ST-T changes during continuous electrocardiographic monitoring in selected unstable patients. *American Heart Journal, 103,* 4-12.

Biblo, I. A., & Waldo, A. L. (1986). Supraventricular arrhythmias. In A. Moss & A. Stern (Eds.), *Noninvasive electrocardiology—clinical aspects of Holter monitoring.* London: Saunders Co.

Bronzino, J. D. (2000). Regulation of medical, device innovation. In J. D. Bronzino (Ed.), *The biomedical engineering handbook.* Boca Raton, FL: CRC Press.

Bronzino, J. D., Flannery, E. J., and Wade, M. L. (1990a) "Legal and Ethical Issues in the Regulation and Development of Engineering Achievements in Medical Technology," Part I *Engineering in Medicine and Biology Magazine, IEEE* vol. 9, no. 1, pp. 79-81

Bronzino, J. D., Flannery, E. J., and Wade, M. L. (1990b) "Legal and Ethical Issues in the Regulation and Development of Engineering Achievements in Medical Technology," Part II *Engineering in Medicine and Biology Magazine, IEEE*, vol. 9 no. 2, pp. 53-57

Cosby, R. S., & Herman, L. M. (1962). Sequential changes in the development of the electrocardiographic pattern of left ventricular hypertrophy in hypertensive heart disease. *American Heart Journal, 63,* 180.

CSE Working Party. (1985). Recommendations for measurement standards in quantitative electrocardiography. *European Heart Journal, 6,* 815-825.

Cuomo, S., Marciano, F., Migaux, M. L., Finizio, F., Pezzella, E., Losi, M. A., & Betocchi, S. (2004). Abnormal QT interval variability in patients with hypertrophic cardiomyopathy. Can syncope be predicted? *Journal of Electrocardiology, 37*(2), 113-119.

Dobbs, S. E., Schmitt, N. M., & Ozemek, H. S. (1984). QRS detection by template matching using real-time correlation on a microcomputer. *Journal of Clinical Engineering, 9,* 197-212.

Dower, G. E. (1984). The ECGD: A derivation of the ECG from VCG leads. *Journal of Electrocardiology, 17*(2), 189-191.

Extramiana, F., Neyroud, N., Huikuri, H. V., Koistinen, M. J., Coumel, P., & Maison-Blanche, P. (1999a). QT interval and arrhythmic risk assessment after myocardial infarction. *American Journal of Cardiology, 83,* 266-269.

Fisch, C. (2000). Centennial of the sting galvanometer and the electrocardiogram. *Journal of the College of Cardiology, 36*(6), 1737-1745.

Franchini, K. G., & Cowley, A. E., Jr. (2004). Autonomic control of cardiac function. In D. Robertson, I. Biaggioni, G. Burnstock, & P. A. Low (Eds.), *Primer on the autonomic nervous system* (2nd ed., pp. 134-138). Englewood Cliffs, NJ: Elsevier Academic Press.

Friesen, G. M., Jannett T. C. et al. (1990). A comparison of the noise sensitivity of nine QRS detection algorithms. *IEEE Transactions on Biomedical Engineering, 37*(1), 85-98.

Fumo, G. S., & Tompkins, W. J. (1982). QRS detection using automata theory in a battery-powered microprocessor system. *IEEE Frontiers of Engineering in Health Care, 4,* 155-158.

Gaita, F., Giustetto, C., Bianchi, F., Wolpert, C., Schimpf, R., Riccardi, R., Grossi, S., Richiardi, E., & Borggrefe, M. (2003). Short QT syndrome a familial cause of sudden death. *Circulation, 108,* 965-970.

Garibyan, L. and L. S. Lilly (2006). The electrocardiogram. In L.S. Lilly (Ed.) Pathophysiology of Heart Disease,: *A Collaborative, Project of Medical Students and Faculty*, fourth ed.. pp. 80-117. Lippincott Williams & Wilkins, Philadelphia.

Gulrajani, R. M. (1998). The forward and inverse problems of electrocardiography. Gaining a better qualitative and quantitative understanding of the heart's electrical activity. *IEEE MBE Magazine, 17*(5), 84-101.

Hamilton, P. S., & Tompkins, W. J. (1986) Quantitative investigation of QRS detection rules using the MIT/BIH arrhythmia database. *IEEE Transactions on Biomedical Engineering, 33,* 1157-1165.

Hull, E. (1961). The electrocardiogram in pericarditis. *American Journal of Cardiology, 7,* 21.

IEC 60601-2-51. (2003). Medical electrical equipment: Particular requirements for the safety, including essential performance, of ambulatory electrocardiographic systems. First edition 2003-02, International Electrotechnical Commission, Geneva,

Iyer V., Edelman E. R. & Lilly L. S. (2006). Basic cardiac structure and function. In L.S. Lilly (Ed.) *Pathophysiology of Heart Disease: A Collaborative Project of Medical Students and Faculty*, fourth ed.. pp. 1-28. Lippincott Williams & Wilkins, Philadelphia.

Klingeman, J., & Pipberger, H. V. (1967). Computer classification of electrocardiograms. *Computers and Biomedical Research, 1,* 1.

Kohler, B., Hennig, C., & Orglmeister, R. (2002). The principles of software QRS detection. *IEEE Engineering in Medicine and Biology Magazine, 21*(1), 42-57.

Lass, J., Kaik, J., Karai, D., & Vainu, M. (2001). Ventricular repolarization evaluation from surface ECG for identification of the patients with increased myocardial electrical instability. *Proceedings of the 23rd Annual International Conference of the IEEE Engineering in Medicine and Biology Society* (pp. 390-393).

Levkov, C. L. (1987). Orthogonal electrocardiogram derived from limb and chest electrodes of the conventional 12-lead system. *Medical and Biological Engineering and Computing, 25,* 155-164.

Lombardi, F. (2001). Frequency domain analysis of heart rate variability In W. Zareba, P. Maison-Blanche, & E. F. Locati (Eds.), *Noninvasive electrocardiology in clinical practice.* Armonk, NY: Futura.

Macfarlane, P. W., Lorimer, A. R., & Lowrie, T. D. V. (1971). 3 and 12 lead electrocardiogram interpretation by computer. A comparison in 1093 patients. *British Heart Journal, 33,* 226.

Malik, M. (1995). Effect of ECG recognition artefact on time-domain measurement of heart rate variability. In M. Malik & A. J. Camm (Eds.), *Heart rate variability.* Armonk, NY: Futura.

Malik, M., & Camm, A. J. (2004). *Dynamic electrocardiography.* Armonk, NY: Blackwell Futura.

Malik, M., Farbom, P., Batchvarov, V., Hnatkova, K., & Camm, J. (2002). Relation between QT and RR intervals is highly individual among healthy subjects: Implications for heart rate correction of the QT interval. *Heart, 87,* 220-228.

Malik, M., Farrell, T., Cripps, T., & Camm, A. J. (1989). Heart rate variability in relation to prognosis after myocardial infarction: Selection of optimal processing techniques. *European Heart Journal, 10,* 1060-1074.

Marcus, F. I. (1986). Ventricular arrhythmias In A. Moss & S. Stern (Eds.), *Noninvasive electrocardiology—clinical aspects of Holter monitoring.* London: Saunders Co.

McPherson, C. A. & Rosenfeld L. E. (1999). Heart rhythm disorders. In B.L. Zaret, M. Moser and Cohen L. S., (Eds.) *Yale University School of Medicine Heart Book*, pp. 195-204. Hearst Books. New York. Available online at http://www.med.yale.edu/library/heartbk/ (accessed in November 2008).

Milliez, P., Leenhardt, A., Maison-Blanche, P., Vicaut, E., Badilini, F., Siliste, C., Benchetrit C., & Coumel, P. (2005). Usefulness of ventricular repolarization dynamicity in predicting arrhythmic deaths in patients with isquemic cardiomyopathy (from the European Myocardial Infarct Amiodarone Trial). *American Journal of Cardiology, 95,* 821-826.

MIT-BIH Database Distribution. (n.d.). *MIT/BIH ECG database.* Cambridge, MA: Massachusetts Institute of Technology.

Moody, G. B., & Mark R. G. (1990). The MIT-BIH arrhythmia database on CD-ROM and software for use with it. *Computers in Cardiology, 17,* 185-188.

Moody, G. B., Mark, R. G., Zoccola, A., & Mantero, S. (1986). Derivation of respiratory signals from multilead ECGs. *Computers in Cardiology, 13,* 113-116.

Morlet, D. (1986). *Contribution a l'analyse automatique des electrocardiogrammes—algorithmes de localisation, classification et delimitation precise des ondes dans le systeme de Lyon* (in French). PhD Thesis, INSA-Lyon, France.

Morlet D, Rubel P, Arnaud P, Willems JL. (1988) An improved method to evaluate the precision of computer ECG measurement programs. *Int J Biomed Comput. 22*(3-4), 199-216

Moss, A. J. (1986). Clinical utility of ST segment monitoring. In A. Moss & S. Stern (Eds.), *Noninvasive electrocardiology—clinical aspects of Holter monitoring.* London: Saunders Co.

Moss, A. J., Bigger, J. T., & Odoroff, C. L. (1987). Postinfarction risk stratification. *Progress in Cardiovascular Disease, 29,* 389-412.

Moss, A. J., Schnitzler, R., Green, R., & DeCamilla, J. (1971). Ventricular arrhythmias 3 weeks after acute myocardial infarction. *Annals of Internal Medicine, 75,* 837-841.

Nelson, S. D., Kou, W. H., & Annesley, T. (1989). Significance of ST segment depression during paroxysmal superventricular tachycardia. *Journal of the American College of Cardiology, 13,* 804.

Pan, J., & Tompkins, W. J. (1985). A real-time QRS detection algorithm. *IEEE Transactions on Biomedical Engineering, 32*(3), 230-236.

Parker J.O., di Giorgi S., & West R.O (1966) A hemodynamic study of acute coronary insufficiency precipitated by exercise. *American Journal of Cardiology* 17: pp. 470-483,

Pellerin, D., Maison-Blanche, P., Extramiana, F., Hermida, J. S., Leclercq, J. F., Leenhardt, A., & Coumel, P. (2001). Autonomic influences on ventricular repolarization in congestive heart failure. *Journal of Electrocardiology, 34*(1), 35-40.

Pordy, L., Jaffe, H., Chesky, K. et al. (1968). Computer diagnosis of electrocardiograms IV, a computer program for contour analysis with clinical results of rhythm and contour interpretation. *Computers and Biomedical Research, 1,* 408-433.

Pottala, E. W., Bailey, J. J., Horton, M. R., & Gradwohl, J. R. (1989). Suppression of baseline wander in the ECG using a bilinearly transformed, null-phase filter. *Journal of Electrocardiology, 22*(suppl), 243-247.

Rolls H. K., Stevenson W. G., Strichartz G. R.& Lilly L. S. (2006) Mechanisms of cardiac arrhythmias. In L.S. Lilly, (Ed.) *Pathophysiology of Heart Disease: A Collaborative Project of Medical Students and Faculty* , fourth ed.. pp. 269-289. Lippincott Williams & Wilkins, Philadelphia.

Sörnmo, L., & Laguna, P. (2005). *Bioelectrical signal processing in cardiac and neurological applications.* Englewood Cliffs, NJ: Elsevier Academic Press.

Stern, S., & Tzivoni, D. (1974). Early detection of silent ischemic heart disease by 24-hour electrocardiographic monitoring of active subjects. *British Heart Journal, 36,* 481-486.

Stramba-Badiale, M., Locati, E. H., Martinelli, A., Courvillet, J., & Schwartz, P. J. (1997). Gender and the relationship between ventricular repolarization and cardiac cycle length during 24-h Holter recordings. *European Heart Journal, 18,* 1000-1006.

Swiryn, S., McDonough, T., & Hueter, D. C. (1984). Sinus node function and dysfunction. *Medical Clinics of North America, 68,* 935-954.

Task Force of the ESC/ASPE. (1996). Heart rate variability: Standards of measurement, physiological interpretation, and clinical use. *European Heart Journal, 17,* 354-381.

Tayler, D. I., & Vincent, R. (1985). Artefactual ST segment abnormalities due to electrocardiograph design. *British Heart Journal, 54,* 11-28.

Thakor, N. V. (1978). Reliable R-wave detection from ambulatory subjects. *Biomedical Sciences Instrumentation, 14,* 67-72.

Thakor, N. V., Webster, J. G., & Tompkins, W. J. (1980). Optimal QRS filter. *Proceedings of the IEEE Conference on Frontiers of Engineering in Health Care* (vol. 2, pp. 190-195).

Thakor, N. V., Webster, J. G., & Tompkins, W. J. (1983). Optimal QRS detector. *Medical & Biological Engineering & Computing, 21,* 343-350.

Thakor, N. V., Webster, J. G., & Tompkins, W. J. (1984a). Design, implementation, and evaluation of a microcomputer-based portable arrhythmia monitor. *Medical & Biological Engineering & Computing, 22,* 151-159.

Thakor, N. V., Webster, J. G., & Tompkins, W. J. (1984b). Estimation of QRS complex power spectra for design of a QRS filter. *IEEE Transactions on Biomedical Engineering, 31,* 702-706.

Valensi, P. E., Extramiana, F., Johnson, N. B., Motte, G., Maison-Blanche, P., & Coumel, P. (2002). Influence of cardiac autonomic neuropathy on heart rate dependence of ventricular repolarization in diabetic patients. *Diabetes Care, 25*(5), 918-923.

Van Mieghem, C., Sabbe, M., & Knockaert, D. (2004). The clinical value of the ECG in noncardiac conditions. *Chest, 124,* 1561-1576.

Vera, Z., & Mason, D. T. (1981). Detection of sinus node dysfunction: Consideration of clinical application of testing methods. *American Heart Journal, 102,* 308-312.

Wagner, G. S., & Marriott, H. J. (1994). *Marriott's practical electrocardiography* (9th ed.). Lippincott Williams & Wilkins, Philadelphia

Weisner, S. J., Tompkins, W. J., & Tompkins, B. M. (1982a). A compact, microprocessor-based ECG ST-segment monitor for the operating room. *IEEE Transactions on Biomedical Engineering, 29,* 642-649.

Weisner, S. J., Tompkins, W. J., & Tompkins, B. M. (1982b). Microprocessor-based, portable anesthesiology ST-segment analyzer. *Proceedings of the Northeast Bioengineering Conference* (pp. 222-226).

Willems J. L., The CSE Working Party. (1985). Recommendations for measurement standards in quantitative electrocardiography. Eur Heart J. 6:815–825.

Willems, J. L. (1990). *Common standards for quantitative electrocardiography: 10th CSE progress report.* Leuven, Belgium: ACCO.

Willems, J. L., Arnaud, P., van Bemmel, J. H., Bourdillon, P. J., Degani, R., Denis, B., Graham, I., Harms, F. M., Macfarlane, P. W., Mazzocca, G. et al. (1987). A reference data base for multilead electrocardiographic computer measurement programs. *Journal of the American College of Cardiology, 10*(6), 1313-1321.

Yan, G. X., & Antzelevitch, C. (1998). Cellular basis for the normal T wave and the electrocardio-graphic manifestations of the long-QT syndrome. *Circulation, 98,* 1928-1936.

Yap, Y. G., & Camm, A. J. (2003). Drug induced QT prolongation and torsades de pointes. *Heart, 89,* 1363-1372.

Yasuma, F., & Hayano, J. (2004). Respiratory sinus arrhythmia. Why does the heartbeat synchronize with respiratory rhythm? *Chest, 125,* 683-690.

Zaret B.L., Moser M. & Cohen L. S. (medical editors) (1999). Yale, University School of Medicine Heart Book. Hearst Books. New York. Available online at http://www.med.yale.edu/library/heartbk/ (accessed in November 2008)

Chapter III
Background 2: Telemedical Solutions in Cardiac Diagnostics: Current Issues

This chapter presents basic facts about the social impact and frequency of cardiovascular diseases in aging societies. Being the primary cause of mortality in developed countries, cardiovascular abnormalities receive the most of the attention in the medical world. The problem is particularly observed in developed countries with a significantly longer life expectancy (Japan, Canada) and leading in healthcare organization and research. Also considering the acuteness of a typical cardiac failure gives proper attention to why cardiology is given so much importance in the treatment of life-threatening situations. Making progress in cardiac diagnosis and treatment, including modern and wide-range surveillance, is potentially beneficial to whole societies and countries. It also influences both life length and comfort, which are today among the most appreciated of human values.

In the context of improving everyday life, the Holter technique is introduced, highlighting the extended features resulting from a continuous recording of patients' ECGs in true to life conditions. These benefits include the opportunity for risk stratification in the real patient's environment, much more reliable than laboratory examinations. The Holter technique, although invented 50 years ago (Holter, 1961), is from its beginning and still today a source of new inspiration for both medical and technical research. Medical science has discovered new aspects and diagnostic possibilities based on the cooperation of the cardiovascular, nervous, endocrine, and respiratory systems in the organism, represented by a correlation of representative vital signs. This research broadens the insight of the doctor to a patient and the healthcare manager with regard to aging populations. At the same time the quality of diagnostics improves and the diagnostic itself becomes less invasive and more accepted as an element of everyday life.

The progress would not be possible without the parallel development of healthcare technology. The traditional recording tape has been replaced by digital storage media or digital data transmission, removing technological frontiers (e.g., the maximum examination duration), improving data quality, and presenting the opportunity of seamless surveillance for the outpatient. The term "technology" also includes an emerging and rapidly developing domain of medical signal processing aimed at sustained assistance of a problem-oriented automat in the interpretation of biological signs. The advantages of this approach include easier management of the rapidly increasing data flow, pre-selection and highlighting of abnormalities, and standardization of diagnostic procedures worldwide. Cardiology is here again a leading application of biomedical signal processing, because of the number of automatically recognizable diseases and the number of scientists involved in relation to the number of people benefiting in their everyday lives.

The achievements of contemporary digital wireless transmission are presented in the context of continuous cardiac surveillance. The opportunity for immediate interaction with the patient with heart failure adds value, compared with regular long-term recording. Various aspects of interaction, including distant drug and activity messages, are discussed. The concept of interaction is further exploited and extended to the interaction of distant cooperating software.

CARDIOVASCULAR DISEASES AS A CIVILIZATION ISSUE

As is commonly known, cardiovascular diseases are life-threatening. Virtually all diseases could be life-threatening, but analyzing the background of that belief, we found two major foundations:

- Cardiovascular diseases are very common in our society. Everyday life brings us into contact with cardiac-disabled people, and the common awareness about the importance of cardiac failure is fairly high. Unfortunately this awareness does not influence the lifestyle of the people potentially exposed to danger (e.g., genetic preconditions, diet, stress).
- Cardiovascular diseases may develop silently and manifest their symptoms as an emergency. The sudden cardiac arrest and consequent complete impairment of blood transportation function causes irreversible mortal changes in cells

in the first two minutes. Therefore every rescue action must be undertaken promptly in such cases.

Many diseases and also the aftermath of accidents meet one of the criteria above. Because cardiovascular diseases meet both of these criteria, their common reception is very serious.

The Role of the Cardiovascular System

Simple forms of life are based on independent cells. Each cell fulfills all life-oriented tasks—basically metabolism and procreation. Complicated organisms evolved towards the specialization of cells. They form systems of task-oriented structures and functionality. Cells are no longer independent; on the contrary, they benefit from the life of other cells and vice versa their lives support the life of the other cells. This is best reflected in the common etymology of the words 'organism' and 'organization'.

Particularly in the human body, not every cell is near enough to the environment to easily exchange substances (including nutrients, oxygen, carbon dioxide, and the waste products of the metabolism), energy (including heat), and momentum (Schneck, 2000). The *cardiovascular system* fulfills the task of a general transportation network. It is purposely organized to make available thousands of miles of access pathways for the transport to and from a different neighborhood of any given cell and any material needed to sustain its life.

The cardiovascular system consists of (Hurst, 2002):

- *blood vessels*—a complex branching configuration of distributing and collecting pipes and channels;
- *the heart*—being a main and unique propeller of the working fluid;
- *the blood*—the working fluid fulfilling many other functions, for example, immunological; and
- *sophisticated means for both intrinsic (inherent) and extrinsic (autonomic and endocrine) control.*

The *vascular system* is divided by a microscopic capillary network into:

- an upstream, high-pressure, efferent arterial side consisting of relatively thick-walled, viscoelastic tubes that carry the blood away from the heart; and
- a downstream, low-pressure, afferent venous side, consisting of correspondingly thinner (but having a larger caliber) elastic conduits that return the blood back to the heart.

Except for their differences in thickness, the walls of the largest arteries and veins consist of the same three distinct, well-defined, and well-developed layers:

- *tunica intima*—the innermost and the thinnest continuous lining,
- *tunica media*—the middle thickest layer composed of numerous circularly arranged elastic fibers, and
- *tunica adventitia*—the outer medium-sized vascular sheath consisting entirely of connective tissue.

The largest blood vessels, such as the aorta, the pulmonary artery, the pulmonary veins, and others, have such thick walls that they require a separate network of tiny blood vessels—the *vasa vasorum*—just to service the vascular tissue itself.

Blood vessel structure is directly related to its function (Caro, Pedley, Schroter, & Seed, 1978). The thick-walled large arteries and main *distributing branches* are designed to withstand the pulsating blood pressure of 80 to 130 mmHg (10.66-17.33 kPa). The smaller elastic *conducting vessels* need only operate under steadier blood pressures in the range of 70 to 90 mmHg (9.33-12 kPa), but they must be thin enough to penetrate and course through organs without affecting the anatomic integrity of the mass involved. Controlling arterioles operate at blood pressures between 45 and 70 mmHg (6-9.33 kPa), but are heavily supported with smooth muscle tissue so that they may be actively closed when the flow to the subsequent capillary is to be restricted; the smallest capillary *resistance vessels* (which operate at blood pressures on the order of 10 to 45 mmHg - 1.33-6 kPa) are designed to optimize conditions for the material transportation between blood and the surrounding interstitial fluid.

At the venous side, one encounters a relatively steady blood pressure continuously decreasing from around 30 mmHg (4 kPa) all the way down to near zero, so these vessels can be thin-walled without disease consequence. However, the low blood pressure, slower, steady flow, thin walls, and larger caliber that characterize the venous system cause blood to tend to “pool” in veins, allowing them to act somewhat like reservoirs. Therefore at any given instant, about two-thirds of the total human blood volume is residing in the venous system, and the remaining one-third is divided among the heart (6.5%), the microcirculation (7% in systemic and pulmonary capillaries), and the arterial system (19.5 to 20%).

The *human heart*, having an approximate size of the clenched fist, is a conically shaped muscular organ occupying a small region between the third and sixth ribs in the central portion of the thoracic cavity of the body. Its dimensions are within 12 to 13 centimeters from base (top) to apex (bottom) and 7 to 8 centimeters at its widest point, and the weight is approximate 300 grams—about 0.5% of the individual’s body weight. It rests on the diaphragm, between the lower part of the two lungs, its base-to-apex axis leaning mostly toward the left side of the body and slightly forward. The heart is divided by a strong muscular wall—the interatrial-interventricular septum—into right and left sides, each being a self-contained two-stage pumping device. The left side of the heart drives oxygenated blood through the aortic semilunar outlet valve into the *systemic circulation,* which carries the fluid to a differential neighborhood of each cell in the body—from which it returns to the right side of the heart low in oxygen and rich in carbon dioxide. The right side of the heart then drives this deoxygenated blood through the pulmonary semilunar (pulmonic) outlet valve into the *pulmonary circulation,* which carries the fluid to the lungs—where its oxygen supply is replenished and its carbon dioxide content is purged before it returns to the left side of the heart to begin the cycle all over again. Because of the anatomic proximity of the heart to the lungs, the right side of the heart does not have to work very hard to drive blood through the pulmonary circulation, so it functions as a low-pressure (physiologically 40 mmHg) pump, compared with the left side of the heart, which does most of its work at a high pressure (physiologically up to 140 mmHg) to drive the blood through the entire systemic circulation to the furthest extremes of the organism.

Each side of the heart is further divided into two chambers separated by a one-way valve:

- *atrium*—a small upper receiving chamber; and
- *ventricle*—a lower discharging chamber, which is about twice the size of its corresponding atrium.

In order of size, the somewhat spherically shaped left atrium is the smallest chamber—holding about 45 ml of blood (at rest), operating at pressures on the order of 0 to 25 mmHg, and having a wall thickness of about 3 mm. The pouch-shaped right atrium is next (63 ml of blood, pressure 0 to 10 mmHg (1.33 kPa), 2-mm wall thickness), followed by the conically/cylindrically shaped left ventricle (100 ml of blood, up to 140 mmHg (18.66 kPa) of pressure, variable wall thickness up to 12 mm) and the crescent-shaped right ventricle (about 130 ml of blood, pressure up to 40 mmHg (5.33 kPa), and a wall thickness on the order of one-third that of the left ventricle, up to about 4 mm). The heart chambers collectively have a capacity of about 350 ml, what makes about 6.5% of the nominal total blood volume. In order to put the blood in the unidirectional motion, the heart chambers are separated by valves of different anatomy. In the low pressure right heart, the 3.8-cm-diameter tricuspid valve separates the right atrium from the right ventricle and the 2.4-cm-diameter pulmonary valve separates the right ventricle from the pulmonary vessel. In the high-pressure left heart, the 3.1-cm diameter bicuspid or mitral valve separates the left atrium from the left ventricle; and the outlet valve, the 2.25-cm-diameter aortic semilunar valve, separates the left ventricle from the aorta.

During its perpendicular action the organ alternately fills and expands, contracts, and then empties as it generates a *cardiac output*. The heart action has two phases:

- diastolic of the average duration of 480 ms, the inlet valves of the two ventricles are open, and the outlet valves are closed—the heart ultimately expanding to its *end-diastolic-volume* (EDV), which is on the order of 140 ml of blood for the left ventricle; and
- systolic of the average duration of 270-ms electrically induced vigorous contraction of cardiac muscle drives the intraventricular pressure up, forcing the one-way inlet valves closed and the unidirectional outlet valves open as the heart contracts to its *end-systolic-volume* (ESV), which is typically on the order of 70 ml of blood for the left ventricle.

The principal mechanical effectiveness of the heart, called the *stroke volume* (SV), is measured as the volume of blood expelled from the heart during each systolic interval. Because the ventricles normally empty only about half their contained volume with each heartbeat, the SV is the difference between the *actual* EDV and the *actual* ESV. The ratio of SV to EDV is called the *cardiac ejection fraction*—its nominal values range*s* from 0.5 to 0.75, whereas 0.4 to 0.5 signifies mild cardiac damage, 0.25 to 0.40 implies moderate heart damage, and below 0.25 is a warning of severe damage to the heart's pumping ability.

The blood, accounting for about 8 ± 1% of total body weight, averaging 5200 ml, is a complex, heterogeneous suspension of formed elements—the blood cells, or hematocytes—suspended in a continuous, straw-colored fluid called plasma. Nominally, the composite fluid has a mass density of 1.057 ± 0.007 g/cm^3, and it is three to six times as viscous as water. The hematocytes include three basic types of cells: red blood cells (erythrocytes, totaling nearly 95% of the formed elements), white blood cells (leukocytes, averaging <0.15% of all hematocytes), and platelets (thrombocytes, on the order of 5% of all blood cells). Hematocytes are all derived in the active ("red") bone marrow (about 1,500 grams) of adults from undifferentiated stem cells called hemocytoblasts, and all reach ultimate maturity via a process called hematocytopoiesis.

The primary function of erythrocytes is to aid in the transport of blood gases—about 30 to 34% (by weight) of each cell consisting of the oxygen—and carbon dioxide, carrying protein hemoglobin and a small portion of the cell containing the enzyme carbonic anhydrase, which catalyzes the reversible formation of carbonic acid from carbon dioxide and water. The primary function of leukocytes is to endow the human body with the ability to identify and dispose of foreign substances such as infectious organisms that do not belong there—agranulocytes (lymphocytes and monocytes) essentially doing the 'identifying' and granulocytes (neutrophils, basophils, and eosinophils) essentially doing the 'disposing'. The primary function of platelets is to participate in the blood clotting process.

Some 6.5 to 8% of plasma by weight consists of the plasma proteins, of which there are three major types—albumin, the globulins, and fibrinogen—and several of lesser prominence. The primary functions of albumin are to help maintain the osmotic (oncotic) transmural differential pressure that ensures proper mass exchange between blood and interstitial fluid at the capillary level, and to serve as a transport carrier molecule for several hormones and other small biochemical constituents (such as some metal ions). The primary function of the globulin class of proteins is to act as transport carrier molecules for large biochemical substances, such as fats (lipoproteins) and certain carbohydrates (muco- and glycoproteins) and heavy metals (mineraloproteins), and to work together with leukocytes in the body's immune system.

The *cardiovascular system control* is optimized for the better performance of the transportation task (Dawson, 1991). Blood flows through organs and tissues either to nourish and sanitize them or to be itself processed (e.g., oxygenated in pulmonary circulation). Thus any given vascular network normally receives blood according to the metabolic needs of the region it perfuses and/or the function of that region as a blood treatment plant and/or thermoregulatory pathway. However, it is not feasible to expect that our physiologic transport system can be all things to all cells all of the time—especially when resources are scarce and/or time is a factor. Thus the distribution of blood is further prioritized according to three basic criteria:

1. how essential the perfused region is to the maintenance of life itself,
2. how essential the perfused region is in allowing the organism to respond to a life-threatening situation, and
3. how well the perfused region can function and survive on a decreased supply of blood.

The control of cardiovascular functions is accomplished by mechanisms that are based on two mechanisms:

- *intrinsic control*—inherent physicochemical attributes of the tissues and organs themselves; and
- *extrinsic control*—attributed to the effects on cardiovascular tissues of other organ systems in the body, mainly the autonomic nervous system and the endocrine system.

The *control of blood pressure* is accomplished primarily by adjusting at the arteriolar level the downstream resistance to flow—an increased resistance leading to a rise in arterial backpressure, and vice versa. Normally, the total systemic peripheral resistance is 15 to 20 mmHg/liter/min of flow but can increase significantly under the influence of the vasomotor center located in the medulla of the brain, which controls arteriolar muscle tone. The *control of blood volume* is accomplished mainly through the excretory function of the kidney.

In addition to prioritizing and controlling the *distribution* of blood, physiologic regulation of cardiovascular effectiveness is directed mainly at four other variables: cardiac output, blood pressure, blood volume, and blood composition. The cardiac output can be increased by increasing the heart rate (a chronotropic effect), increasing the end-diastolic volume (allowing the heart to fill longer by delaying the onset of systole), decreasing the end-systolic volume (an inotropic effect), or doing all three things at once. Indeed, under the extrinsic influence of the sympathetic nervous system and the adrenal glands, HR can triple, to some 240 beats/minute if necessary; EDV can increase by as much as 50%, to around 200 ml or more of blood; and ESV can decrease a comparable amount (the cardiac reserve), to about 30 to 35 ml or less. The combined result of all three effects can lead to more than a sevenfold increase in cardiac output—from the normal 5 to 5.5 liters/minute to as much as 40 to 41 liters/minute or more for a very brief period of strenuous exertion.

The purpose of the consideration above is the presentation of a very complicated system of transportation and also the information exchange the human is endowed with. This system is designed to support many challenges humans have had to face during years of development. Several mechanical, electrical, and information-related dependencies allow the extreme flexibility of the cardiovascular system and its adaptation to the particular life condition of humans. Also a review of a large variety of mammals, whose cardiovascular systems are very close to that of humans, shows that many descriptive parameters depend on species size, weight, and life conditions.

Among the highest risk factors for humans are the unprecedented length of life, stress, and lack of physical exercise. Within the last hundred years, the adaptability of the cardiovascular system in humans has grown, and currently this system could be considered as a most vulnerable part of the human organism. Therefore humans are expected to modify their behavior according to the known limits of the cardiovascular system adaptation. Fortunately, humans are rational beings, capable of doing this.

The cardiology-oriented medical devices and software we are developing commonly raise the connotation of life-threatening illness, long treatment, pain, and fear. A second association is that of the sophisticated tool which, in the hands of a doctor, gives him or her in better insight and imagination for each particular disease which are the backdrop for optimal therapy. Our wish as biomedical engineers is also to provide society with an everyday wearable device designed to assist lifestyle surveillance and relay knowledge of that most vulnerable point of the human organism.

The Facts About the Social Impact of Cardiovascular Diseases

Table 3.1 shows the most frequent causes of mortality in the United States, according to National Center for Health Statistics data.

Heart disease and cancer were the first and second leading causes of death, respectively, of both men and women. The four major race groups—White, Black or African American, American Indian or Alaska Native (AIAN), and Asian or Pacific Islander (API)—shared seven of the 10 leading causes of death. Only for the API population was heart disease (25.3%) slightly preceded by cancer (26.2%) as the top killer (Heron & Smith, 2003; National Center for Health Statistics, 2005).

In a common belief, a heart attack victim is a middle-aged man, perhaps a little paunchy, most likely a workaholic executive type. It is a stereotype that has been reinforced by the media and by the medical profession itself, which in the past has focused much of its research on heart disease of this type of patient. The reason that so much more attention has been focused on men is that they are much more likely to be stricken with heart disease in their prime middle years, whereas women tend to get it 10 to 20 years later (Healthsquare, 2007).

The facts show that 9% of women between the ages of 45 and 64 have some form of cardiovascular disease, ranging from coronary artery disease to stroke or renal vascular disease (American Heart Association, 2005). By the time a woman reaches 65, she has a 1 in 3 chance of developing cardiovascular disease. For most women, it is only after menopause that heart disease becomes a problem. But a

Table 3.1. Most frequent mortality causes in the United states (Heron & Smith, 2003)

Cause of Death (based on the International Classification of Diseases, Tenth Revision, 1992)	Deaths (number)	Percent of Total Deaths
Diseases of heart (I00-I09,I11,I13,I20-I51)	685,089	28.0
Malignant neoplasms (cancer) (C00-C97)	556,902	22.7
Cerebrovascular diseases (I60-I69)	157,689	6.4
....	....	....
Total	2,448,288	100.0

woman of 60 is about as likely to get heart disease as a man of 50, and by the time they are in their seventies, men and women get heart disease at equal rates.

The following statistics confirm that heart disease, in its various forms, is the leading killer of Americans:

- One-third of all deaths of Americans each year are attributable to heart disease. Heart disease kills more people each year than cancer, accidents, and diabetes combined.
- All forms of cardiovascular disease kill nearly 900,000 Americans a year. Stroke alone kills 157,000.
- Myocardial infarction, commonly known as a heart attack, kills 244,000 American women a year.
- Forty percent of citizens in developed countries with heart disease will eventually die of it; in other countries the contribution of heart diseases in total mortality is slightly lower, however the percentage of heart diseases that end-up with a death is even higher due to improper therapy.
- About 8.9% of all white men, 7.4% of black men, and 5.6% of Mexican American men live with coronary heart disease.
- The average age of a first heart attack for men is 66 years.
- Almost half of the men who have a heart attack under age 65 die within eight years.
- Results from the Framingham Heart Study suggest that men have a 49% lifetime risk of developing coronary heart disease after the age of 40.
- Between 70% and 89% of sudden cardiac events occur in men.

The significance of these facts is clear when you consider the aging American population. By the year 2000, 35% of American men and 38% of women were 45 years of age or older. By 2015, those percentages will rise to 42% and 45% respectively. This means that heart disease will be an even bigger problem in the future than it is now.

One of the problems is that until now, treatment of women with heart disease has been based primarily on what is known about men. This is not satisfactory, provided many factors unique to women's health. Separate studies are postulated to evaluate sex-specific heart diseases and normal values (e.g., age-dependent borderline values), since current treatment-based corrections of only some coefficients are claimed not adequate. In fact, some studies have shown that despite the fact that women with heart disease are often sicker than men with the same disease, they are frequently treated less aggressively.

Fortunately, heart disease is both preventable and treatable, and as doctors learn more about what causes the problem, it is becoming increasingly apparent that there is much that a prospective patient can do to prevent it from ever occurring. Diet and lifestyle changes can be very effective preventive efforts for some forms of heart disease. To work best, these efforts should begin early in life, long before you perceive yourself to be at risk. And if heart disease does strike, modern science and technology have an ever-growing arsenal of weapons available to successfully fight it and restore its victims to healthy and productive lives.

Statistics reflect an encouraging trend. Better understanding of preventative measures and increasing sophistication in diagnosis and treatment have resulted in decreasing rates of heart disease in both men and women. For example, in the United States in the 1980s, death rates from heart disease went down 27% for white women and 22% for African American women (Healthsquare, 2007).

The prevention, self-consciousness, and knowledge of basic medical facts are today considered a most straightforward and cost-effective way to limit the social impact of cardiovascular disease. Therefore many world organizations and governments are joining efforts to inform people about how to recognize sudden cardiac events and how to behave in case if you are a subject or witness of it. Unfortunately, this first-line pre-medical help currently has no instrumentation at all. This justifies a need for a vital sign recorder and interpreter as widespread and not much more sophisticated than a cell phone today.

LONG-TERM AND PERVASIVE CARDIAC MONITORING TO IMPROVE OF QUALITY OF LIFE

Electrocardiography has been in use for a century and still evolves towards new applications, methodologies, and interpretation of the recorded data (Macfarlane & Lawrie, 1989). Although the pioneers of electrocardiography did not imagine current technology, and we too cannot imagine future development, the physical principle remains the same: recording and analyzing the electrical representation of heart activity. Development is made in three parallel and mutually dependent areas:

- Medical methodology of the examination allows formerly impossible medical tests to be supported by today's technology, creating new challenges for engineers.
- Recording electronic technology, including all the hardware involved in the physiological measurements, biosensors, recorders, microprocessors, storage, and transmission media, respond to current medical demands, are verified by medical practice, and create a backdrop for development of new medical investigation methods;

- Signal and data management and processing benefits from the development of the hardware and tries to respond to the augmenting requisites of medical demand. On the other hand verified software automates routine procedures and allows medical staff to focus on patient diseases and future investigations.

Four different electrocardiographic techniques are recently changing its contribution thanks to the use of modern telecommunication technologies. The transportation of the patient is replaced whenever possible by data transmission that moves the diagnosis to the patient's natural environment and extends it in time. The hospital is therefore reserved for the most complicated and unstable cases, as its real advantages are: controlled conditions (e.g., nutrition, respiration, drug delivery), the immediate access to rare and expensive equipment, and the possibility of surgical intervention. Besides economic aspects, home care and diagnosis have several methodological advantages. First, the metrological principle should be recalled by saying that the measurement should have minimum influence for the observed object. In the case of cardiac diagnosis, this prerequisite means keeping the patient as much as possible in his or her everyday living conditions and recording the heart response to all activity he or she normally undertakes. The second advantage is the simulation of the continuous presence of medical assistance, which is of particular importance in case of a sudden event, but it also has a very reasonable justification in modeling lifestyle to the physical conditions imposed by a cardiac disease or prevention program. This advantage is a novelty, rarely found in telemedical devices since the

Table 3.2. Summary of main properties of cardiac reporting systems

Category	12-Lead Bedside Electrocardiographs	Digital Holter Recorders	Event Recorders	Distributed Surveillance Systems
Detailed Diagnosis	yes	limited	no	yes
Long-Term Monitoring	no	yes	yes	yes
Patient-Independent Diagnosis	yes	yes	no	yes
Home Care Conditions	no	yes	yes	yes
Immediate Interpretation	yes	no	yes	yes
Interaction with the Patient	yes	no	limited	yes

majority of them are designed to transmit the data from the patient to the doctor, but not vice versa. Table 3.2 presents a summary of the main properties of various cardiac reporting systems.

Bedside ECG Recorders with Interpretation Features

Clinical cardiologists foresee the in-hospital use of the classic 12-lead ECG will continue for rate, rhythm, and conduction disturbances; for diagnosing myocardial ischemia; for further analysis of the P wave; for scrutinizing the delicate structure of the QRS complex; for understanding thus far hidden significance of heart rate variability beyond the traditional time and frequency domain methods, such as by analysis of fractal correlation properties and nonlinear heart rate dynamics; and for examination in even more detail of the T waves with their peculiar sensitivity to foresee arrhythmias before they are manifested otherwise (Bayes de Luna & Stern, 2001).

In general, the resting ECG is excellent at diagnosing arrhythmias, but it is often not helpful in diagnosing patients with structural heart disease. It is common to see a neonate with a major congenital heart defect and a normal ECG. Right heart hypoplasia syndromes, such as tricuspid atresia, pulmonary atresia (with intact ventricular septum), and Ebstein's anomaly, and children with atrioventricular canal defects have an abnormal leftward axis on the ECG. Most other structural heart defects are associated with a normal ECG. Careful scrutiny of the P wave axis can help diagnose the rare patient with *situs in versus* of the atria. The presence of two distinct P waves, with flipping of the rhythm from one to the other, may point toward the rare patient with heterotaxy syndromes, where the patient may have bilateral morphological right or left atriums. These conditions, however, are also usually associated with extremely complex structural defects (Moss, 1987; Wagner, 1994; de Chazal, 1996; Daskalov, 1999; Sörnmo, 2005).

Ambulatory Recorders

Ambulatory recorders may be divided into continuous recorders (Holters), which provide between 6 and 72 hours of continuous recording, and event monitors, which record segments of seconds or a few minutes' duration surrounding periods of interest (Mueller, 1978; Tompkins, 1982; DiMarco, 1990). Historically, Holter recorders have used analog tape for storing electrogram data, with typically a standard 60-minute audiotape being used to record for a period of 24 hours. Almost all manufacturers are now moving to digital storage, usually using solid state memory cards. For reporting, the tape, solid state memory card, or the entire recorder are plugged into a computer port and the data is transferred onto the hard disk of the interpreting and reporting workstation. This can be a specifically developed computer, but it is typically a modified PC or other commercially available computer workstation. Holter recordings are automatically analyzed to facilitate identification of zones of interest, but manual editing and checking are needed. Irrespective of the analysis method, the speed and quality of both automated and manual analyses are dependent on the recording quality. Finally, a report comprising printouts of zones of interest, supplemented by tabular reports of the frequency of ectopics, runs of tachycardia, and pauses, is issued. The reporting facility will automatically add representative ECG strips from zones of interest, and additional strips can be added manually.

Palpitations, reported as one the most frequent cardiac symptoms that occur on a daily basis or more often, may reasonably be expected to be captured on 24-hour Holter recordings. It is crucial that the reporting of the recording also documents the concordance between symptoms (as captured by activating the event button of the recorder and/or entries on a diary sheet) and arrhythmias. Most nocturnal bradyarrhythmias may be ignored if they have occurred during sleep. Sinus bradycardia, sinus arrest, sinus node exit block, and Wenckebach AV block are all frequently seen during the night in fit young subjects and in those undergoing Holter monitoring for unrelated reasons. Even third-degree AV block may occasionally be seen, but this degree of conduction block should prompt further evaluation if syncope or dizziness are the original reason for the Holter study. Ventricular pauses of significant duration are another common finding that prompt concern and confusion as to the best course of action. Pauses of more than three seconds were found in 0.8% of Holter recordings (Hilgard, Ezri, & Denes, 1985).

Asymptomatic tachycardia is often likewise neglected when found incidentally in subjects who have monitoring performed for unrelated reasons. However, ventricular arrhythmias, particularly in those with structural heart disease, may have important implications for prognosis. For symptoms that occur very infrequently, Holters have a low diagnostic yield, but may still be of value in the diagnostic evaluation of subjects through the detection of asymptomatic arrhythmias. These may guide further evaluation, with findings such as sinus arrest or chronotropic incompetence triggering evaluation for sinus node disease, while detection of short runs of tachycardia suggest more prolonged or rapid episodes of the same arrhythmia as the cause of symptoms.

In patients with frequent arrhythmias or ectopy, Holter monitoring is useful to judge the efficacy of drug therapy. The percentage of total QRS complexes represented by ectopic beats can be a useful index of the efficacy of the drug in suppressing symptomatic premature ventricular contractions.

Event Recorders

Event recorders may be looping or non-looping. A looping recorder will store in memory a period of the preceding ECG so that when the event button is pressed, not only electrocardiographic events from that point on are recorded, but also a period of the preceding ECG. Consequently, looping event recorders must be worn continuously, while the electrodes of non-looping recorders need to be applied to the skin only when symptoms occur. Event recorders have used solid state memory for some time since their memory requirement is much less, making this option financially and practically feasible. Looping event recorders are significantly smaller than Holter recorders, but are worn in a similar fashion, usually on a belt clip. Some event recorders take novel approaches, however, such as being worn on a necklace or on the wrist. Devices applied at the time of symptoms are simply carried in a pocket or bag, and patients must open their upper garments to apply the device electrodes to the skin when symptoms occur. For event recording, automated analysis is somewhat superfluous, as recordings are of short duration and thus zones of interest can be identified manually. Although the principles involved in the analysis and reporting equipment are similar to those for Holter monitoring, the emphasis is different, with other requirements such as facilities for transtelephonic reception and databasing of records being more important (Thakor, Webster, & Tompkins, 1982). Numerous studies have shown that patient-activated, long-duration monitoring provides a high diagnostic yield and is very cost effective for the evaluation of palpitations (Fogel, Evans, & Prystowsky, 1997; Zimetbaum et al., 1997, 1998), and is superior to Holter recordings (Kinlay et al., 1996). The diagnostic yield for syncope and presyncope is lower.

Looping event recorders may be worn continuously for one to four or more weeks, but a period of two weeks has been suggested as optimal (Zimetbaum et al., 1998). Non-looping recorders that are applied to the skin only at times of symptoms may be used over much longer periods of time, but the yield is lower, particularly for presyncope and brief palpitations. Furthermore, documentation of the arrhythmia onset will be absent, so any QRS morphology change is missed. Clearly the yield from non-looping event recorders in those with typical Stokes-Adams attacks will be very low since any transient arrhythmia will have passed by the time the patient can apply the device. Even application by a relative or partner may often miss the episode and can be misleading since moderate bradycardia or tachycardia is a normal reflex response to a range of events that cause syncope.

Although not strictly noninvasive, the role of implantable loop recorders (and the recording facilities of pacemakers and implantable cardioverter-defibrillators where in situ already) should not be overlooked because they allow event recording over much longer periods than is feasible using adhesive electrodes and external recorders. The implantable loop recorder is currently marketed for the diagnosis of infrequent syncope after an appropriate range of noninvasive tests have failed to yield a diagnosis

Monitoring Equipment Manufacturers Survey

Tele-cardiology has already been recognized as a valuable tool for the distant assessment of patient status. The diagnosis is cardiac-oriented, but also includes several vital parameters such as blood oxygenation and respiration. This set of parameters is frequently used in home care conditions to monitor the overall status, physical load, sleeping conditions, and so forth.

The remote monitoring of cardiac function is present in commercial offerings of several manufacturers, as well as in scientific interests of many research groups. In fact, these two fields cannot be clearly distinguished, since what the research and development departments of companies are doing is actually on the same scientific level as university research teams. Therefore it is rather a formal classification depending on whether the equipment manufacturer prefers to maintain its own R&D department, or cooperate with an external research institution, commercial or public.

Some initiatives from medical companies are also visible. They cooperate with insurance agencies or public healthcare providers and complement their offer. The benefit of such cooperation to each side is:

- The hospital can release the patient earlier, speeding up the resources recycling.
- The patient returns home with practically hospital-equivalent quality of monitoring.
- The insurance agency saves on expenses, since even prolonged home care monitoring is much cheaper than hospital treatment.

For the purpose of this book, we created a short survey of the actual telecare offer, but having three sources of information of different characteristics, we do not attempt to compare them:

- Scientific reports focus on the novelty aspects and interoperability of solutions, and often include a sophisticated description of methods and functions. This offer is directed to healthcare managers and manufacturers, but unfortunately, not to the patients.
- Commercial advertising of the manufacturers highlights the technical parameters, but hides the details—particularly the methods that are best protected

and often patented. This offer is targeted to healthcare providers and rarely to patients, because the doctor-end must be serviced by professionals.

- Healthcare offers provide few technical parameters, as these offers focus on patients. Sometimes the commercial healthcare provider does not even disclose the equipment manufacturer name, and the instrumentation bears the providers' trademarks as if they were purchased or leased on original equipment manufacturer (OEM) license.

Below is a short survey of offers available on the Internet (please note, the manufacturer selection and order is random, with no relation to the authors; the description may contain trademarks belonging to the owners, given as examples of solutions):

- **PDSHeart Cardiac Monitoring Service:** PDSHeart provides leading edge technology in the area of non-looping and looping event monitors with auto trigger capability. PDSHeart also supplies the most modern and versatile digital Holter monitors for diagnostic capability at no cost to the cardiology practice. All necessary Holter supplies are tailored and packaged conveniently in individual Holter kits. Pacemaker Monitoring Service allows patients to test the overall functionality of their pacemakers over the telephone, at any time. Certified cardiac technicians supervise pacemaker follow-up on the telephone by contacting the patient according to a preset schedule. The service is economical and reassuring to the patient.
- **Healthfrontier's ecg@Home:** The ecg@Home records and stores the electrical heart signal obtained from the first or second standard ECG leads in a non-invasive manner. This device acquires a 10-second signal strip from lead (I) using the two built-in electrodes on which the thumbs are placed and lead (II) by using the right thumb and a third external electrode on the left leg. The ecg@Home also stores three important ECG parameters: (1) deviation of the ST segment of the wave, (2) duration of the QRS complex, and (3) abnormalities of the T wave. The recorded data is sent to a data warehouse via the Internet, wireless device, e-mail, or via the built-in trans-telephonic coupler to the provider tele-health center, where it can be immediately tracked, scanned, and analyzed or alternatively transmitted to a caregiver of the patient's choice.
- **CardioComm:** CardioComm Solutions is a medical software company with a decade of experience in building ECG management systems used for event monitoring and pacemaker follow-up. In 1999, CardioComm created its own product line, the Global ECG Management System (GEMS), for pacemaker/ICD and arrhythmia follow-up. After establishing an international customer base, CardioComm began direct sales and marketing in the United States in

2000. GEMS and GEMS Lite are the answers to the ever-increasing volume of confidential patient data management in the fields of arrhythmia, pacemaker, and ICD patient follow-up. The GEMS products are efficient, scalable, and filled with unique and valuable features. GlobalCardio is an FDA-cleared, ASP Internet-based software application. GlobalCardio provides physicians and caregivers with the ability to transmit, store, retrieve, and analyze ECG data securely over the Internet for all of their cardiac patients.

- **Pulse Biomedical Inc.'s QRS-Card(TM)/232:** Pulse Biomedical Inc. (PBI) is a manufacturer of computer-based electrocardiogram products. PBI designs, develops, manufacturers, and markets both the hardware and software components of a 12-lead, diagnostic-quality ECG device for use with an IBM-compatible personal computer. The company received FDA clearance to market its Resting QRS-Card ECG product in November 1991 and Stress ECG in July 1998. The initial product consisted of a separate card that was inserted into the PC with DOS-based software running in the PC. Through R&D, the product (QRSCard™/232) has evolved to an external hardware module about the size of a small cellular phone with communication to the PC via the serial port. The system is a fully integrated Windows® 98/2000 product, and works with Windows CE Handheld (hpc) and Palmtop (ppc) devices. In addition to software to monitor current resting and stress ECGs, the company is now developing software for signal-averaged, high-resolution ECGs. PBI's resting, stress, and high resolution ECGs use the same QRSCard™/232 hardware components.
- **GE Medical Systems:** GE Healthcare's comprehensive product portfolio provides solutions for all care areas in the field of diagnostic cardiology and patient monitoring. The GE Resting ECG Solution is a complete package of algorithms and features like gender-specific 12SL, ACI TIPI, 15-lead, and P wave Signal Averaging, along with the latest technology for mobile data transfer to MUSE (MobileLink). CASE/CardioSoft systems deliver highly scalable multifunctional solutions for stress and resting ECGs, as well as for ambulatory BP and spirometry. All systems can be networked and configured to meet your information management requirements. The ultra-light SEER Light recorder (70 g) and the most advanced algorithms for cardiac risk prediction provide the patient with a superior Holter completely integrated to our network solutions. For customers demanding telemetry excellence, the Apex Pro and TELEGUARD telemetry systems deliver. They collect and distribute non-invasive cardiac data from different sources, supporting network connectivity scalable to your needs. MUSE provides comprehensive data storage, management, and statistical analysis with easy access from virtually anywhere.

- **Quinton-Burdick ECG Solutions:** For more than 45 years Burdick has been recognized as a leading brand of ECGs in the primary care market. Today Burdick electrocardiographs continue to set the industry standard and offer a wide range of related cardiopulmonary diagnostics including PC-based tests. The Burdick brand provides solutions to meet the ever-changing challenges associated with the practice of medicine, practice management, and patient management.
  Cardiac Science's Burdick brand has a long history in Wisconsin and is well known for instruments that provide both performance and lasting dependability for physicians throughout the country. In its early years, it was an early explorer and inventor of electrocardiography technology. With its customer-oriented designs, Burdick quickly became the preferred brand for accurate ECG recording, and now, as a part of Cardiac Science Corporation, remains the preferred brand today. Verified technology provides solutions ranging from single-channel ECGs to PC-based devices with advanced communications. In addition to ECGs, the Burdick product line includes ABP systems, defibrillators, Holters, PC-based diagnostics, pulse oximeters, spirometers, and exercise stress systems. These products are known as clinically superior, easy-to-use, networked solutions for diagnostic cardiology.
- **Spacelabs:** Spacelabs continues a distinguished record of innovation that started in 1958 when Spacelabs helped design the first systems to monitor astronauts in space. In the 1960s, Spacelabs developed medical telemetry systems for hospitals. Today, Spacelabs provides flexible systems that allow hospitals to respond easily to varying levels of acuity. As a leading global provider of patient monitoring systems, Spacelabs systems support time-saving, informed decision making for care teams in critical care, emergency, and perioperative areas. Developed in partnership with caregivers, monitoring systems focus on making the most efficient use of valuable staff time and on improving standards of patient care. Integrated solutions include wired and wireless networks and clinical information connectivity. With its first of many 608-614 MHz telemetry installations occurring in October 1999, Spacelabs Healthcare was the first to provide products that operate in the new frequency bands. Ultraview Digital Telemetry is now installed in hospitals across the United States and Canada. Spacelabs representatives can help caregivers change a current telemetry system based on Private Land-Mobile Radio (PLMR) to one that operates in the WMTS.
- **Card Guard Ltd. Selfcheck and Instromedix Products:** Card Guard is a leading provider of innovative telemedicine technologies and telehealth services. The Card Guard Ltd. remote patient monitoring solutions are designed for high-risk and chronically ill patients, homecare and disease management

programs, ordinary consumers of health products, and the wellness community. Card Guard offers a complete patient monitoring solution for routine examinations in the home, as well as monitoring patients with one or more chronic diseases such as asthma, chronic obstructive pulmonary disease, coronary disease, congestive heart failure, diabetes, or hypertension.

Card Guard's PMP4 Web-based medical center and suite of vital sign monitors allow any home healthcare giver to quickly and accurately capture patient data on a PDA for on-the-spot review. The medical data is easily uploaded to a dedicated Web-based medical center for immediate analysis and follow-up action by a healthcare professional in a remote location. Electronic patient monitoring is an exciting development for home healthcare providers. Driven by an aging population suffering from any number of chronic diseases and a 'stay-at-home' mindset, healthcare payers will capitalize on accessible at-home monitoring tools and services. The PMP4 user-friendly interface and immediate reporting ability allows almost anyone to perform and transmit a medical test for review and follow-up.

- **HeartLine Products from Aerotel:** Aerotel provides complete solutions for telemedicine, telehealth, and telecare applications. Their patient monitoring systems consist of medical call center software and compact, reliable, transtelephonic and digital monitoring devices that effectively transfer vital medical or lifestyle data over the telephone, the Internet, or wireless networks. Whether it is an ECG, blood pressure values, blood glucose level, pulse oximeter, weight, or other vital sign, the modular monitoring systems reliably transfer essential data to a monitoring center, enabling accurate diagnosis. The patient information and the transmitted data can be viewed locally or via the Internet. Aerotel Medical Systems offers various remote monitoring solutions for telehealth, telecare, and teleassistance call centers.

  These solutions are designed to enable medical professionals at remote locations to view, analyze, and react to medical information received from mobile users via wireless monitoring devices.
- **Welch Allyn:Micropaq + Cardio Control:** Welch Allyn has brought significant innovations to frontline care providers, strengthening their position as the market leader in core physical exam products, while expanding their reach further into digital and connected products. Welch Allyn offers the convenience and efficiency of a patient monitor that is wireless and wearable, that is ideal for monitoring vital signs of higher-acuity overflow patients and ambulating patients, and for administering medications at the bedside.

  The small patient device displays heart rate, one or two ECG leads, motion-tolerant SpO2, and pulse bar. It continues monitoring with alarms even when out of telemetry range for up to the 25-hour battery life when fully charged. The remote recorder uses a wireless link to communicate with Welch Allyn's Acuity and Acuity LT Central Monitoring Stations, and warns when it is out of range or not connected to the wireless network. It uses two-way communication between Micropaq and the Acuity Central Station in order to enhance monitoring decisions and reduce human error.

- **CardioNet:** CardioNet is the world's leading supplier of mobile cardiac outpatient telemetry. CardioNet provides the next-generation ambulatory cardiac monitoring service with beat-to-beat, real-time analysis; automatic arrhythmia detection; and wireless ECG transmission. CardioNet's Mobile Cardiac Outpatient Telemetry (MCOT) system was developed to address physicians' challenges in diagnosing arrhythmias and patients' need for an easy-to-use automated system. CardioNet monitors every heartbeat, non-invasively, during the patient's normal daily activities, for up to 21 days, and detects, records, and transmits event data automatically to the prescribing physician.
  The system merges patient monitoring technology, wireless communications, and the Internet to allow targeted cardiac rhythm-related problems to be quickly identified, quantified, and communicated to the prescribing physician. The physician selects patient-specific monitoring thresholds and response parameters.
  The CardioNet Monitoring Center reports events, analysis, and symptoms to the physician daily by fax or via the Internet, according to physician preference. Daily telemetry reports incorporate heart rate trends and A Fib burden information, sample strips of detected arrhythmias, and other important diagnostic information. Urgent telemetry reports are sent to the physician immediately when critical events occur, and when directed, the CardioNet Monitoring Center helps arrange emergency medical services.
- **Medtronic:** Medtronic provides clinicians who treat heart failure with simple access to tailored heart failure information stored in its many ICD and CRT-D devices. CardioSight Service offers direct access to exclusive, device-derived information tailored to the management of heart failure, better enabling clinicians to quickly identify issues and respond to significant clinical events. The CardioSight Reader—based on proven Medtronic CareLink® technology—is quick and easy to use, providing flexibility in clinic workflow. Much like existing tools for measuring patients' vital signs, the CardioSight Reader can be used to conveniently obtain important details on patient status. Within minutes of downloading device information using the reader, a Heart Failure Management Report or Cardiac Compass™ Trends Report is faxed to the clinic and can be added to the patient chart before the physician consults with the patient. The CardioSight Reader gives insight into a patient's condition

without using a device programmer. It provides simple, one-touch operation, enabling access to read-only information without the possibility of changing device parameters.

- **Cardiomedix:** Cardiomedix offers over a decade of excellence and leadership in providing comprehensive ambulatory cardiac monitoring nationwide by an expert, highly qualified team. The company is also known for its 25 years of pioneering work in the field of cardiac telemedicine. This vast experience resulted in the development of unique procedures to facilitate and maximize the benefits of the system. Cardiomedix is recognized for its excellence and customer satisfaction, and is keeping its leadership role in telemedicine by further developing patented, next-generation technology. One of Cardiomedix's missions is to assist patients in the very early stages of a heart attack, while they are far away from immediate medical help: at home, at work, or on the golf course. It is imperative that heart attack patients be under immediate medical supervision, preferably within the first hour from the initiation of symptoms. It has been amply proven that early, specialized, medical intervention within this timeframe—'the golden hour'—can save lives, diminish the damage to the heart, and expedite recovery. A patient enrolled in the Cardiomedix service can contact a highly qualified cardiac nurse at the Cardiomedix control center at any time of day or night from any telephone worldwide. The patient will be asked to describe his or her symptoms and transmit their ECG. This helps the experienced nurse identify the warning signs and the need for immediate medical emergency care.
- **Cardiobeat:** Cardiolert Systems is a development stage company prototyping efficient technologies and services to improve therapy for heart failure victims and improve the quality of their lives. The Cardiolert System is a cost-effective tool that enhances caregiver effectiveness in diagnosing and treating heart failure at all stages. Caregivers utilizing this technology can significantly improve cardiovascular condition. Early studies demonstrate the potential for a 50% reduction in hospitalization with a corresponding improvement in patients' quality of life. The Cardiolert System is a cost-effective, portable impedance cardiograph (ICG) system for diagnosing and treating heart failure.

  The CT2014 is about the size of a personal data assistant. It connects to a PC for data collection and local reporting. The PC transmits test information to a central site for backup, additional processing, and e-mail transmission. E-mail transmission supports homecare and disease management applications where evaluation occurs remote from the patient. Internet communication is near instantaneous, permitting collaboration of caregivers to determine the best possible therapy.

- **Cardiocom LLC (weight and symptom monitor):** Cardiocom has created entirely new value in disease management by developing intervention and management processes that are more efficient and more effective. Cardiocom's targeted solutions improve patient care and reduce unnecessary medical costs. Cardiocom focuses expensive clinical resources so they know who, when, and why to intervene each day. Cardiocom's patient management tools drive case ratios to new levels that provide a sustainable competitive market advantage.
  Cardiocom's solutions are more than just biometric monitoring devices. The products and services operate as an integrated system for a specific disease state. They integrate state-of-the-art monitoring technology with targeted, personalized care management services and advanced rule-based software, including multiple disease-specific question sets.
  Cardiocom also provides the option of turn-key clinical call center services, including: identification, stratification, enrollment, intake assessment, health survey screening, coaching, intervention, high-risk management, education materials, and outcome reporting.
- **QRS Diagnostic LLC:** QRS manufactures highly portable and affordable PC-based and handheld medical devices. The QRS product line includes electrocardiograms, spirometers, pulse oximeters, blood pressure meters, and vitals. With its patented PC-card technology, QRS delivers affordable, reliable, and completely portable medical devices. These products include complementary patient management software to simplify the management of physiological data.
  The Biolog is a complete 12-lead ECG capable of recording one, six, or twelve channels of diagnostic ECG data. For an instant single-channel ECG, anyone can press the Biolog to the patient's chest for a quick 'window on the heart'. The other option is to connect the 6-lead or 12-lead ECG cable for a complete diagnostic ECG. The Biolog ECG is mobile, compact, and simple to use. Ideal for emergency situations, the Biolog is just as practical for routine on-the-spot checks as it is for acquiring and analyzing 12-lead ECG data.

Issues of Home-Care Cardiac Monitoring

Holter and event recorders have a central role in diagnosing and monitoring arrhythmias, but to provide optimal diagnostic yield, the device most appropriate for the symptom frequency should be chosen. Event recorders are superior for the diagnosis of palpitations and syncope in most patients, but numerous specific indications remain for Holter. These include the detection of asymptomatic arrhythmia (whether diagnostically or for risk stratification), assessment of patients with very frequent symptoms, and monitoring of rate control. Other advances that are either available or pending include autotrigger capabilities of event recorder devices, allowing the detection of asymptomatic arrhythmias. The implantable loop recorder is also likely to have extended capabilities in future versions.

The main issue of the event recorder is the stability of electrode contact. In a nonlooping recorder the standardized electrode position for every recording is hardly to be expected in home care conditions. On the contrary, the operation time of a looping recorder significantly extends the electrode stability period, and prolonging the monitoring time raises the probability of the patient action that influences the electrodes contact.

Despite careful collection of recordings, artifacts still occur and can at times be difficult to discriminate from cardiac abnormalities. Recorded signals of noncardiac origin can arise from several sources. Typically the artifacts are classified into one of the following ranges:

- *biological*—sinusoidal VT-like signals may be recorded in Parkinson's disease or another tremor, regional muscle activity may be intentional or reflect the sensation of cold;
- *electromagnetic*—induced by a wide range of external electrical appliances (electric toothbrushes, electric razors, and electric blankets, with either the ECG leads or the patient's body acting as an antenna for the electromagnetic fields); and
- *conductance artifacts*—usually due to poor electrical contact in the recording circuit (typically at the skin-electrode interface, skin activity, transpiration, etc.).

These issues are particularly difficult to avoid when in home care conditions, an untrained person or a patient himself/herself is applying the electrodes without signal quality control. Every conventional 12-lead recorder and most Holter recorders are applied by a qualified technician, and in most systems the immediate assessment of the signal quality is provided by the system. In home care conditions, signal verification is done automatically and the electrocardiogram is rarely displayed by the device. In such cases the benefit of interactive systems emerges: the signal quality may be assessed by a distant center or supervising cardiologist.

THE USE OF MODERN TELECOMMUNICATION SOLUTIONS FOR CARDIAC MONITORING

Telecommunication Technology

The long anticipated information age is taking shape at the cross-section of multimedia signal processing and telecommunications-based networking (Onaral, 2001). The physical constraints of location have naturally led, over the centuries, to the creation of conventional patient care services and facilities. As the "information superhighway" is laid out with branches spanning the world via wired and wireless communication channels, we will come closer to a bold new era in healthcare delivery, namely, the era of remote monitoring, diagnosis, and intervention.

Forward-looking medical industries are engaging in research and development efforts to capitalize on the emerging technologies. Medical institutions in particular recognize the transforming power of the impending revolution. A number of hospitals are undertaking pilot projects to experiment with the potential of the new communication and interaction media that will constitute the foundations of futuristic healthcare systems. There is a consensus among healthcare administrators that the agility and effectiveness with which an institution positions itself to fully embrace the new medical lifestyle will decide its viability in the next millennium.

Although multimedia communication is yet in its infancy, recent developments foretell a bright future. Many agree that multimedia networking is becoming a reality thanks to advances in digital signal processing research and development. Trends towards the implementation of algorithms by fewer components are leading to decreasing hardware complexity while increasing processing functionality (Halpern et al., 1992).

The vast and vibrant industry producing multimedia hardware and software ranging from application-specific digital signal processors and video chip sets to videophones and multimedia terminals heavily relies on digital signal processing know-how.

As in the case of generic digital signal processing, biomedical signal processing is expected to play a key role in mainstreaming patient care at a distance. Emerging methods in biomedical signal analysis that promise major enhancements in our ability to extract information from vital signals were introduced above. This chapter provides a glimpse of the future—when biomedical signals will be integrated with other patient information and transmitted via networked multimedia—by examining trends in key communications technologies, namely, public switched-network protocols, wireless communications, and so forth (Duisterhout, Hasman, & Salamon, 1991).

Wireless communication is the fastest growing sector of the telecommunications industry (Wireless, 2007). Progress in this direction is closely monitored by the healthcare community because the technology holds the potential to liberate ambulatory patients who require long-term monitoring and processing of biomedical signals for timely intervention. Wireless and interactive access by medical personnel to physiologic multimedia information will no doubt be a symbol of future distributed healthcare delivery systems.

The term 'wireless network' may technically be used to refer to any type of network that is wireless, although it is most commonly used to refer to a telecommunications network whose interconnections between nodes is implemented without the use of wires, such as a computer network, which is a type of communications network. Wireless telecommunications networks are generally implemented with some type of remote information transmission system that uses electromagnetic waves, such as radio waves, for the carrier, and this implementation usually takes place at the physical level or "layer" of the network.

Since then wireless networks have continued to develop and their applications have significantly grown. Cellular phones are part of huge wireless network systems. People use these phones daily to communicate with one another. The global number of GSM users was estimated to reach three billion by the end of 2007 across more than 212 countries and territories. Sending information overseas is possible through wireless network systems using satellites and other signals to communicate around the world. Emergency services such as police departments employ wireless networks to communicate important information quickly. People and businesses use wireless networks to send and share data quickly, whether it be in a small office building or across the world. Another important use for wireless networks is as an inexpensive and rapid way to be connected to the Internet in countries and regions where the telecommunication infrastructure is poor or there is a lack of resources, like in most developing countries.

Though very prominent with its new features, wireless communication shows considerable drawbacks:

- Compatibility Issues—Different components not made by the same manufacturer may not work together at all, or might require extra work to fix compatibility issues.
- Speed Issues—Wireless networks, in terms of Internet connections, are typically slower than those that are directly connected through an Ethernet cable.
- Security Issues—A wireless network is more vulnerable because anyone can try to break into a network broadcasting a signal. Many networks offer WEP (wired equivalent privacy) or WPA (Wi-Fi protected access). WPA provides more security to wireless networks than a WEP security setup. The use of

firewalls helps to fix security problems in some wireless networks that are more vulnerable.

Wireless communication may use different technologies depending on required bandwidth, range, and acceptable costs.

The *Wi-Fi* (Wireless Fidelity) Alliance is a consortium of separate and independent companies agreeing to a set of common interoperable products based on the family of IEEE 802.11 standards (Wi-Fi, 2007). Wi-Fi certifies products via a set of established test procedures to establish interoperability. A Wi-Fi-enabled device such as a PC, cell phone, or PDA can connect to the Internet when within range of a wireless network connected to the Internet. The area covered by one or more interconnected access points is called a hotspot. Hotspots can cover as little as a single room with wireless-opaque walls or as much as many square miles covered by overlapping access points. Wi-Fi also allows connectivity in peer-to-peer (wireless ad-hoc network) mode, which enables devices to connect directly with each other. This connectivity mode is useful in consumer electronics and mobile industrial applications. Wi-Fi allows LANs to be deployed without cabling for client devices, typically reducing the costs and time of network deployment and expansion. Wi-Fi is a global set of standards. Unlike mobile telephones, any standard Wi-Fi device will work anywhere in the world. Wi-Fi is widely available in more than 250,000 public hotspots and tens of millions of homes and corporate and university campuses worldwide. The drawbacks of Wi-Fi technology are:

- lack of worldwide consistency on spectrum assignments and operational limitations,
- weak data encryption strength provided by WEP and the need for configuration for each new device, and
- high power consumption compared to other low-bandwidth standards and relative low range.

WiMAX (Worldwide Interoperability for Microwave Access) is a telecommunications technology aimed at providing wireless data over long distances in a variety of ways, from point-to-point links to full mobile cellular type access (WiMAX, 2007). It is based on the IEEE 802.16 standard, which is also called WirelessMAN. WiMAX allows the user, for example, to browse the Internet on a laptop computer without physically connecting the laptop to a router, hub, or switch via an Ethernet cable. The name WiMAX was created by the WiMAX Forum, which was formed in June 2001 to promote conformance and interoperability of the standard. The forum describes WiMAX as "a standards-based technology enabling the delivery of last mile wireless broadband access as an alternative to cable and DSL." As opposed to Wi-Fi, WiMAX is a long-range system covering many kilometers that typically uses licensed spectrum to deliver a point-to-point connection to the Internet from the ISP to the end user. Different 802.16 standards provide different types of access, from mobile (analogous to cell phone access) to fixed (an alternative to wired access, where the end user's wireless termination point is fixed in a location).

Mobile WiMAX networks comprise mostly indoor customer premise equipment (CPE) such as desktop modems, laptops with integrated Mobile WiMAX, or other Mobile WiMAX devices. Mobile WiMAX devices typically have an antenna design that is of lower gain by nature due to their inherent omni-directional (and portable) design. In practice this means that in a line-of-sight environment with a portable Mobile WiMAX CPE, symmetrical speeds of 10 Mbit/s at 10 km could be delivered, but in urban environments it is more likely that these devices will not have a line-of-sight and therefore users may only receive 10 Mbit/s over 2 km. Higher-gain directional antennas can be used with a Mobile WiMAX network, with range and throughput benefits but the obvious loss of practical mobility.

Cellular companies report the research on WiMAX as a means of increasing bandwidth for a variety of data-intensive applications. Simultaneously emerges the technological ability to serve as a high bandwidth alternative for the Internet or cellular phone traffic from remote areas back to an Internet backbone. Although the cost per user/point of WiMAX in a remote application will be higher, it is not limited to such applications. Given the limited wired infrastructure in some developing countries, the costs to install a WiMAX station in conjunction with an existing cellular tower or even as a solitary hub are likely to be small in comparison to developing a wired solution. Areas of low population density and flat terrain are particularly suited to WiMAX and its range. For countries that have skipped wired infrastructure as a result of prohibitive costs and unsympathetic geography, WiMAX can enhance wireless infrastructure in an inexpensive, decentralized, deployment-friendly, and effective manner.

GSM is a cellular network, which means that mobile phones connect to it by searching for cells in the immediate vicinity (GSM, 2007). GSM networks operate in four different frequency ranges. Most GSM networks operate in the 900 MHz or 1,800 MHz bands. Some countries in the Americas (including Canada and the United States) use the 850 MHz and 1,900 MHz bands because the 900 and 1,800 MHz frequency bands were already allocated. Cell horizontal radius varies depending on antenna height, antenna gain, and propagation conditions from a couple of hundred meters to several tens of kilometers. The longest distance the GSM specification supports in practical use is 35 kilometers (22 miles). The transmission power in the handset is limited to a maximum of 2 watts in GSM850/900 and 1 watt in GSM1800/1900. The maximum data rate (Full Rate) of a single channel is 12.2 kbit/s. Its ubiquity makes international roaming very common between mobile phone operators, enabling subscribers to use their phones in many parts of the world. GSM differs from its predecessors in that both signaling and speech channels are digital call quality, and also data communication was built into the system. Release '97 of the GSM standard added packet data capabilities by means of General Packet Radio Service (GPRS).

GPRS data transfer is typically charged per megabyte of transferred data, while data communication via traditional circuit switching is billed per minute of connection time, independent of whether the user has actually transferred data or has been in an idle state (GPRS, 2007). GPRS can be used for services such as Wireless Application Protocol (WAP) access, Short Message Service (SMS), Multimedia Messaging Service (MMS), and for Internet communication services such as e-mail and World Wide Web access.

GPRS is packet switched, which means that multiple users share the same transmission channel, only transmitting when they have data to send. Thus the total available bandwidth can be immediately dedicated to those users who are actually sending at any given moment, providing higher use where users only send or receive data intermittently. Web browsing, receiving e-mails as they arrive, and instant messaging are examples of uses that require intermittent data transfers, which benefit from sharing the available bandwidth. GPRS speed is a direct function of the number of TDMA (Time Division Multiple Access) time slots assigned, which is limited by the particular cell capacity and the maximum capability of the mobile device expressed as a GPRS multislot class. For example the device class 10 supports up to four downlink slots, up to two uplink slots, but no more that five simultaneously active slots.

GPRS is packet based. When TCP/IP is used, each phone can have one or more IP addresses allocated. GPRS will store and forward the IP packets to the phone during cell handover (when you move from one cell to another). A radio noise-induced pause can be interpreted by TCP as packet loss and cause a temporary throttling in transmission speed. The maximum speed of a GPRS connection offered in 2003 was similar to a modem connection in an analog wire telephone network, about 32 to 40 kbit/s, depending on the phone used. Latency is very high; a round-trip ping is typically about 600 to 700 ms and often reaches 1s. GPRS is typically prioritized lower than speech, and thus the quality of connection varies greatly.

Computer Networking

Computer technology is considered a main area of development in healthcare delivery centers throughout the world (Sengupta, 2001). Information technology gradually improves the basic practice of medicine through the quality and quantity of information used by clinicians and administrators. Similarly to personal communication, *computer networking* is a technological support for transparent and efficient digital data flow from the creators of the information to the ultimate end users (Tanenbaum, 1988).

In the early 1980s computers in a medical center were targeted to administrative needs. Central mainframe computers were employed for financial data processing. Quite soon thereafter, first attempts were made towards the automation of laboratory functions, and personal computers became cost effective to collect both departmental data for billing purposes and clinical data for clinical purposes. Today computers are used for many purposes: in ancillary departmental settings such as in laboratories, pharmacies, and radiology and pathology departments; in administrative contexts such as billing, patient management, transportation, and payroll; for clinical and scholarly purposes such as electronic medical records, imaging, and searches for medical references; and in basic research functions such as for molecular modeling, genetics, and robotics surgery (Rennels & Shortliffe, 1987; Duisterhout et al., 1991).

The concept of distributed computing is fast becoming a reality in medical domains, and it deals with the collection, integration, and presentation of data distributed over several computers (Rennels & Shortliffe, 1987). Seamless information exchange requires the ubiquitous presence of a network, which—composed of hardware and software components or layers—interconnects these computers. Communication protocols as definitions of data exchange rules between computers are often subject to worldwide standards. A collection of specific layers and implementations of corresponding protocols is known as a communication standard. Several communication standards are in clinical use today. The proprietary standards usually better fit the specific needs of a particular application but limit the possibility of data exchange. Open standards are provided for unlimited data exchange but must consider various application specificity. Historically, individual departments experimented with networking and succeeded in creating local solutions. Today, one of the most important issues is the integration of medical data when networks came to be appreciated as institutional resources and the local islands of information had to be rearranged for the larger institutional goals of networking efficiency and reliability.

Another area of development is a result of replacement of traditional paper-based patient charts by electronic health records (EHRs). Since computers are far more efficient and accurate in organizing, maintaining, and disseminating these records, unprecedented quality of service is offered by data management and protection. Similarly, automated decision-making applications (Cimino et al., 1994) may start to be developed and put into practice, thanks to the concept of a purely electronic medical record.

The variety of *healthcare dataforms* requires the highest performance of electronic storage and transmission systems and media (McDonald & Hammond, 1989). Regardless of their size, records are important in patient care. One byte of the laboratory result code has often even more life-critical influence to the treatment than a whole CT-scan image. Since clinical data originate at many diagnostic systems, collecting the data at a single, physically central repository requires designing a comprehensive clinical information system and implementing a logically integrated repository of all clinical information for each patient. A data review application, integrated in the hospital information system, supports querying the central repository for all data over the network. The topic of clinical and hospital data interchange (DICOM, HL7, etc.) is developed in Chapter IV. However, visual data type is worth mentioning here as raising particular requirements from the network infrastructure. All radiology tests (Halpern et al., 1992) are performed as visual interpretation of images and video sequences (X-ray images, CAT scans, PET scans, SPECT scans). To a lesser degree, ultrasound sonograms, pathology slides, gated blood pool studies, and neurology are other sources of these data. A network that can support multiple-thread real-time video streaming requires special consideration and design, and is also more expensive.

In academic institutions, a large amount of computer-based educational information is graphical and video based. Many stand-alone educational products are being actively used today, and in the future, these educational materials with real patient data will be available over the same network and on demand to all students, faculty, and practitioners.

The *Internet reference model* or TCP/IP (Transmission Control Protocol/Internet Protocol) model is a layered abstract description for communications and computer network protocol design. It was created in the 1970s by DARPA for use in developing the Internet's protocols, and the structure of the Internet is still closely reflected by the TCP/IP model. The original TCP/IP reference model consists of four layers, but is now presented as a five-layer model, mainly for educational purposes and to reflect real-world protocol architecture. The layers near the top are logically closer to the user application (as opposed to the human user), while those near the bottom are logically closer to the physical transmission of the data. Viewing layers as providing or consuming a service is a method of abstraction to isolate upper-layer protocols from the technical details of transmitting bits over the Ethernet and collision detection, while the lower layers avoid having to know the details of each and every application and its protocol. The following is the layer order with a short description of each:

1. The *application layer* is used by most programs for network communication. Data is passed from the program in an application-specific format, then

encapsulated into a transport-layer protocol. From there, the data is passed down into the lower-layer protocol of the transport layer.

2. The *transport layer*'s responsibilities include end-to-end message transfer capabilities independent of the underlying network, along with error control, fragmentation, and flow control. The transport layer can be considered as a transport mechanism or medium whose responsibility is to make sure that its contents (passengers/goods) reach its destination safely and soundly, unless a higher or lower layer is responsible for safe delivery. Some applications, such as voice over IP (VOIP), can tolerate dropped packets; a reliable transport would prevent delay or reordering. The transport layer provides this service of connecting applications together through the use of ports. Since IP provides only a best-effort delivery, the transport layer is the first layer of the TCP/IP stack to offer reliability.
3. The *network layer*, as originally defined, solves the problem of getting packets across a single network. For the purpose of the concept of internetworking, additional functionality was added to this layer, consisting of routing the packet across a network of networks. All routing protocols are also part of the network layer.
4. The *data link layer*, which is the method used to move packets from the network layer on two different hosts, is not really part of the Internet protocol suite, because IP can run over a variety of different link layers. The processes of transmitting packets on a given link layer and receiving packets from a given link layer can be controlled both in the software device driver for the network card, as well as on firmware or specialist chipsets. These will perform data link functions such as adding a packet header to prepare it for transmission, then actually transmit the frame over a physical medium. On a local wired network, Ethernet is usually used, and on local wireless networks, IEEE 802.11 is usually used. For wide-area networks, either PPP over T-carrier or E-carrier lines, Frame relay, ATM, or packet over SONET/SDH (POS) are often used.
5. The *physical layer* is responsible for encoding and transmission of data over network communications media. It operates with data in the form of bits that are sent from the physical layer of the sending (source) device and received at the physical layer of the destination device. Ethernet, Token Ring, SCSI, hubs, repeaters, cables, and connectors are standard network devices that function at the physical layer. The physical layer is also considered the domain of many hardware-related network design issues, such as LAN and WAN topology and wireless technology.

The *Open Systems Interconnection* Basic Reference Model is another layered, abstract description for communications and computer network protocol design, developed as part of the Open Systems Interconnection (OSI) initiative. It is also called the *OSI seven-layer model*. The layers are, from top to bottom: Application, Presentation, Session, Transport, Network, Data Link, and Physical. A layer is referred to as a collection of related functions that provides services to the layer above it and receives service from the layer below it.

A *local area network* (LAN) topology is the layout of networking segments (copper cables, fiber cables, or the transparent/electromagnetic environment in the case of wireless) and their interconnections by devices such as repeaters, bridges, and routers. Traffic estimates and patterns, redundancy, isolation and security, physical plant including building and cabling layout, and organizational structure must be considered by the topology design. A medical center LAN needs to accommodate heterogeneous sets of computers and consequently needs to support several higher-layer protocols. The choice of higher-layer protocols also influences the choice of bridges and router devices. Although initially driven by the integration of existing systems, a medical center LAN settles on a small subset of protocols for most of its mainstream communication, which is practically motivated by support and maintenance issues.

A widely used application on today's PCs is terminal emulation, by which a PC behaves as a terminal to an ancillary or central computer on the network, and thus subsequently has access to all medical applications on that application server computer. LANs, instead of the traditional point-to-point connections, have become the primary medium for computer communication at healthcare practice centers to the extent that all new computers are expected to be LAN compatible. A special group of LAN administrators is required to maintain and service the LANs. Managing networks and distributed applications is orders-of-magnitude harder than managing a single, monolithic system. It is, however, extremely important to invest in and learn how to manage the hundreds of networking and computing components that bring value to the networks. Monitoring of applications helps determine future demands for resources, performance guarantees, and opportunities to make a system more reliable.

Wide area networks (WANs) are applied by healthcare centers for three main purposes:

- to connect networks at physically distant buildings, offices, or clinics;
- to connect networks to different organizations (affiliated hospitals, insurance agencies, government regulatory bodies) or services (Internet, disaster recovery backup locations); or
- to provide dial-in and dial-out capabilities for employees.

The difference between the first two purposes is that of control and security: access to medical information requires better control when connected to an external organization. The concept of a firewall as a part of networking topology has become popular when connecting to the Internet in order to deter unwarranted access. A physician's office may connect to insurance networks for billing, as well as to online services to connect to the large Internet. In all cases, an external telecommunications carrier's service is used to provide underlying long-distance, point-to-point communications capability.

The aggregate bandwidth in a WAN connection is typically much smaller than the LAN's bandwidth because of the higher costs of WAN connections. It is common to extend the LAN protocols to run over the WAN connections, so that applications run transparently regardless of location, but perhaps at a slower speed due to the restricted bandwidth.

For many applications requiring low datastream, a sufficient dial-in and dial-out access is provided over asynchronous phone lines with speeds ranging up to 28.8 Kbits/s. Instead of cable modems, for wireless applications GSM (Global Solution for Mobile Communication) modems are used. They are fully transparent to the application because of using the AT-command set (Hayes). Further development of the wireless solution is offered by GPRS (General Packet Radio Service) technology that multiplies up to four GSM communication channels to provide a flexible-bandwidth link of a throughput up to 40 kbps. With implementations of the point-to-point protocol (PPP) standard, the dialing-in PC will become a full peer node on the organizational network, instead of becoming a terminal to some computer or going through a surrogate PC on the network.

Recently, data interconnections through WAN have exploded among care facilities, private physicians' offices, nursing homes, insurance agencies, health maintenance organizations, research institutions, and state and federal regulatory agencies. The problem of security has become ever more important in this new world of accessible yet confidential patient information—including issues of who owns the data, how to protect the data, how to convert it securely to meet societal needs for statistical information, and so on. Smart cards, encryption digital signatures, guaranteed authentication and authorization, and constant accounting and auditing are several techniques being considered in intense discussions addressing the security aspects of medical information networking (U.S. Congress, 1993).

The *use of networks* at healthcare practice centers has provided value by increasing data availability, flexibility, and efficiency of operations. As our studies show, the main advantage of the distributed data processing and management has not yet been applied. As such it is considered ubiquitous and pervasive surveillance of citizens' health through the telemetry monitoring of principal vital signs and their interpretation in distributed systems. As has been demonstrated in this chapter, all technological issues have already been solved.

REFERENCES

American Heart Association. (2005). *Heart disease and stroke statistics—2005 update.* Dallas.

Bayes de Luna, A., & Stern, S. (2001). The future of noninvasive electrocardiology In W. Zareba, P. Maison-Blanche, & E. H. Locati (Eds.), *Noninvasive electrocardiology in clinical practice.* Armonk, NY: Futura.

Caro, C. G., Pedley, T. J., Schroter, R. C., & Seed, W. A. (1978). *The mechanics of the circulation.* New York: Oxford University Press.

Cimino, J. J., Clayton, P. D., Hripcsak, G. et al. (1994). Knowledge-based approaches to the maintenance of a large controlled medical terminology. *Journal of the American Medical Informatics Association, 1,* 35.

Daskalov, I. K., & Christov, I. I. (1999). Electrocardiogram signal preprocessing for automatic detection of QRS boundaries. *Medical Engineering and Physics, 21,* 37-44.

Dawson, T. H. (1991). *Engineering design of the cardiovascular system of mammals.* Englewood Cliffs, NJ: Prentice Hall.

de Chazal, P., & Celler, B. G. (1996). Automatic measurement of the QRS onset and offset in individual ECG leads. *Proceedings of the 18th Annual IEEE International Conference on Engineering in Medicine and Biology Society,* Amsterdam.

DiMarco, J. P., & Philbrick, J. T. (1990). Use of ambulatory electrocardiographic (Holter) monitoring. *Annals of Internal Medicine, 113,* 53-68.

Duisterhout, J. S., Hasman, A., & Salamon, R. (Eds.). (1991). *Telematics in medicine.* Amsterdam: Elsevier Science.

Fogel, R. I., Evans, J. J., & Prystowsky, E. N. (1997). Utility and cost of event recorders in the diagnosis of palpitations, presyncope, and syncope. *American Journal of Cardiology, 79,* 207-208.

GPRS. (2007). *General Packet Radio Service.* Retrieved from http://en.wikipedia.org/wiki/General_Packet_Radio_Service

GSM. (2007). *Global System for Mobile Communications.* Retrieved from http://en.wikipedia.org/wiki/Global_System_for_Mobile_Communications

Halpern, E. J., Newhouse, J. H., Amis, E. S. J. et al. (1992). Evaluation of teleradiology for interpretation of intra-venous urograms. *Journal of Digital Imaging, 5*(2), 101.

Healthsquare. (2007). *Heart disease.* Retrieved from http://www.healthsquare.com/heartdisease.htm

Heron, M. P., & Smith, B. L. (2003). *Deaths: Leading causes for 2003.* Hyattsville, MD: National Center for Health Statistics.

Hilgard, J., Ezri, M. D., & Denes P. (1985) Significance of ventricular pauses of three seconds or more detected on twenty-four-hour Holter recordings. *American Journal of Cardiology, 55,* 1005-1008.

Holter, N. (1961). New method for heart studies: Continuous electrocardiography of active subjects over long periods is now practical. *Science, 134,* 1214-1220.

Hurst, W. (2002). *The heart, arteries, and veins* (10th ed.). New York: McGraw-Hill.

Kinlay, S., Leitch, J. W., Neil, A., Chapman, B. L., Hardy, D. B. et al. (1996). Cardiac event recorders yield more diagnoses and are more cost-effective than 48-hour Holter monitoring in patients with palpitations: a controlled clinical trial. *Annals of Internal Medicine, 124,* 16-20.

Macfarlane, P. W., & Lawrie, T. D. V. (Eds.). (1989). *Comprehensive electrocardiology. Theory and practice in health and disease* (vols. 1-3). Oxford: Pergamon Press.

McDonald, C. T., & Hammond, W. E. (1989). Standard formats for electronic transfer of clinical data. *Annals of Internal Medicine, 110,* 333.

Moss, A. J., Bigger, J. T., & Odoroff, C. L. (1987). Postinfarction risk stratification. *Progress in Cardiovascular Diseases, 29,* 389-412.

Mueller, W. C. (1978). Arrhythmia detection program for an ambulatory ECG monitor. *Biomedical Sciences Instrumentation, 14,* 81-85.

National Center for Health Statistics. (2005) *Health, United States, 2005 with chartbook on the health of Americans.* Hyattsville, MD.

Onaral, B. (2001). Future directions: Biomedical signal processing and networked multimedia communications. In J. D. Bronzino (Ed.), *The biomedical engineering handbook.* Boca Raton, FL: CRC Press.

Rennels, G. D., & Shortliffe, E. H. (1987). Advanced computing for medicine. *Scientific American, 257*(4), 154.

Schneck, D. J. (2000). An outline of cardiovascular structure and function. In J. D. Bronzino (Ed.), *The biomedical engineering handbook.* Boca Raton, FL: CRC Press.

Sengupta, S. (2001). Computer networks in health care. In J. D. Bronzino (Ed.), *The biomedical engineering handbook.* Boca Raton, FL: CRC Press.

Sörnmo, L., & Laguna, P. (2005). *Bioelectrical signal processing in cardiac and neurological applications.* Englewood Cliffs, NJ: Elsevier Academic Press.

Tanenbaum, A. S. (1988). *Computer networks* (2nd ed.). Englewood Cliffs, NJ: Prentice Hall.

Thakor, N. V., Webster, J. G., & Tompkins, W. J. (1982). A battery-powered digital modem for telephone transmission of ECG data. *IEEE Transactions on Biomedical Engineering, 29,* 355-359.

Tompkins, W. J. (1982). Trends in ambulatory electrocardiography. *IEEE Frontiers of Engineering in Health Care, 4,* 201-204.

U.S. Congress. (1993). *Protecting privacy in computerized medical information* (Office of Technology Assessment, OTA-TCT-576). Washington, DC: U.S. Government Printing Office.

Wagner, G. S., & Marriott, H. J. (1994). *Marriott's practical electrocardiography* (9th ed.). Lippincott Williams & Wilkins, Philadelphia

Wi-Fi. (2007). *Wi-Fi.* Retrieved from http://en.wikipedia.org/wiki/Wi-Fi

WiMAX. (2007). *WiMAX.* Retrieved from http://en.wikipedia.org/wiki/WiMAX

Wireless. (2007). *Wireless network.* Retrieved from http://en.wikipedia.org/wiki/Wireless_network

Zimetbaum, P., Kim, K. Y., Ho, K. K., Zebede, J., Josephson, M. E. et al. (1997). Utility of patient-activated cardiac event recorders in general clinical practice. *American Journal of Cardiology, 79,* 371-372.

Zimetbaum, P. J., Kim, K. Y., Josephson, M. E., Goldberger, A. L., & Cohen, D. J. (1998). Diagnostic yield and optimal duration of continuous-loop event monitoring for the diagnosis of palpitations: A cost-effectiveness analysis. *Annals of Internal Medicine, 128,* 890-895.

ONLINE REFERENCES

http://www.aerotel.com/en/

http://www.burdick.com/products/

http://www.cardguard.com/newsite/index.asp

http://www.cardiocom.net/

http://www.cardiocomm.com/

http://www.cardiolertsystems.com/

http://www.cardiomedix.com/cardiomedix.htm

http://www.cardionet.com/

http://www.gehealthcare.com/euen/products.html

http://www.healthfrontier.com/

http://www.medtronic.com/

http://www.monitoring.welchallyn.com/

http://www.pdsheart.com/about.html

http://www.qrscard.com/

http://www.qrsdiagnostic.com/

http://www.spacelabshealthcare.com/company/index.html

Chapter IV
Background 3: Databases in Cardiology:
Current Issues

Databases are commonly understood as reservoirs of data storage, retrieval, and interchange systems. The specificity of medical databases applications is a result of the modality multitude and the role that databases play in current information technology-based societies. In this application, database formats and standardization have a direct impact on health monitoring and prevention in society. They also play an important role in global range scientific investigation in the area of medicine.

This chapter defines the set of standard diagnostic parameters and metadata expected from cardiac examinations. Rest ECG, exercise ECG, and long-term recording techniques are compared with regard to method-appropriate hierarchies of diagnostic results. This summary is approaching the idea of high redundancy in the dataset influencing data transmission and database operations. As far as the paper record was concerned, these spare data were useful in the validation and correction of human errors. Nowadays, automatic error detection and correction codes are widely applied in systems for storage and transmission of digital data.

Basic issues about DICOM and HL7, two widespread medical information interchange systems, are presented thereafter. These general-purpose systems integrate multi-modal medical data and offer specialized tools for the storage, retrieval, and management of data. Both standards originate from the efforts of standardizing the description of possibly wide aspects of patient-oriented digital data in the form of electronic health records. Certain aspects of data security are also considered here.

Following this, the reader's attention is focused on cardiology-oriented data specifications: SCP-ECG and MFER. These two examples provide ECG-specialized tools, data formats, and management methods. Some of the specifications (e.g., local signal decimation) are based on medical findings derived from the signal by diagnostic procedures and already anticipate the presentation of the authors' proposal of data-dependent reporting formats.

The interoperability of diagnostic equipment is presented as an important aspect of patient safety. Since many diagnostic techniques are based on trends and time-series analysis rather than on isolated measurements, the independence of data from the equipment- or manufacturer-specific technical issues is crucial. The international initiative Open ECG is mentioned as an example of efforts towards the interoperability. The consortium consists of researchers, medics, and industry representatives with the aim of widening the impact of common data exchange in the public health sector. Besides the promotion of the SCP-ECG standard, Open ECG is a non-commercial platform for volunteers to exchange tools and ECG interpretation procedures, viewers, format converters, and other cardiology-related software.

STANDARD REPORT OF A CARDIAC DIAGNOSIS

Modalities in Cardiac Diagnostics

Electrocardiography, although the most widespread cardiac functional examination and the most known electrophysiological test, does not pretend to be the only examination in cardiology. The variety of modalities reflects almost the full range of diagnostic methods applied in medicine, and consequently the use of medical data varying in their origin, nature, and volume is common in the description of the heart. Particular modalities are based on different phenomena triggering the action, directly included in the action, resulting from the action or accompanying the action of the heart. Therefore, these techniques are used as complementary depending on patient status and history.

Electrocardiography is focused on the generation and conduction of electrical activity stimulating the heart muscle contraction and accompanying the subsequent refraction. All sources of the heart action and the stimulus conduction pathways are represented in the ECG. Conduction conditions are also reflected in the electrical relations in the cellular level (drugs or ischemiae) or by the muscle tissue alterations resulting from the infarction. The principal advantages of the ECG are its very low price, frequency of use, feasibility in home-care conditions by untrained personnel (or even the patient himself), low invasiveness, and high informative value.

Ultrasonography (USG) reveals a static image of moving tissues, and as a cardiology-oriented application it is useful in monitoring muscle contraction and valve functions. The average displacement of the muscle tissue yields a rough estimate of the stroke volume and the volume of blood flow per heartbeat. The impaired mobility is interpreted as heart tissue damage determined with a higher precision than in the ECG. The time-motion (TM) presentation in the USG is used to determine the heart rate, amplitude, and velocity of the moving valves. Doppler ultra-sonic examinations provide a direct insight into the blood flow and reveal anatomic defects or injury-caused leakages. The technology allows precise measurements of blood volume temporal relations and the spatial distribution of the flow in the vessel section.

Unfortunately, professional training is necessary for correct measurements, the equipment is rather expensive, and the examination conditions are limited to the cases of the resting subject. Functional imaging of the heart is the source of the most precise spatial information about the heart muscle tissue and its activity, and may reveal muscle diseases in the earliest phases. Despite its high resolution, the volume and price of the accompanying equipment as well as the professional skills required from the personnel significantly limit the possible applications to well-prepared patients. The resulting volume of data also limits tele-medical use of functional cardiac imaging.

Coronarography is the isotope radiation-based technology of monitoring the blood flow in the coronary arterias. The blood transports the marker throughout the vessels, and subsequent frames of recorded moving images are a background for calculations of the volume and speed of the blood flow. The unexpected deceleration of the blood is interpreted as flow obturation caused by a narrowing of the vessel or calcification impairing the transportation of oxygen and nutritive products to the heart muscle. Due to its invasiveness, the coronarography is currently rarely employed in functional heart imaging. The circulating isotope is influencing organs before it disappears.

Thorax-impedance measurements are based on modulation of electrical properties of the thorax, including the heart during the cardiac cycle. The drawback of this method is the influence of electrical property changes due to the respiration. The heart rate and global information about variations of properties of the heart muscle tissue are easily derived from thoracograms, however the precise location of the impaired regions is not possible to determine. The method is also suitable for rough estimations of heart volume stroke.

Rheography is a blood inertion-based mechanical technique based on turbulent blood flow during the heart contraction. Thanks to the known anatomy of the aorta arc, the sudden flow of a considerable amount of blood causes a compensatory motion in the body whose amplitude can be measured as a representation of the stroke volume. Mechanical rheography requires precise measurement equipment and patient positioning, but it is the only non-image-based methodology for measuring the circulatory effects of the heart activity. Due to its nature, the rheography requires the patient to be at rest, so the application area is limited.

Magnetocardiography is a non-invasive measure of the variation in magnetic field strength above the thorax and can be used to detect electromagnetic phenomena in the heart (Smith et al., 2006). The magnetic field sensors used to record magnetocardiograms (MCGs) are superconducting quantum interference devices (SQUIDs; Zimmerman, Theine, & Harding, 1970) that require liquid helium cooling (Hart, 1991; Cohen, Edelsack, & Zimmerman, 1970). The detectors are extremely sensitive and can measure the weak magnetic fields generated by the electrical activity of the heart. Because of their expense and the need for magnetic shielding, the diagnostic usefulness of MCG systems needs to be carefully assessed. Many studies have demonstrated the potential benefit of magnetocardiography over electrocardiography for some clinical applications (Fenici, Brisinda, & Meloni, 2005; Mori & Nakaya, 1988; Nomura et al., 1994). Magnetocardiograms have been found to be more accurate than ECGs for the diagnosis of right atrial hypertrophy and right ventricular hypertrophy, and have been used to determine the location of conduction pathways in the heart non-invasively, making MCGs potentially beneficial for the localization of arrhythmia sources for catheter ablation (Mori & Nakaya, 1988; Nomura et al., 1994). Magnetocardiography can also detect circular vortex currents, which give no ECG signal. As a result, MCGs may show ischaemia-induced deviations from the normal direction of depolarization and repolarization better than or in a different way than ECGs. The technique also offers a simple non-invasive method for examination of the foetal electrophysiological signal, which is difficult to obtain from the surface ECG and may be useful in antenatal assessment, identifying and classifying clinically relevant arrhythmias (Van Leeuwen et al., 1999; Kandori et al., 2002; Quartero, Stinstra, Golbach, Meijboom, & Peters, 2002; Wakai, Strasburger, Li, Deal, & Gotteiner, 2003; Van Leeuwen, Lange, Klein, Geue, & Gronemeyer, 2004).

Seven different basic techniques are briefly presented above as a review of cardiac functional reporting methods and their outputs as multi-modal records containing:

- a voltage time series representing an endogenous or artificially paced electrical stimulus;
- static images resulting from mechanical wave-based or radiation isotope-based imaging;

- motion images resulting from mechanical wave-based frequency-differential measurements, thorax impedance tomography, or radiation isotope-based serial imaging;
- a displacement time series representing the stroke blood mass of the body weight ratio; and
- magnetic fields measurement time series.

Reporting Standards and Variants in Electrocardiology

Electrocardiography at its beginning existed as a single technique. For the specificity of the diagnostic needs, it evolved towards various methodologies applied today. The most common electrocardiographic examination is still used as a control test, but other modalities are used in specific medical domains:

- the exercise test,
- the tilt test,
- the Holter recording,
- ubiquitous monitoring, and
- event recording.

Some elements of diagnostic reporting are common for every electrocardiological finding, whereas others depend on the examination being appropriate to limited subset techniques or specific techniques.

The common parameter featured in all cardiac electrodiagnostic systems is the heart rate. The reason for this is twofold:

1. The heart rate is quite easy to compute, and even a simple automated recorder can do this task whereas sophisticated interpretive recorders issue the heart rate at the initial stage of processing.
2. Due to the automatic regulation of the heart action by the ANS, the heart rate is representative of the overall patient status.

The heart rate is issued by a wide range of diagnostic devices. Besides electrocardiographs, this parameter is typical for cardiotocographs, ultrasonographs with a time-marked presentation, Doppler ultrasound devices, blood saturation detectors (SpO2), and blood pressure monitors. The heart rate could be derived in such a sophisticated manner as through the measure of the divergence of eye globe-reflected infrared beams (see Chapter VI). This method is based on variations of eye globe pressure caused by blood stoke rhythm and enables reliable measurements without physical contact and the subject's knowledge.

The other parameter common to almost every electrophysiological measurement in cardiology is the ST segment evaluation. Elevation or depression of the ST segment is a primary indicator of pathological repolarization of the heart muscle caused by (Armstrong & Morris, 1983; Badilini, Zareba, Titlebaum, & Moss, 1986; Moss, 1986; Akselrod et al, 1987):

- insufficient oxygenation that indicates impaired oxygen exchange or transportation (low efficiency or diseases of the lungs, low partial pressure of oxygen in the hemoglobin, obturated bronchial tubes or coronary arteries); or
- the influence of drugs that may affect electrical phenomena at the cell level which changes the stimulus conduction path.

ST changes are also widely used to assess the stage of myocardial infarction. The infarction is quite a rapid process of deoxygenation and death of cells in a given region of the heart muscle. The subject immediately requires therapy, which depends on the progress of the infarction. The method is based on the global description of repolarization abnormality caused by the electrochemical changes in the presence of ischemia and local cells death. This makes the most rapid, however not the most accurate assessment of the infarction stage (acute, recent, old) sufficiently reliable for the appropriate treatment. However, in an emergency the sensitivity and specificity are sufficient to classify the subject correctly.

Unfortunately, the ST level is very prone to measurement conditions such as skin-electrode contact and skin perspiration. It is controversial as to how the same amplitude rules and decision threshold values are recommended for all populations regardless of body shape, possible skin moisture, different recording channels, and even various QRS amplitudes.

Most, but not all automatic systems for interpretation of electrocardiograms feature the classification of heartbeats in order to distinguish sinus-originated and ectopic beats. The true definition of a sinus rhythm is too complex to be verified by simple systems in real time, but a rough estimation aimed at detecting the ectopic beat is performed. Various approaches are used in the interpretive systems. These are:

- based on a measure of QRS complex lengths that may not exceed a specified duration (usually 120 ms),
- based on the expected shape of the QRS wave defined separately for each lead, or
- based on the approximate determination of heart electrical axis and the measurement of its beat-to-beat variance.

The occurrence of ectopic beats is used as a statistic parameter in the rest ECG report, as an alert during the exercise test, and as an inhibitor of some calculations (e.g., ST level assessments) applicable only to sinus rhythm.

Very simple in use, and consequently popular in home care use, are small devices designed for everyday wearing by healthy people in the prevention of cardiac failures. These recorders, which are similar in shape to a cell phone, require pressing two buttons simultaneously with both thumbs for a few seconds in regular intervals. The actual measures made are: blood oxygenation, heart rate, and ST depression. From these basic vital signs, the processor computes diagnostic parameters, but the outcome is simplified to a text message displayed on the screen. Such systems are intended to modulate lifestyles by indicating potentially dangerous conditions: stress, overwork, drug overdose, and so forth.

Several diagnostic parameters are specific to ECG recording techniques:

- Detailed measurement of the waves is typical for the rest ECG; Holter techniques rarely use sufficient sampling rates, while stress tests usually records signals with motion and muscular interferences affecting the measurement accuracy.
- Determination of rhythm origin is possible in all techniques, but typical for Holter recordings featuring signal strips of adequate length; rest ECG usually is too short to notice escape beats, and the stress test should not be performed in the presence of escape beats.
- Analysis of heart rate variability (HRV) aims at diagnosing the ANS and is performed only in Holter techniques; in the stress test, the heart rate depends on the workload, the influence of the ANS is masked, and the rest ECG is too short to notice the rhythm changes modulated by the ANS.
- Analysis of the arrhythmia and pacemaker are based on long sequences of events; the statistical parameters may be reliably calculated from at least a one-hour recording, thus these data are typical for Holter recordings. Nevertheless singular failures may be detected from the rest ECG. Patients with persistent arrhythmia or pacemakers are definitely excluded from the exercise test, at least as it is usually carried out nowadays.

In order to systematize our considerations, three groups of parameters can be defined using the data origin as a criterion:

1. rhythm analysis, derived from RR intervals and rhythm origin (arrhythmia, heart rate variability, heart rate turbulence, pacemaker series, etc.);
2. contour analysis, estimated from a single beat, usually the most representative heartbeat in a considered record strip (detection of conduction defects, hypertrophy, infarct, ventricular late potentials, etc.); and

Table 4.1 Excerpt from Minnesota Code Table

1-1-1	Q/R amplitude ratio ≥ 1/3, plus Q duration ≥ 0.03 sec in lead I or V6.
1-1-2	Q duration ≥ 0.04 sec in lead I or V6.
1-1-3	Q duration ≥ 0.04 sec, plus R amplitude ≥ 3 mm in lead aVL.
1-2-1	Q/R amplitude ratio ≥ 1/3, plus Q duration ≥ 0.02 sec and < 0.03 sec in lead I or V6.
1-2-2	Q duration ≥ 0.03 sec and < 0.04 sec in lead I or V6.
	……
9-8-2	Technical problems which do not interfere with coding.

3. cardiac series analysis, being representative of beat-to-beat changes of selected parameters (ST-change, QT-variability, T wave alternans).

The major diagnostic findings are standardized under the Minnesota Code Classification System for Electrocardiographic Findings (Prineas, Crow, & Blackburn, 1982). Each code consists of one to three digits according to the finding position in a diagnostic tree. The examples of the codes are displayed in table 4.1.

Code definition is completed by a table of incompatible and concurrent codes. The standard also contains Categories of the Minnesota ECG Abnormalities supporting the abnormal behavior of the interpretation software including the absence of the signal.

MEDICAL DATABASES AND THE INTEGRATION OF MEDICAL DATA

Patient- and Hospital-Oriented Health Records

The patient health record (PHR), also extended to a personal health record, is a description of all parameters necessary to identify the patient and to reveal his or her diagnostic data (Pryor, 2000). Although many in-hospital recordings are currently stored in digital databases, PHRs usually have a paper format when the patient is discharged. The non-machine-readable form causes additional workload when the patient is next directed to another health provider. The manual retrieval of electronic data is a potential source of human error and degrades the value of historical records. This is a serious limitation for a serial comparative assessment of a disease evolution because this valuable method is based on patient auto-reference. As the use of HL7 becomes more widespread, some electronic data can be partly retrieved in an electronic way by matching corresponding data fields in source and destination records.

In some developed countries PHRs are available as magnetic strip cards; this form, as far as it is supported by health providers, creates an opportunity for efficient and complete data exchange. The early applications employed the storage of a complete record on a magnetic strip, however this solution has been recently abandoned for two reasons: data volume and data security.

Due to the very limited capacity of the magnetic strip, it is more suited to storing identification data (like on credit cards) than to supporting long-term records of signals or images. The alternative solution is the centralized management of patient data by the commercial PHR provider or insurance agency without the right to access or modify medical data. The centralized management solution consists of granting access rights to particular records to various healthcare providers after correct patient and institution identification. Such systems are transparent enough to guarantee privacy because each access to the database is logged with the client digital identification system. The patient is independent in granting the authorization to access his or her medical data for a particular "transaction" with a healthcare provider.

The PHR provider manages the PHR, guarantees its continuous accessibility to authorized institutions, and provides protection from unauthorized access. Each time the authorized health provider makes a request, the PHR management system creates new records for the storage or release of a report and all the data necessary for further treatment.

Simultaneously with patient discharge, the health record is updated by any relevant medical data; however, the discharging hospital has granted modification rights only to the own-created records. The update consists of copying the subset of integrated patient data from his or her longitudinal files to a remote database. The detailed data filters depend on the patient status and on the policy of the healthcare provider, but must to comply with some minimum requirements. Copying insufficient or inappropriate data leads to incomplete patient records, which are not useful in further treatment. In such cases if the health record update was explicitly or by default included in the healthcare contract, the patient may claim his or her rights were violated. On the other hand, copying too much data causes an unnecessary management expense to the PHR provider and may defeat the performance of the database retrieval engines.

The concept of the hospital information system (HIS) consists of integration and dissemination of the patient or hospital information (Pryor, 2000). Such a system must meet the global needs of those it is to serve. In this context, if we look at the hospital as the customer of the HIS, then the HIS must be able to provide global and departmental information on the state of the hospital. If an HIS function were the recording of patient treatment cost, then the system must record all patient costs no matter which department they originate from. Likewise, all clinical information about the patient must reside within the HIS database so that it is available to all clinical sources. It is the totality of function that differentiates the HIS from the departmental or restricted clinical system, and not the particular functions provided to a department or clinical support incorporated within the system.

The development of an HIS can take many architectural forms. It can be accomplished through interfacing of a central system to multiple departmental or clinical information systems. A second approach that has been developed assumes the implementation of departmental or clinical system applications, in addition to a set of global applications. Because of the limitations of all existing systems, any comprehensive HIS will in fact be a combination of interfaces to departmental/clinical systems and the applications/database of the HIS purchased by the hospital. With regard to the functionality, clinical and departmental systems have many common features of the HIS. They all require a database for recording patient information. Both types of systems must be able to support the data acquisition and the reporting of patient data. The communication of information to other clinical or administrative departments is required. Some form of management support can also be found in all the systems. Thus, again looking at the basic functions of the system, one cannot differentiate the clinical/departmental systems from the HIS.

The first HISs were considered only as an extension to the financial and administrative systems in place in the hospital. With this simplistic view many early systems developed database strategies that were limited in their growth potential. Their databases mimicked closely the design of the financial systems that presented a rigid structure with well-defined fields. Although those fields were adequate for recording the financial information used by administrators to track the patient treatment costs, they were unable to easily adapt to the requirement of recording the clinical information being requested by healthcare providers. Today's HIS databases should be designed to support longitudinal patient records (the entire clinical record of a patient covering multiple inpatient and outpatient encounters), support integration of all clinical and financial data, and provide decision support functions.

The support of longitudinal patient records is now a requirement of the HIS. Traditionally, the databases of the HISs were encounter based. They were designed to manage a single patient visit to the hospital, in particular to create a financial record of the visit and make data recorded during the visit available to the care provider. Unfortunately, with regard to those systems, care providers were unable to view the progress of a patient over a number of visits, even to the point that in some HISs, critical information such as patient allergies needed to be entered with each new encounter. From a clinical perspective, the management of a patient must at least be considered in the context of a single episode of care. The care provider, to properly manage the patient, must have access to all the information recorded from those multiple encounters. The need for a longitudinal view requires that the HIS database structure both allow for access to patient data independent of an encounter and still provide for encounter-based access to adapt to the financial and billing requirements of the hospital.

Besides the longitudinal requirement, the need for integration of patient data is also important. Usually, the clinical information tended to be stored in separate departmental files. With this structure it was easy to report from each department, but the creation of reports combining data from the different sources is complicated. In particular, in those systems where access to the departmental data was provided only though interfaces with no central database, it was impossible to create an integrated patient evaluation report. Using those systems, care providers would view data from different screens at their terminal and extract using pencil and paper the information from each department that are necessary to properly evaluate a patient. With the integrated clinical database, the care provider can directly view, on a single screen, information from all departments formatted in a way that facilitates patient evaluation.

Today's HIS is no longer a database and communication system, but it is 'an assistant' in patient management. Clinical knowledge bases have been included as an integral part of the HIS. These knowledge bases contain rules and/or statistics with which the system can provide alerts or reminders leading to the implementation of clinical protocols. Execution of the information is highly dependent on the structure of the clinical database.

These enhanced features of the HIS database are necessary if the HIS is going to serve the needs of the digital era hospital. Beyond these inpatient needs, the database of the HIS is part of an enterprise's clinical database that will include not only clinical information about inpatient encounters, but also clinical information recorded in the physician's office or the patient's home during outpatient encounters. Subsets of these records will become part of state and national healthcare databases. Therefore, in properly selecting an HIS, the most critical factor is understanding the structure and functionality of its database.

In its principal role, the HIS must support an integrated patient record. Therefore, its ability to acquire clinical data from a variety of sources directly affects its ability to support patient evaluation and management functions. All HIS systems provide for direct terminal entry of data and interfacing with other systems which are necessary to compute a complete patient record. Physical interface with those systems is straightforward with today's technology. The potential difficulty results from incompatibility of data transmitted between systems, particularly when coded information from different systems is transmitted. In spite of many efforts, there are few medical standards for either the medical vocabulary or the coding systems. Thus, each manufacturer may have chosen an entirely different terminology or coding system to describe similar medical concepts. In building the interface, therefore, it may be necessary to build unique translation tables to store the information from each specific system into the databases of the HIS. This requirement has limited the building of truly integrated patient records.

The acquisition of data from patient monitors used in the hospital can either be directly interfaced with the HIS or recorded through an interface with an ICU system. Otherwise the monitoring data must be entered manually by the nursing personnel. It should be noted that whenever possible automated acquisition of data is preferable to manual entry because it is more accurate and reliable and less resource intensive. In early HISs without interfaces with patient monitors, the frequency of data capture is much lower. This affects the ability of the HIS to implement real-time medical decision logic to monitor the status of the patient. That is, in the ICU where decisions need to be made in a very time-restricted manner, the information on which the decision is based must be entered promptly. Without automatic entry of the data, the critical data needed for decision making may be outdated or not present at all, thus the computer-assisted management of the patient is seriously affected.

Besides administrative and financial functions, the patient admitting service supports the master patient index (MPI) and the longitudinal clinical file to allow the HIS to meet its critical clinical functions. The MPI contains a unique identifier for the patient and other entries necessary for the admitting staff to identify the patient (name, sex, birth date, Social Security number). This information will be used by the program to select potential patient matches in the MPI from which the administration can link to the current admission. If no matches are detected by the program, the system creates a new record in the MPI. This identification is very prone to human error (e.g., the matching record is not found because the wrong data was entered). In earlier HISs where no longitudinal record existed, this problem was not critical, but in today's system, errors in matching can have serious clinical consequences. Therefore, several approaches were implemented to eliminate this problem, including probabilistic matching, auditing processes, and post-admission consolidation.

The longitudinal record may contain either a complete clinical record of the patient or only those variables that are most critical in subsequent admissions. Among the data that have been determined as most critical are key demographic data, allergies, surgical procedures, discharge diagnoses, and radiology reports. Beyond these key data elements, modern systems provide computational power and data storage resources large enough to store complete clinical records. In those systems the structure of the records of the longitudinal file contain information regarding the encounter, admitting physician, and any other information that may be necessary to view the record from an encounter point of view or as a complete clinical history of the patient.

The purpose of patient evaluation programs supervised by or incorporated in the HIS is to provide the care provider with complete information about the patient which assists in evaluating the medical status of the patient. In their simplest form these applications are departmentally oriented. Thus, laboratory reports, radiology reports, pharmacy reports, nursing records, and the like can be displayed or printed on hospital terminals. This form of evaluation functionality is commonly called *results review* because it only allows for the results of departmental tests to be displayed, with no attempt to integrate patient data or issue a consistent patient evaluation report.

Provided the HIS is using a central integrated patient database, the issued patient reports can be much more sophisticated. In this form the care provider has, within a single report correlated by the computer, the clinical information necessary to evaluate the patient's status rather than looking for data on reports from the laboratory system, the pharmacy system, and the nurses' notes. As the amount and variety of data recorded by the HIS increases, the system can produce purpose-specific patient evaluation reports. Integrated reports issued by contemporary HIS applications summarize on one to two screens all the patient's clinical records captured by the system. These reports shorten the information access time and present data in a more intuitive and clinically useful form.

Patient evaluation is usually followed by prescribed therapy that ensures an optimal outcome for the patient. The HIS records the order in the patient's computerized medical record and transmits the order to the appropriate department for execution. In those hospitals where departmental systems are interfaced with the HIS, the electronic transmission of the order to the departmental system is a natural part of the order entry system. Unfortunately, current order-entry applications are rarely accepted by the physician because of their inconvenient interface. The use of order sets, allowing the physician to enter multiple orders from a single screen, has improved its acceptability, but several problems still prevent universal acceptance of such systems. One of them is that the order set is rarely sufficiently complete to contain all the orders that a physician would want to request.

The other problem is the lack of integration of the application into the intellectual tasks of the physician. Newer systems are incorporating the ordering task into other applications assisting the physician throughout the entire intellectual effort of patient evaluation and management.

Beyond simple test ordering, many newer HISs are implementing decision support packages. Such systems can incorporate medical knowledge usually as rule sets to assist the care provider in the management of patients. The execution of the rule sets can be performed in the foreground through direct calls from an executing application or in the background with the storage of clinical data in the patient's computerized medical record. This latter mode is called data-driven execution and provides an extremely powerful method of knowledge execution and alerting. After execution of the rule sets, the HIS will alert the care provider of any outstanding information that may be important regarding the status of the patient or suggestions about patient management. New implementations of HIS notification methods include electronic messages directed to appropriate personnel on duty, regardless of physical distance.

The use of decision support has ranged from simple laboratory alerts to complex patient protocols. The responsibility of the HIS is to provide the tools for creation and execution of the knowledge base. Hospital experts are responsible for the actual logic that is entered into the rule sets. The inclusion of decision support functionality in the HIS requires that the HISs be designed to support a set of knowledge tools. In general, a knowledge-based system will consist of a knowledge base and an inference engine. The knowledge base will contain the rules, frames, and statistics that are used by the inference applications to substantiate a decision. In the healthcare area, the knowledge base should be sufficiently flexible to support multiple forms of knowledge. The tasks of the application manager are to provide a human interface with the application, control the functional capabilities of the application, and invoke the appropriate inference engine for the support of any artificial intelligence functionality.

The role of the HIS has recently evolved towards the advisory tasks concerning patient care. With this extension into clinical care, the HIS has not only added new functionality to its design, but has enhanced its ability to serve the traditional administrative needs of the hospital as well. The creation of these global applications, which go well beyond those of the departmental/clinical systems, is now making the HIS a patient-oriented system. It provides global information for the accurate analysis of hospital efficiency in the operation of both the administrative and medical care aspects. This knowledge allows for continuous optimization of healthcare provided to patients at the least cost to the hospitals. The considerations above and anticipated benefits increase the role of HIS as an analytic tool fulfilled thanks to the use of institution-integrated databases and the implementation of medical knowledge bases complementing the traditional functionality of the HIS.

The Health Level Seven (HL7) Protocol

A group of healthcare computer systems users in 1987 started developing the HL7 protocol to create a common communication platform that allows healthcare applications to share clinical data with each another. This project later developed into the establishment of the Health Level Seven organization. Over time the HL7 interoperability protocol became a nationally, internationally, and globally accredited standard.

The name "Level Seven" refers to the highest level of the ISO communications model for open systems interconnection (OSI). This application level contains a definition of the data to be exchanged, the interchange timing, and the error messaging to the application. Examples of the functions supported by the seventh level are: security checks, participant identification, availability checks, exchange mechanism negotiations, and most importantly, data exchange structuring.

The aims of the HL7 organization focus on the interface requirements of the entire healthcare institution, while most other efforts focus on the requirements of a particular department. HL7 undertakes ongoing developments of protocols on the fastest possible track that is both responsive and responsible to its members. The group addresses the unique requirements of the already installed hospital and departmental systems, some of which use mature technologies. HL7 develops specifications, the most widely known being a messaging standard that enables disparate healthcare applications to exchange clinical and administrative data. HL7's mission is:

"To provide (global) standards for the exchange, management and integration of data that supports clinical patient care and the management, delivery and evaluation of healthcare services. Specifically, to create flexible, cost effective approaches, standards, guidelines, methodologies and enable healthcare information system interoperability and the sharing of electronic health records." (Dolin, Alschuler, Boyer, & Beebe, 2004).

Members of Health Level Seven are known collectively as the Working Group, which is organized into technical committees (TCs) and special interest groups (SIGs). The technical committees are directly responsible for the content of the standards. Special interest groups serve as a testbed for exploring new areas that may need coverage in HL7's published standards. A list of the technical committees and special interest groups, as well as their missions, scopes, and current leadership, is available on the HL7.org Website.

While HL7 focuses on addressing immediate needs, the group continues to dedicate its efforts to ensuring concurrence with other U.S. and international standards development activities. HL7 aims at identifying and supporting the diverse requirements of each of its membership constituencies: users, vendors, and consultants. According to their specific needs, requirements, priorities, and interests, HL7 supports all groups as they make important contributions to the quality of the organization.

The messages in HL7 v2.x have a variable-length, positional format and consist of lines of ASCII text. Each line of text is a fixed sequence of data fields separated by delimiters. In the HL7 standards document, each data item is well defined. HL7 v2.5 contains approximately 1,700 data items. Each data element is usually separated by vertical bar (or pipe "|") characters, may have components (separated by "^" characters), and may repeat (e.g., for multiple patient IDs, phone numbers, etc.).

An example HL7 message follows:

```
MSH|^~\&|PATH||GP123||200407161745||ORU^R01|101|P|2.5^AUS|34
567||AL|NE|AUS||en<cr>PID|||KNEE123||Knees^Nobby^J^^Mr||
19331215|M|||23 Shady Lane^LIGHTNING RIDGE^NSW^2392|||||||
219171803<cr> OBR|1|PMS66666|956635.9|LFT^LIVER FUNCTION
TEST^N2270<cr> OBX|1|NM|1751-7^S Albumin^LN
||38|g/L|35-45||||F<cr> OBX|2|NM|1779-8^S Alkaline Phosphatase^LN||
52|U/L|30-120||||F<cr>
```

The version 2.x standards are widely used in hospital and medical campus settings. National HL7 standards exist for patient administration, pathology (standard and handbook), medications, disease registries, and discharge/referral. Global HL7 versions 2.1 to 2.5.1 have been published, and work on V2.6 was expected to be published by the end of 2007.

The Clinical Document Architecture (CDA) is an HL7 standard for the creation of clinical documents using XML (eXtensible Mark-up Language). XML is a process for adding non-printable characters to text documents to allow the computer system to process the text (e.g., change the format). The use of the bracket structure as <instruction> is the method of embedding instructions in the text.

By leveraging the use of XML, the HL7 Reference Information Model (RIM), and coded vocabularies, the CDA makes documents both *machine readable,* so they are easily parsed and processed electronically, and *human readable,* so they can be easily retrieved and used by the people who need them. CDA documents can be displayed using XML-aware Web browsers or wireless applications such as cell phones.

The Clinical Document Architecture is an HL7 standard for the representation and machine processing of clinical documents in a way that makes the documents both human readable and machine processable, and guarantees the preservation of the content by using the eXtensible Markup Language (XML) standard. It is a useful intuitive approach to the management of documents which make up a large part of the clinical information processing arena.

The CDA specifies the structure and semantics of clinical documents in healthcare (Dolin et al., 2004). A document can be defined as a piece of text or information that would usually be authenticated by a signature, for example, a progress note, a pathology request, a radiology report, or an account. The CDA document may contain text, images and multimedia, and coded data. It can be handled in following ways:

- stored either permanently or temporarily as a document in a computer system; or
- transmitted as the content of a message using e-mail, HL7, or any other messaging system.

CDA was created recognizing that much of healthcare is involved in creating and managing documents and that the document paradigm is well understood by clinicians and administrators.

A clinical document has the following features, which form the framework for the CDA:

- persistence,
- stewardship,
- authentication,
- wholeness and context, and
- human readability.

CDA aims to give priority to documents generated by clinicians in order to:

- standardize the format of the many thousands of types of clinical documents,
- support the exchange of clinical information for human readability and information processing,
- promote longevity of information by separating data from the systems that store it (to avoid obsolescence as it occurs with technological processes and by being computer platform independent), and
- allow for the appropriate local adaptation of the standard to meet national or specific user requirements.

The CDA document consists of:

- *Header*—This contains key descriptive information about the document (metadata) such as who wrote it, who is it intended for, and type of document.
- *Body*—This contains the text of the document which may be structured at least under key headings or sections. It is possible for the text to contain coded

values. It is also possible to have no text information in the body such as an image of an X-ray (using the DICOM standard representation).

CDA has been developed in three stages: Level 1 through Level 3. Level 1 has a structured header and structured body message with limited coding capacity for content. Levels 2 and 3 impose more structure to allow for the representation of 'context' or constrained fields and more coded data. The standard has been published for Level 1, and Levels 2 and 3 are currently in draft stages. CDA Level 2 and 3 documents (along with the standard electronic health record architecture) require the use of templates and archetypes, which define key information in the context of complex health concepts such as family history or blood pressure.

Digital Imaging and Communications in Medicine

Digital Imaging and Communications in Medicine (DICOM) is a standard for handling, storing, printing, and transmitting information in medical imaging (NEMA, 2007a, 2007b). It includes a definition of the file format as well as a network communications protocol. A communications protocol is an application protocol based on TCP/IP to communicate between systems. DICOM files can be exchanged between two entities that are capable of receiving image and patient data in DICOM format. It was developed by the DICOM Standards Committee, whose members are also partly members of the National Electrical Manufacturers Association (NEMA), which owns the copyright to the DICOM.

In early 1980s emerged a need to exchange computed tomography or magnetic resonance images between devices from various manufacturers. Radiologists wanted to use the images for dose-planning for radiation therapy. After two years of work, the first standard was released in 1985 as ACR/NEMA 300. Very soon after its release, many clarifications and improvements were needed due to internal contradictions in the specifications.

The second release in 1988 gained more acceptance among vendors. Image transmission was specified as being over a dedicated 50-pin DICOM cable. The first commercial equipment supporting ACR/NEMA 2.0 was presented at the annual meeting of RSNA in 1990 by GE Healthcare and Vortech. As a response to the need for improvement, several extensions to ACR/NEMA 2.0 were created, like Papyrus (developed by the University Hospital of Geneva, Switzerland) and SPI (Standard Product Interconnect, driven by Siemens Medical Solutions and Philips Medical Systems).

In the third version of the standard released in 1992, the name DICOM was first used. New service classes were defined, network support added, and the Conformance Statement was introduced. Officially, the latest version of the standard is still 3.0, however it has been constantly updated and extended since 1992. Instead of using the version number, the standard is often version-numbered using the release year, for example, "the 2007 version of DICOM."

The DICOM standard aims at the integration of scanners, servers, workstations, printers, and network hardware from multiple manufacturers into a picture archiving and communication system. The different devices come with DICOM conformance statements, which clearly state the DICOM classes they support. DICOM has been widely adopted by hospitals and is making inroads in smaller applications like dentists' and doctors' offices.

The specific feature of DICOM among other data formats used in medicine is collecting information into data sets. That means that any image file actually contains patient IDs within the file, so that the image can never be separated from this information by mistake.

The DICOM format header describes image dimensions and retains other text information about the scan. The size of this header varies depending on how much header information is stored. The image data follows the header information (the header and the image data are stored in the same file). DICOM requires a 128-byte preamble (these 128 bytes are usually all set at zero) followed by the letters D, I, C, M. This is followed by the header information, which is organized into 'groups'.

DICOM uses data objects consisting of a number of attributes, including items such as name, ID, and so forth, and also one special attribute containing the image pixel data (i.e., logically, the main object has no 'header' as such—it is merely a list of attributes, including the pixel data). A single DICOM object can only contain one attribute containing pixel data. For many modalities, this corresponds to a single image. But note that the attribute may contain multiple "frames," allowing for the storage of cine loops or other multi-frame data. Another example is NM data, where an NM image by definition is a multi-dimensional multi-frame image. In these cases three- or four-dimensional data can be encapsulated in a single DICOM object. Pixel data can be compressed using a variety of standards, including JPEG, JPEG Lossless, JPEG 2000, and run-length encoding (RLE). LZW (zip) compression can be used for the whole data set (not just the pixel data), but this is rarely implemented.

The same basic format is used for all of the applications, including network and file usage, but when written to a file, usually a true 'header' is added containing copies of a few key attributes and details of the application that wrote it.

DICOM consists of many different services (tab. 4.2), most of which involve the transmission of data over a network, and the file format below is a later and relatively minor addition to the standard.

DICOM restricts the filenames on DICOM media to eight characters. This is a historical requirement to maintain compatibility with older existing systems. It also mandates the presence of a media directory, the DICOMDIR file, which provides index and summary information for all DICOM files on the media. The DICOMDIR information provides substantially greater information about each file than any filename could, so there is less need for meaningful file names.

The DICOM, despite its name, supports not only imaging data interchanges. The data frame may contain raw or processed ECG signals, breathing curve, and many

Table 4.2 Basic DICOM services

Store	The DICOM store service is used to send images or other persistent objects (structured reports, etc.) to a PACS or workstation.
Storage Commitment	The DICOM storage commitment service is used to confirm that an image has been permanently stored by a device (either on redundant disks or on backup media, e.g., burnt to a CD). The service class user (modality, workstation, etc.) uses the confirmation from the service class provider (archive station) to make sure that it is safe to delete the images locally.
Query/Retrieve	This enables a workstation to find lists of images or other such objects and then retrieve them from a PACS.
Modality Worklist	This enables a piece of imaging equipment (a modality) to obtain details of patients and scheduled examinations electronically, avoiding the need to type such information multiple times (and the mistakes caused by retyping).
Modality Performed Procedure Step	A complementary service to the modality worklist, this enables the modality to send a report about a performed examination including data about the images acquired, the start time, the completion time, the duration of a study, the dose delivered, and so forth. It helps give the radiology department a more precise handle on resource (acquisition station) use. Also known as MPPS, this service allows a modality to better coordinate with image storage servers by giving the server a list of objects to send before or while actually sending such objects.
Printing	The DICOM printing service is used to send images to a DICOM printer, normally to print an "x-ray" film. There is a standard calibration (defined in DICOM Part 14) to help ensure consistency between various display devices, including hard copy printouts.
Off-Line Media	The off-line media files correspond to Part 10 of the DICOM standard. It describes how to store medical imaging information on removable media. Except for the data set containing, for example, an image and demography, it is also mandatory to include the file meta information.

other kinds of one-dimensional data. Among its modalities, three have particular importance with regard to cardiology:

- CD = Color Flow Doppler,
- EC = Echocardiography, and
- ECG = Electrocardiogram.

DICOM is an evolving standard, and it is maintained in accordance with the Procedures of the DICOM Standards Committee. Proposals for enhancements are forthcoming from the DICOM Committee member organizations based on input from users of the standard. These proposals are considered for inclusion in future editions of the standard. A requirement in updating the standard is to maintain effective compatibility with previous editions.

CARDIOLOGY-ORIENTED DATABASES AND COMMUNICATION FORMATS

Serial Communication Protocol ECG

The SCP-ECG is a standard specifying the interchange format and a messaging procedure for ECG cart-to-host communication and for the retrieval of SCP-ECG records from the host (to the ECG cart). The basis for the SCP standard was developed during a European AIM R&D project in 1989-1991 (Willems et al., 1987; Van Bemmel & Willems, 1990; Willems, 1991). During this project an inventory of existing ECG compression methods was made and a new approach for quality assured ECG signal compression was developed.

During the design of the interchange format, basic results from an early American development— the so-called *Universal Veterans Administration Protocol*—were considered; one of the co-workers in the CEN Project Team that finally edited the SCP standard document came from a large American company and made many valuable contributions. In 1993 the *SCP Standard Communication Protocol* was approved by CEN as a pre-standard ENV 1064.

This standard was then implemented by a couple of European and American manufacturers. Practical experience during implementation and in the field confirmed its usability for telemetric applications, as well as for effective data volume storage and retrieval (demonstrated in the OEDIPE project). However, the originally desired high flexibility with (too) many manufacturer-specific implementation options and a few ambiguities within the text resulted in insufficient interoperability between devices of different manufacturers. As a consequence, this document was reviewed by an AAMI committee (now with participants from Europe), and the revised version was then balloted positively and became in 2000 the AAMI Standard EC71.

Meanwhile, communication technology has changed significantly, and larger memory capacities are available today. In some applications data compression and transmission of the relatively large ECG raw data records are less critical. So, for compatibility with the increasing use of HL7/XML messaging in electronically supported healthcare applications, an object-oriented approach with the application of a standardized nomenclature appears to have become a further solution. Nevertheless, for many real-time applications in telemedicine, the SCP interchange format, with its high potential for flexible and—if properly implemented—still interoperable data records, remains one of the best solutions, as so much consensus on necessary accompanying ECG information has been documented.

The SCP standard specifies that the information must be structured into sections as follows (Fisher & Zywietz, 2001):

Mandatory	2 BYTES - CHECKSUM - CRC - CCITT OVER THE ENTIRE RECORD (EXCLUDING THIS WORD)
Mandatory	4 BYTES - (UNSIGNED) SIZE OF THE ENTIRE ECG RECORD (IN BYTES)
Mandatory	(Section 0) POINTERS TO DATA AREAS IN THE RECORD
Mandatory	(Section 1) HEADER INFORMATION - PATIENT DATA/ECG ACQUISITION DATA
Optional	(Section 2) HUFFMAN TABLES USED IN ENCODING OF ECG DATA (IF USED)
Optional	(Section 3) ECG LEAD DEFINITION
Optional	(Section 4) QRS LOCATIONS (IF REFERENCE BEATS ARE ENCODED)
Optional	(Section 5) ENCODED REFERENCE BEAT DATA IF REFERENCE BEATS ARE STORED
Optional	(Section 6) "RESIDUAL SIGNAL" AFTER REFERENCE BEAT SUBTRACTION IF REFERENCE BEATS ARE STORED, OTHERWISE ENCODED RHYTHM DATA
Optional	(Section 7) GLOBAL MEASUREMENTS
Optional	(Section 8) TEXTUAL DIAGNOSIS FROM THE "INTERPRETIVE" DEVICE
Optional	(Section 9) MANUFACTURER SPECIFIC DIAGNOSTIC AND OVERREADING DATA FROM THE "INTERPRETIVE" DEVICE
Optional	(Section 10) LEAD MEASUREMENT RESULTS
Optional	(Section 11) UNIVERSAL STATEMENT CODES RESULTING FROM THE INTERPRETATION

Each section is divided into two parts: the section ID header and the section data part:

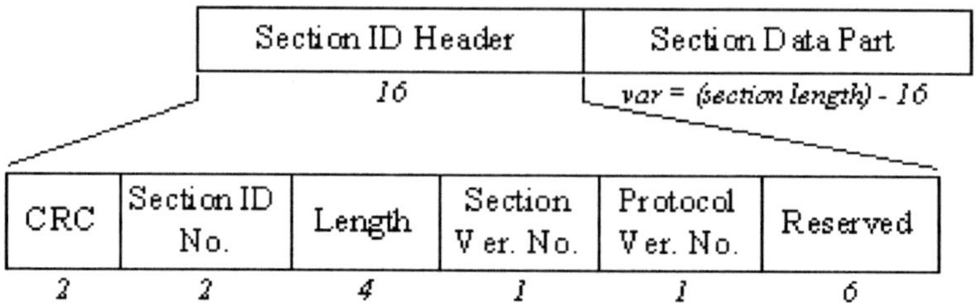

While the section ID header always has a length of 16 bytes, the section data part is variable. Note that the complete section length (relevant for the section length information) includes the length of the ID header.

The SCP standard allows for a rather large number of options to store and format the ECG data. ECG data may be acquired at different sampling rates, with different quantization levels; they may be not compressed or be compressed by selectable methods, and an SCP-ECG record may or may not contain an analysis and over-reading results. Also, the number of leads, the length of the recording interval, and even the simultaneity of leads is left open to the manufacturer.

The pointer section essentially represents the table of contents of the SCP-ECG record under consideration. The pointer section is therefore a useful means to identify what the content of a transmitted SCP record will be. The header section has structured in up to 35 different tags. It carries the essential information like patient ID (name, ID number, age, date of birth, height, weight, gender, etc), drugs and referral information, acquiring and analyzing device information, and many other kinds of information. This section also accepts a free-text medical history. Optional section 2 contains information about which way the ECG data are encoded as part of this specific SCP-ECG record (in section 5 and section 6). Section 2 is not mandatory, and when present it states that the ECG signal in sections 5 and 6 (if they exist) was also Huffman coded (entropy encoded). Section 3 contains the ECG lead definition. The SCP standard allows an SCP-ECG record to include data from 1, …, 255 leads. The standard contains a code list for all common leads as well as for specific lead sets. This specification also contains information about whether leads are recorded simultaneously or sequentially. Finally, in section 3 the length of the recording for each of the leads is contained by specifying the starting and ending sample number. The standard specifies that the lead data are sequentially ordered.

Considering the application of an SCP-ECG protocol in a simple recording system, it is possible to build the record length information (by means of the CRC check) and, by using sections 0, 1, (2), 3, and 6, a fully interoperable SCP-ECG record. Apart from all demographic patient information, this record would contain device and recording ID and the ECG raw data without any processing of the ECG signal itself. Only if some compression by Huffman entropy encoding is desired does the data need to be processed accordingly. Filling sections 4, 5, 7, and all other ones requires gradually increasing more ECG analysis. For the support of section 4, an algorithm for ECG beat detection is necessary; for section 7, a measurement algorithm is also necessary; and for filling section 8, a diagnostic classification algorithm must be applied. These sections, together with sections 10 and 11, are designed for sophisticated interpreting devices because of high computational requirements.

The SCP-ECG besides standard Huffman-based coding of raw data implements its specific ECG-oriented method for waveform compression (Zywietz, Joseph, & Degani, 1990). This method requires some analysis of the ECG signal, in particular the beat localization and beat typing. The compression has been proven to issue reliable results only if particular minimum requirements of analysis accuracy are met. In most cases the ECG is a quasi-stationary time series with repetitive ECG cycles. In this situation it is possible to calculate a so-called "reference beat" as the median or average of the most frequent ECG cycles. It is then possible to subtract this reference beat from all locations where a beat has been detected within the ECG record, which requires a precise beat alignment. As a result, the residual data record has only very small amplitudes in all samples. By then computing second differences and carrying out Huffman encoding, compression ratios of more than 25 may be obtained.

Measurements and diagnostic classification are performed on the reference beat. This reference beat is for the reconstruction of a raw data ECG record stored with redundancy reduction only (in section 5). The residual data are sample decimated and somewhat truncated outside the region of the detected (and subtracted) QRS complex.

Medical Waveform Format Encoding Rules (MFER)

Medical waveforms such as electrocardiograms and electroencephalograms are widely utilized in physiological examinations, healthcare information, and other areas in the clinical field. Signal processing technology has extended the utilization of waveform data to various fields including research and investigation. However, there is no commonly used standard format for waveform data, only proprietary standards. HL7 and DICOM formats enable the description of medical waveforms, but the scope of application is limited. IEEE 1073 provides some stipulations, but it is specialized at the medical device level and is not always easy to apply. To make physiological information easy to handle, medical waveform data should be described separately from other information, and thus it is desirable to have a universal standard description format for medical waveforms. If such a standard format is popularly used, physiological information could be utilized more efficiently and the effective use of waveform data can be expected for healthcare information such as electronic health records and physiological research.

The aims of medical waveform description format encoding rules are displayed in table 4.3 (Hirai & Kawamoto, 2004).

It is expected that MFER will be used in keeping with the following basic policy.

- MFER must not impede features of each individual system and must not prevent technological development.
- MFER aims at enabling easy conversion of historic databases of medical waveforms, accurate encoding of present waveform information, and the sufficient description of possible new medical waveforms in the future.
- MFER does not exclude other rules.

MFER is used for the storage of any waveforms in temporal frames. Thus, its major components are sampling and frame information. Sampling information consists of two attributes: (1) sampling frequency or sampling interval, and (2) sampling resolution. The frame information describes how waveform data are aligned, and it has three major components which are data block, channel, and sequence.

The definitions of MFER are classified into three levels: (1) basic specification, (2) extended specification, and (3) auxiliary specification. It is recommended that MFER describes level 2 and a level 3 information in the host protocol such as HL7 or DICOM.

The header and waveform data shall be encoded based on the encoding rules and shall be composed of the type, length, and value (TLV). The type, represented by a predefined tag, indicates the attributes of the data.

- The tag (T) consists of one or more octets and indicates the attributes of the data value. The tag is composed of a class, primitive/context (P/C), and a tag number. The tag is sorted into four classes. Class 0 is MFER level 1, class 1 is MFER level 2, class 2 is MFER level 3, and class 3 is for private use.
- The data length (L) is the length of data values indicated in one to four octets (the number of octets used for the data length section is up to five). In the case that the data value section uses 128 octets or more, the total data length is encoded using multiple octets. The first octet identifies the number of octets used to indicate the total data length. However, MFER allows for the representation of a data length using multiple octets even if the value section uses 127 octets or less. MFER allows for the designation of an infinite data

length by encoding 0x80 for the data length. This infinite length designation is terminated by encoding the end-of-contents.

- Value (V) is the contents, waveform data, or the like of the attribute identified by the tag.

MFER applies data encoding rules for maximum format flexibility. In order to suffice with minimum definitions for ordinary uses, all definitions in MFER are optional. All tags have default values defined, and as long as a tag uses the default value, the item need not be defined. Multiple definitions can be made for any item. Depending on items, a new definition overrides an old definition or all definitions.

Table 4.3 Principal aims of medical waveform description format encoding rules

Simple and Easy Installation	MFER is aiming at utmost simplification; for example, MFER enables simple encoding of standard 12-lead ECG. Simplification facilitates understanding, installation, trouble shooting, and decreases implementation costs.
Harmonization with Other Standards	MFER is specialized in medical waveforms. For encoding information other than medical waveforms, it is recommended to use the HL7, DICOM, or IEEE 1073 format, whichever is suitable for the specific non-waveform information. In principle, therefore, it is considered more effective to encode information such as patient information and examination information, excluding medical waveforms, using a format which is desirable for such information rather than using MFER for both waveforms and patient information.
Separation of Application and Provider	With MFER, providers of medical waveforms concentrate on the description of waveforms as accurately as possible using the entire set of rules. Applications are not obliged to wholly install the specifications, but might understand and utilize only the necessary information for each individual purpose. Depending on the system design, unnecessary tips in the information supplied by providers may be ignored or regarded as errors to suspend processing.
Human Interface Specification	Medical waveform information must be encoded in such a manner as to enable users to cope with diversified purposes and differences among patients. MFER not only encodes data in a definite form, but also has a structure to enable the transmission of important information using messages to users.

Each definition is interpreted in a definition order. If an item has related definitions, definitions shall be made in correct order. The root definition is effective for all channels. The channel definition is effective only for the relevant channel and overrides the root definition. If the data length is defined as zero (no data) in the definition of an item, the content in the definition is reset to default. If a definition is made without the necessary preceding definition, the definition is ignored.

Although MFER can describe original data or processed data, it is preferable that original data are described in MFER in order to allow each processing application to make its specific transformation of data in an independent way.

MFER can describe all medical waveforms, not only standard 12-lead ECGs, but also Holter ECGs, monitoring ECGs, intra-cardiac ECGs, VCGs, EEGs, monitoring waveforms, and so on. Since MFER specification is simple, anyone can easily develop a new viewer or a research program. Also, the viewer can display all MFER waveforms as Internet applications because of executing an IE plug-in module.

INTEROPERABILITY ISSUES

Standards and Concepts

For computerized electrocardiography, the ECG Standard Communications Protocol CEN ENV 1064 (http://www.centc251.org) specifies the exchange of data between ECG devices/carts and related computer systems. It provides a flexible data exchange format, a comprehensive coding scheme, and features like data compression and so forth. Due to the relevance of ECG data in numerous medical procedures and domains, however, diverse communication standards had to encompass ECG communication capabilities. Motivated by intensive care and operation theatre requirements, CEN standards ENV 13734/35 (http://www.centc251.org)—commonly known under the acronym "VITAL"—and related IEEE 1073 (http://www.ieee1073.org) documents have been aligned and extended to build the CEN ISO/IEEE 11073 family of standards (http://www.iso.ch/tc215). It aims at real-time 'plug-and-play' medical device interoperability for a wide range of medical devices, including real-time ECG data communication. It addresses:

- transports (e.g., cable-connected or wireless);
- general application services (e.g., polled vs. 'event-driven' services);
- device data (specifying an object-oriented data model, terminology, nomenclature, and coding scheme optimized for vital signs information);
- optional components for specific communication need or device functionalities ("Application Profiles"/"Device Specializations"); and

- internetworking and gateway standards (e.g., a gateway from 11073-based messaging and data representation to HL7 or DICOM).

For off-line vital signs representation and exchange, particularly among sleep labs, CEN prENV 14271 "File Exchange Format" was inherited from VITAL.

The HL7 (http://www.hl7.org) has no practicable generic (ECG) waveform representation, but utilizes external representation schemes that are 'embedded' in (OBX) segments. The DICOM 3.0 Supplement 30 (http://medical.nema.org) provides "Waveform Object Definitions" for general ECG, ambulatory ECG, 12-lead ECG, and cardiac electrophysiology. DICOM image-related (sequence-related) waveform objects enable the combined processing of DICOM images and related waveforms, and are—in combination with coded diagnostic information—subject to DICOM "Structured Reporting." Similar semantic concepts are also applied by joint IEEE/ISO/HL7 activities to meet recent FDA requirements for provision of original ECG data for clinical studies.

Interoperability and Communication Formats

Until today, departmental/clinical information systems are mostly historically grown 'communication islands' with inconsistent patient-related/medical information representation (Norgall, 2004). They are linked together using (proprietary) one-to-one data conversion. However, the increasing availability of interoperability standards is enabling and driving an ongoing process of transition. Health information integration (e-health) aims at transparency not only among all information systems within one (hospital) enterprise, but between all healthcare-related processes and stakeholders.

Interoperability between medical devices and host systems is a key requirement for the establishment of electronic patient health records. A prerequisite for interoperability is the standardization of message formats and of messaging protocols. Interoperability verification tools are important for the development as well as the compliance testing of SCP-formatted ECG records. They are necessary to promote the interoperability of important non-invasively gathered cardiac function information. This information is increasingly to be integrated into electronic patient health records and to be interchanged between the various healthcare providers.

A comparison of SCP records from different devices of different manufacturers revealed differences in the implementations that made these records not really interoperable. The presence of the manufacturer-specific section is provided for informative purposes, however some applications use this section as a backdoor for the storage of relevant diagnostic data in a manufacturer-specific format. Such a record, despite its formal conformance to the SCP standard, is considerably affected if not inutile at all in terms of interoperability. To identify which of the records resembles the SCP specifications, compliance testing is necessary (Zywietz, 2003). Essentially the compliance tests must cover the following tests:

- the content of the SCP record,
- the format and structure of the SCP record, and
- the messaging mechanisms if records are communicated according to SCP specifications.

There is an interdependence between content and format verification. Because of this interdependence, integrated testing is advisable. Moreover, due to technological progress, the original messaging mechanisms have been changed since 1993 when the SCP-ECG standard was proposed.

The purpose of the content test is to present the content to all parts of an SCP file. The test starts with basic plausibility checks. After reading the input data record, the BIOSIGNA (Fischer & Zywietz, 2004) program verifies the consistency of record length and the length information, and whether the first section is the SCP pointer section.

Subsequently, the validation concerns the content of the SCP pointer section, for example, the section ID, length, and index for each present section in a table. The second part of the content table depicts the content of the SCP section ID headers of all present sections. Comparing the entries for lengths and section identifications of the two tables already allows a visual plausibility check.

Then the content of the other detected sections is verified. The content of these sections depends very much on the format of each specific section. For each section a plausibility check on pointer and length information is to be performed. The information in the output text file is used for the verification and validation of the SCP compression/ decompression and formatting software.

The Open ECG Project

The Open ECG project, a European-funded initiative with global reach, aims to lower the barriers for the seamless integration of ECG devices in e-health services and electronic health record systems (Chronaki, 2004). The Open ECG noted the lack of awareness among the stakeholders, and the absence of consistent and validated implementations for related ECG standards such as the European EN1064 (SCP-ECG). Promoting ECG interoperability standards has been a continuous effort to raise community awareness regarding the key role of standards in achieving plug-and-play ECG device connectivity. So far, the Open ECG portal, online services, and the helpdesk, but also workshops, articles, leaflets, conference participation, and discussions with vendors and users, have contributed to associating Open ECG with a quality trademark.

To consolidate the expertise and interoperability efforts worldwide, Open ECG provides the Web portal collecting data on related projects, together with tools, converters, specifications, and ECG data sets. The open source repository provides best practice in implementation, offering to members an ECG library and tools developed by the community and as part of the Open ECG programming contest (Conforti, Micalizzi, & Macerata, 2004). The Open ECG Industrial Advisory Board—representing associations, national health boards, and the ECG industry, together with the Open ECG community (close to 200 members in March 2004)—provides input on global trends and developments.

The Open ECG helpdesk, a third line of activity, provides information and assistance to developers and integrators. Finally, the Open ECG conformance testing service addresses ECG records and electrocardiographs. ECG record files acquired with different electrocardiographs can be tested online, while successfully tested ECG devices receive an Open ECG interoperability validation certificate.

A common opinion in the Open ECG consortium is that lack of free tools for standard data format handling is one of the main limits to the deployment of standards focused on ECG interoperability. In order to cope with this problem, the consortium decided to adopt and promote, even beyond the project partners, an "open source/free software" strategy for software development and use. Consequently, the consortium decided to create a software repository site that includes Open Source code, and open library software tools intended to be distributed among Open ECG members under a free-software license. This approach provides at least the following advantages:

- a higher degree of independence from the software supply companies,
- absolute warranty of data format accessibility,
- transparency of data-handling procedures, and
- promotion of standards.

The Open ECG consortium disseminates different free tools to encourage and support the use of standards in cardiology. They are accessible through the Web page members' area in two main categories: tools and databases.

In the section "Tools & Converters," different tools are available:

- *SCP to DICOM Converter*—This tool is provided as a Web service and allows any member to submit an SCP-ECG record (version 1.0 or 1.3) for its conversion to DICOM waveform supplement 30 format. The converted file can be immediately viewed through access to a freely available DICOM viewer.

- *SCP-ECG Record Parsing by E-Mail*—This tool is provided as an e-mail service. It is mainly targeted to doctors. Any doctor can submit an SCP-ECG record as an attachment to an e-mail with a specific subject. This record will be automatically parsed, and a graphical and textual report will be sent back to the sender.
- *Link to Useful Tools Available on the Web*—Here there are links to Web sites where are available several tools for different purposes including XML FDA viewers.

There are two sections dedicated to ECG samples:

1. "SCP-ECG Databases" (dedicated to ECG samples in presumed SCP format), and
2. "Other Relevant ECG Formats" (dedicated to other formats like FDA/HL7 Annotated ECG and MFER).

In these sections are information and real samples with some linked comments for the SCP-ECG database to indicate the eventual parts not compliant with the standard.

All the activities of the Open ECG project were dedicated to the interoperability in resting ECGs. In the waveform world this is a very little subset of all the possible clinical examinations, even if quite common and of high volume. The roadmap towards a DICOM-like solution is still very far away, even if significant and helpful steps were accomplished by the Open ECG project. Also for different kinds of medical examinations, where interoperability is an important issue, similar portals would be very helpful.

Unfortunately, in many fields standards do not exist yet (stress ECG, Holter, etc.), thus a speed up of the standardization process would be very welcome for these methods.

In June 2008, OpenECG has more 1000 members (actually 1007 as of June 30, 2008)) and the helpdesk is responding regularly to questions related to the implementation of the SCP-ECG standard (8 in the beginning of 2008).

Supported by the OpenECG community, SCP-ECG has been accepted as a European standard (EN1064:2007). Moreover, the SCP-ECG nomenclature has been aligned to that of IEEE1173, and is currently a Final Draft International Standard (FDIS) in the IEEE 1173 family of standards, and is expected to be promoted to an ISO standard before the end of 2008.

REFERENCES

Akselrod, S., Norymberg, M., Peled, I. et al. (1987). Computerized analysis of ST segment changes in ambulatory electrocardiograms. *Medical and Biological Engineering and Computing, 25,* 513-519.

Armstrong, W. F., & Morris, S. N. (1983). The ST segment during ambulatory electrocardiographic monitoring. *Annals of Internal Medicine, 98,* 249-250.

Badilini, F., Zareba, W., Titlebaum, E. L., & Moss, A. J. (1986). Analysis of ST segment variability in Holter recordings. In A. Moss & S. Stern (Eds.), *Noninvasive electrocardiology—clinical aspects of Holter monitoring.* London: Saunders Co.

Bowman, B. R., & Schuck, E. (2000). Medical instruments and devices used in the home. In J. D. Bronzino (Ed.), *The biomedical engineering handbook.* Boca Raton, FL: CRC Press.

Chronaki, C. E. (2004). Open ECG: Goals and achievements. *Proceedings of the 2nd Open ECG Workshop* (pp. 3-4), Berlin.

Cohen, D., Edelsack, E. A., & Zimmerman, J. E. (1970). Magnetocardiograms taken inside a shielded room with a superconducting point-contact magnetometer. *Applied Physics Letters, 16,* 278-280.

Conforti, F., Micalizzi, M., & Macerata, A. (2004). Collection and development of open tools for ECG interoperability. *Proceedings of the 2nd OpenECG Workshop* (pp. 13-14), Berlin.

Dolin, R. H., Alschuler, L., Boyer, S., & Beebe, C. (2004). *HL7 clinical document architecture. Release 2.0.* HL7 Health Level Seven, Inc., Ann Arbor, MI. Available online at: www.hl7.org (accessed in November 2008)

Fenici, R., Brisinda, D., & Meloni, A. M. (2005). Clinical applications of magneticardiography. *Expert Review of Molecular Diagnostics, 5,* 291-313.

Fischer, R., & Zywietz, C. (2001). *How to implement SCP.* Retrieved from http://www.openecg.net

Fischer, R., & Zywietz, C. (2004). Integrated content and format checking for processing of SCP ECG records. *Proceedings of the 2nd OpenECG Workshop* (pp. 11-12), Berlin.

Hart, G. (1991). Biomagnetometry: Imaging the heart's magnetic field. *British Heart Journal, 65,* 61-62.

Hirai, M., & Kawamoto, K. (2004). MFER—a Japanese approach for medical wave form encoding rules for viewer design. *Proceedings of the 2nd OpenECG Workshop* (pp. 35-37), Berlin.

Kandori, A., Hosono, T., Kanagawa, T., Miyashita, S., Chiba, Y., Murakami, M. et al. (2002). Detection of atrial-flutter and atrial-fibrillation waveforms by fetal magnetocardiogram. *Medical and Biological Engineering and Computing, 40,* 213-217.

Mori, H., & Nakaya, Y. (1988). Present status of clinical magnetocardiography. *Cardiovascular World Report* 1, 78-86

Moss, A. J. (1986). Clinical utility of ST segment monitoring In A. Moss & S. Stern (Eds.), *Noninvasive electrocardiology—clinical aspects of Holter monitoring.* London: Saunders Co.

NEMA (National Electrical Manufacturers Association). (2007a). *DICOM strategic document* (version 7.2). Retrieved from http://dicom.nema.org

NEMA. (2007b). *Digital imaging and communications in medicine (DICOM).* Rosslyn, VA: Author.

Nomura, M., Nakaya, Y., Saito, K., Kishi, F., Watatsuki, T., Miyoshi, H. et al. (1994). Noninvasive localisation of accessory pathways by magnetocardiographic imaging. *Clinical Cardiology, 17,* 239-244.

Norgall, T. (2004). ECG data interchange formats and protocols—status and outlook. *Proceedings of the 2nd OpenECG Workshop* (pp. 25-26), Berlin.

Prineas, R., Crow, R., & Blackburn, H. (1982). *The Minnesota code manual of electrocardiographic findings.* Littleton, MA: John Wright-PSG.

Pryor, T. A. (2000). Hospital information systems: Their function and state. In J. D. Bronzino (Ed.), *The biomedical engineering handbook.* Boca Raton, FL: CRC Press.

Quartero, H. W. P., Stinstra, J. G., Golbach, E. G. M., Meijboom, E. J., & Peters, M. J. (2002). Clinical implications of fetal magnetocardiography. *Ultrasound in Obstetrics and Gynecology, 20,* 142-153.

Smith, F. E., Langley, P., van Leeuwen, P. et al. (2006). Comparison of magnetocardiography and electrocardiography: A study of automatic measurement of dispersion of ventricular repolarization. *Europace, 8,* 887-893.

Van Bemmel, J. H., & Willems, J. L. (1990). Standardization and validation of medical support-systems: The CSE project. *Methods of Information in Medicine , 29* (special issue), 261-262.

Van Leeuwen, P., Hailer, B., Bader, W., Geissler, J., Trowitzsch, E., & Groenemeyer, D. H. (1999). Magnetocardiography in the diagnosis of foetal arrhythmia. *British Journal of Obstetrics and Gynaecology, 106,* 1200-1208.

Van Leeuwen, P., Lange, S., Klein, A., Geue, D., & Gronemeyer, D. H. (2004). Dependency of magnetocardiographically determined fetal cardiac time intervals on gestational age, gender and postnatal biometrics in healthy pregnancies. *BMC Pregnancy Childbirth, 4,* 6.

Wakai, R. T., Strasburger, J. F., Li, Z., Deal, B. J., & Gotteiner, N. L. (2003). Magnetocardiographic rhythm patterns at initiation and termination of fetal supraventricular tachycardia. *Circulation, 107,* 307-312.

Willems, J. L. (1991). *SCP-ECG project manager. Standard communications protocol for computerized electrocardiography. Final specifications and recommendations.* Final Deliverable AIM Project #A1015. Leuven, Belgium: ACCO.

Willems, J. L., Arnaud, P., van Bemmel, J. H. et al. (1985). Assessment of the performance of electrocardiographic computer programs with the use of a reference database. *Circulation, 71,* 523-534.

Willems, J. L., Arnaud, P., van Bemmel, J. H. et al. (1987). A reference database for multilead electrocardiographic computer measurement programs. *Journal of the American College of Cardiology, 6,* 1313-1321.

Zimmerman, J. E., Theine, P., & Harding, J. T. (1970). Design and operation of stable rf-biased superconducting point-contact quantum devices, etc. *Journal of Applied Physics, 41,* 1572-1580.

Zywietz, C., Joseph, G., & Degani, R. (1990). Data compression for computerized electrocardiography. In J. L. Willems (Ed.), *Digital ECG data communication, encoding and storage.* Proceedings of the 1st Working Conference of the SCP-ECG Project (pp. 95-136). Leuven, Belgium: ACCO.

Zywietz, C. (2003). *OpenECG certification and conformance testing process.* Retrieved from http://www.openecg.net

ONLINE REFERENCES

http://medical.nema.org

http://www.centc251.org

http://www.hl7.org

http://www.ieee1073.org

http://www.iso.ch/tc215

Chapter V
General Idea of the Proposed System

After an introduction and three chapters highlighting the present state of the art in computerized electrocardiography (Chapter II), methodological issues of medical and technical nature (Chapter III), and electronic management of medical data storage and exchange (Chapter IV), this chapter is a midway summary. This book might end here if it were a review of present achievements of tele-medical solutions in cardiology.

Fortunately, we are not only witness to the progress, but are also involved in the development of ubiquitous cardiology, so we want to share our ideas, realizations, and results of the research. The review made in previous chapters was not intended to cover the whole domain of computerized cardiology and it does not fulfill such a role. The presentation was done subjectively with a purpose of making foundations for our proposal of an intelligent tele-medical system whose several prototypes were conceived during the last few years. Being bioengineers in our hearts, we are particularly involved in observing nature in its systematic solutions and considering the medical, technical, and sociological observations based on bio-cybernetics.

Having in mind the main goal of technological support for medicine and not challenging current achievements, we observe a significant discrepancy between human and computer ways of "thinking." The example is the development methodology for ECG interpretive software. The outcome of the software under test is compared with the cardiologist outcome, and if the convergence is stated for a limited learning set, it is commonly assumed that the result will be of the same quality for any unknown input signal. Our approach would prefer the software that closely mimics the cardiologists' reasoning. Nevertheless, this cognitive process is hard to extract and is influenced by the standardization of medical procedures. This is in turn driven by the algorithmic approaches close to contemporary computer programs. The first novelty of our proposal, probably hardly accepted, is that we propose the collaboration with doctors not only as advisory experts but also as subjects of our experiments. We hope to be well understood: similarly to the doctor not relying only on the interview and ordering additional examinations, we assume that nobody is able to formulate his or her way of reasoning objectively, and we use various methods of human behavior assessment to discover principles of the data processing during the visual interpretation of the ECG by an expert.

Another novelty of our approach is the use of agile software in the interpretation process. The software may be freely customized by the supervising process in order to provide optimal diagnostic descriptions of the patient. Current systems all use rigid software. Once programmed by the manufacturer, the executable code is only read from the memory and the interpretation flow is the same disregarding sex or race; the only factor sometimes considered is the age of the patient. Consequently, the interpretation process issues many diagnostic parameters not relevant for a particular patient, in order to minimize the risk of missing data. The agile software follows the patient, 'gets accustomed' to his or her features, and is aware of the signs of diseases he or she is suspected of.

The third novelty that should be mentioned is the measurement and use of various relevance coefficients of particular diagnostic parameters. It seems to be obvious and particularly dependent on patient status that some sections of the recorded signals and some variables in the diagnostic outcomes are more important than others. According to our knowledge there is no method to measure and quantify optimal patient description and even doctors' preferences reported previously in the literature.

The technical feasibility of that idea is proven in the chapters that follow. However, its implementation in a wide-sense clinical or home care practice is not very easy because we reveal some unexploited areas that require research. Therefore this chapter ends with suggestions on possible medical investigation areas whose result would be welcomed in development of artificial intelligence-based applications for medicine.

GENERAL OVERVIEW OF THE UBIQUITOUS CARDIOLOGY SYSTEM SCOPE AND STRUCTURE

The tele-medical system providing ubiquitous cardiac surveillance is the scope of research and prototyping in several scientific centers around the world. The subject is worth such attention because of the number of cardiac-impaired people, the sudden course of cardiac events, and the prospective participation of virtually every person in a cardiac prevention program.

According to its name, the ubiquitous cardiology system (UCS) is expected to be accessible without territorial limitations for mobile customers or patients. Therefore, the client terminal (patient electronic device, PED, see Chapter I) must be manufactured as a mobile device, preferably lightweight and small in size. Such a device would not be capable of accumulating the records of all parameters and references, therefore it has to cooperate with a management computer. This station does not have to be mobile, therefore its preferred implementation is on a workstation with a multi-threading operating system. The basic cell of the UCS consists of the supervising server and several client-side remote recorders connected accord-

Figure 5.1. Layered block diagram of the proposed ubiquitous cardiology system

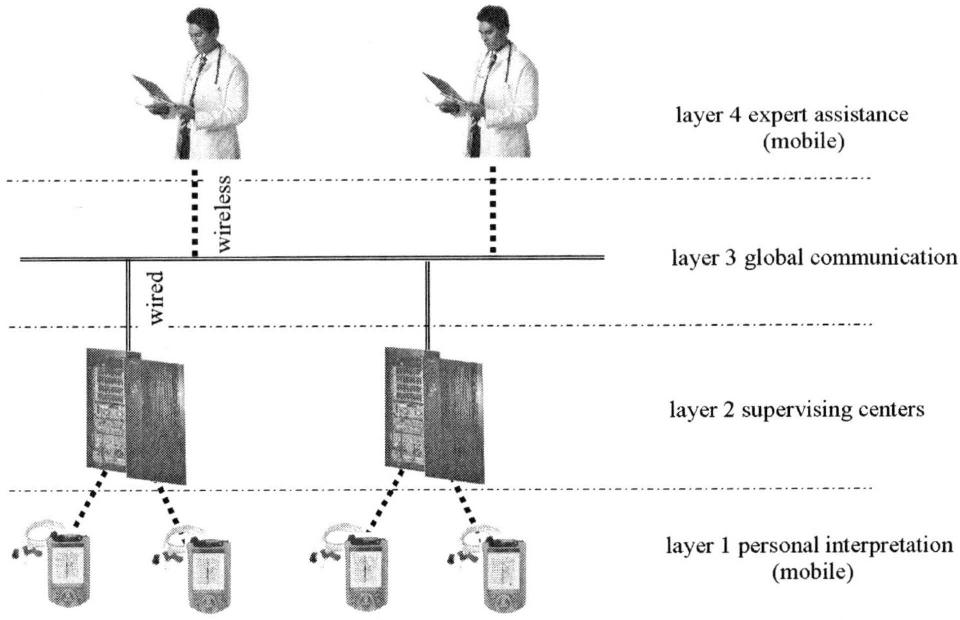

ing to the star topology. The connection may use a wired infrastructure, however the last section must be wireless in order to allow for mobility. The connection is bi-directional, unlike in the prevalence of today's solutions, which assumes that data is transmitted only from the patient to the doctor. The software of a remote recorder contains not only communication, human-interaction, and data acquisition modules, but also basic interpretive procedures (fig. 5.1, layer one, see Chapter I). Unlike in the case of rigid software, the interpretation-oriented procedures are downloadable and commutable within limits of predefined rules. All threads in the supervising center run the same software package (layer two, see Chapter I), including the extended interpretive procedure, data-quality examination process, and remote interpretation supervising module.

The supervising center may be considered as an analogy of the healthcare provider. By default the supervising ends with a fully automated conclusion. In case of any doubts, a human expert on duty is alerted about possible abnormalities (layer three, see Chapter I). The expert may also be mobile, however his access to the network should support higher dataflow in order to transmit images without delay.

Central servers of territorially neighboring nodes of surveillance network are interconnected between them in order to transfer patients (like roaming service in mobile voice communication). They are also connected to the optional servers providing subscriber services of interpretation for unusual or specific cases. The concept of such a service is presented in detail in Chapter VIII. Thanks to the connections of the management center (layer four, see Chapter I), the patient or client does not have to rely on an automatically computed diagnosis and may also freely subscribe to a particular human cardiologist as a first-contact doctor, although contacted virtually. With these measures, our proposal of the UCS fulfills another principal requisite of the home care: it simulates the continuous presence of a human medical expert without limiting patient or customer mobility. Probably you never expect to have the best specialists of the world around you wherever you go!

Thanks to its easy adaptation, the surveillance system follows patient needs and a variety of diagnostic goals. It may be remotely reprogrammed by the server or by the supervising doctor in a wide range of functional features and without the necessity of the physical presence of the patient and doctor in the same place and at the same time. The commutation of the remote software may be performed often—up to 100,000 times—a practical limitation is the flash memory wear. Therefore, 30 different measurements and interpretation protocols may be carried out daily and the re-programming limit will be achieved in approximately 10 years. The agile software opens up a very attractive opportunity to use the same remote device in a personal cardiac prevention program. The promotion of a healthy lifestyle is usually driven by fashion. Like other fashions, the introduction of regular control of principal vital signs needs a considerable amount of money. However, we are convinced that governmental and insurance agencies are likely to invest significant funds in making a small wearable device a part of our everyday life and profit from longer lives due to suppression of occurrence of cardiovascular diseases. The control of our lifestyle based on physiological phenomena may include heart rate, breathing rate, and body motion. These three easily measured parameters are sufficient for a pertinent, medically justified interaction with a subject. This interaction does not refer to the medical knowledge; it consists of textual or voice messages, for example about dangerous physical effort, lack of physical effort, and so forth.

Extension of this idea is an interaction-based pharmacological treatment in home care. The amount of drug is usually prescribed by a doctor with consideration of the expected effect, estimated from the clinical tests. For the reduction of uncertainty, the dose is usually overestimated, unless the doctor has the opportunity to supervise the patient in the hospital and to set the optimal dose interactively with the use of laboratory analyses or other means of therapy validation. Unfortunately, the therapeutic effect is proportional to the necessary dose, while the side effects are proportional to the dose actually taken. Several drugs manifest their effects directly in vital signs, whereas some other pharmacological effects manifest themselves chemically, but these are measurable with the use of transducers in an electrical way. All these patients may be controlled in their homes by a wireless surveillance system issuing a message about the proper dose and when the drug should be taken. For the benefit of elderly people in particular, the interaction may be performed using a full automatic mode by time-optimal delivery of the correct pill by the remotely controlled drug dispenser.

The process of the ECG interpretation is described hereafter as limited to the cooperation of the PED with corresponding thread in the USC server. This cooperation is also based on observations of human relations in cardiology. Rare are cases when two cardiologists perform the same tasks simultaneously. More likely they will share their tasks according to their competences. Similarly, in the proposed system the interpretation process is considered as distributed between the PED and UCS server. The task sharing is asymmetrical, thus the process is always initiated by the PED and continued where possible, and the UCS server takes its execution when necessary and continues to its end. The PED process may be suspended in theory at any stage when its requirements exceed allotted resources and are transferred to the complementary interpretation thread run by the server. In practice, we had to limit possible task transfer points to seven, which demonstrates their feasibility and benefits, while not limiting other approaches.

Another important observation comes from the statistical studies concerning the usage frequency of each particular procedure in the regular ECG interpretation software. Regular cases are the large majority of records, and these signals are easy to interpret. Furthermore, the volume of diagnostic results is very low.

The remaining cases are much more difficult in both medical and computational aspects. It would be unrealistic to expect a reliable analysis of such records in a wearable battery-operated PED. Moreover, for these cases the data reduction ratio is much lower due to several diagnostic parameters important in a description of an ill patient. Finally, these records are more susceptible to errors when interpreted automatically, which increases the necessity of support from a human expert. Consequently, we assumed only primary diagnostic procedures are implemented by default in the PED interpretation software.

REMARKS ABOUT SYSTEM REALIZATION

The cardiac surveillance system for ubiquitous cardiology assumes the optimization of ECG signal interpretation justified on both medical and technical backgrounds. Consequently, with a response to the changes in these aspects, the management software is supposed to continuously revise the interpretation task assignment between the remote PED and the central server. The important criteria for this optimization are:

- the quality and content of patient description,
- the lowest possible datastream transferred through the wireless channel, and
- the lowest possible power consumption by the battery-operated wearable remote recorder.

Contrary to the rigid software, the agile implementation of the interpretation process is able to be adjusted to a specific diagnostic goal. This goal is expressed by the expected optimal patient description, which for every possible patient state takes the form of a list of mandatory, desirable, and optional diagnostic parameters with the attributes of priority, tolerance of value, and validity time. Standard network analysis parameters are selected as a description of the wireless connection use and the transmission quality. Monitoring the connection is necessary to keep the data flow at a reasonably low level, since transmission costs are the primary component of the maintenance expense; thus exceeding some limits will make the ubiquitous cardiology unacceptable for a considerable amount of people. The use of remote recorder resources (CPU, memory, battery, software content, etc.) is also subject to reporting aimed at keeping the management procedure informed about the current capability and reserves of the remote device. The correct estimation of the available resources is a mandatory component of the optimization of the remote ECG interpretation process. Our experiments show that a considerable amount of serious management errors originated from the incorrect estimation of the capacity reserve.

The remote recorder is a programmable device. In the course of our experiments, we try to use a currently available hardware that physically resembles the target product. For scientific purposes, however, the device should be a general-purpose computer with embedded peripherals of external input at least for:

- connections with the ECG acquisition module,
- connections to a bi-directional wireless digital data channel,
- solid or expandable memory sufficient for storage of several minutes of cardiac signal, and
- user interface (graphical communication port).

In our experiments we used personal digital assistant (PDA) class computers (HP Jornada, Assus-565), however we also considered extended mobile telephone sets (Nokia 9500, Nokia N71, and Greenphone). Unfortunately, a frequent obstacle was the lack of reliable documentation. Many of these devices contain peripherals suitable for our task, but the description was rarely detailed enough to create custom applications required to support the desired functions. For the widest range of research, an optimal solution was a development kit for the mobile microprocessor (PXC270), the same as is used in Asus-565. This well-documented testbed equipped with a rich peripherals set complies with all of our assumptions except for the physical size.

The other issue concerning portable computers is the serious limitation of program memory repetitively rewritiable on the run. In the first simulations, we had to load all the procedures to the program memory and switch them on and off by a set of software flags.

The PDA in our figures is often presented as it was displayed on an ECG trace. Such design represents the idea that the device is entirely consecrated to the ECG monitoring task and does not function as a patients' general-purpose PDA. In fact, we never displayed the trace on the PDA screen because of its low quality and also because it is not interesting and may be confusing to the patient. We use the screen of a portable device mainly to communicate with the patient (text messages, menus, icons, etc.).

Initially, it was our intention to integrate all the modules into one case. Unfortunately without having consecrated much more time to the issues of electromagnetic compatibility, we found it reasonable to postpone the realization of this idea to the prototyping phase. The achievement of acceptable ECG record quality needed the radio frequency interferences to be eliminated. Therefore, we decided to separate the ECG amplifiers and converters and the remaining part of the device. This raised another problem that had to be solved: the digital connection between two patient devices. For the reason of physical independence and the galvanic separation of medical and non-medical devices, Bluetooth communication was selected as optimal for short-distance digital ECG transfer.

One of the primary advantages of the proposed UCS is that it uses only existing technology:

- automatic interpretation of the ECG signal,
- dynamically linked libraries and software modification under run (agile software),
- flash memory-based re-programmable hardware structure of the remote device,
- bi-directional data transmission in a global range, and
- multi-threading supported by any workstation using a UNIX-compatible operation system.

Despite the technological feasibility, there is much to be done towards the clinical stage of prototypes. These points are listed in the next section.

SCIENTIFIC RESEARCH AREAS NECESSARY FOR THE REALIZATION OF THE PROPOSED SYSTEM

A big challenge now faces cardiologists. In a classic metrology, the terms systematic error, measurement error, method uncertainty, and data validity time are well defined. The diagnostic parameters issued by humans and current electronic medical equipment do not have such data reliability attributes. Scanning through the data storage and transmission standards (like HL7, see Chapter IV), we hardly found any data field accepting uncertainty measures. Medical science seems not to be accustomed to dealing with limited-reliability data, however this is not true, taking into account the extreme care taken in introducing new methods manifested by the extensive use of statistical tests.

One of the principal concepts introduced in our research is the notion of optimal patient description as it affects the estimation of quality of current diagnostic outcomes. In order to yield a global estimate of diagnosis quality, the values of the difference between measured diagnostic parameters and corresponding references are processed in the context of priority, tolerance, and validity time attributes. As a consequence of the excess of the tolerance margin in the differences between important data, the domain-oriented request is issued for a modification in the corresponding part of the remote recorder software. The data quality and uncertainty factors are thus fundamental for the management of agile software composition and functionality.

Although the prototype was built for the purpose of our limited-scale investigations, the clinical use of the auto-adaptive system should be preceded by a huge research project involving experts from the whole world, aimed at a medically justified consensus with regard to the following new aspects of diagnostic processing and medical data.

- We observe the diagnostic process as an alternate information pursuit and analysis. It is evident that the choice of a subsequent diagnostic step is determined by the precedented result. The tree of the most probable diagnostic sequence in the context of patient status will be of primary importance for the optimization of the automated diagnosis.
- The human expert, depending on previously gathered information and current results, focuses his attention on some diagnostic parameters and neglects others. The parameter hierarchy and relevance coefficients are also important rules for the automated interpretation system to follow.
- When gazing at the ECG printout, the human expert prefers some signal sections over others, which in medical images is known as a "zone of interest." The electrocardiogram provides a set of reliable fiducial points, which can be determined automatically and correlated with the phases of heart evolution. The correlation of such zones in the signal strip in the context of patient disease will be pertinent for the "perceptually lossless" method of ECG compression. This idea follows MP3 perceptual audio coding based on studies of hearing.
- All diagnostic parameters are currently updated at the same moment and are recorded as time series of equal sampling frequency. However, from simple observation and statistics, we know that the variability significantly differs from one parameter to the other. It will therefore be important to attribute each diagnostic data with a validity time, meaning the longest period in which the value should be updated in order to maintain continuity. The other issue is to reveal the very probable dependency of the parameter validity time on patient status.

The postulated areas of medical research will provide opportunities to optimize the diagnostic parameter datastream as an individually selected, irregularly sampled time series and considerably reduce the data volume without significantly affecting the quality of patient description.

These research areas have been put forth at various medical conferences since 2005 in the context of our prototype of an auto-adaptive system as a part of the ubiquitous cardiology concept.

Generally speaking, if computers are rarely used in doctors' offices, it is mainly because of the strange manner of operation they require. The perspective of human-alike, adaptive computers seems to be very attractive, however further investigations of human behavior is needed, along with a systematic, formal description of human reasoning.

Chapter VI
Investigations about the Distributions of Important Information in ECG Signals

This chapter presents an investigation of the distribution of medically relevant information in ECG signal timelines. ECG records clearly represent a cycle of heart evolution; its components, although partly superimposed, follow the time-related dependencies of heart function. During the initial inspection of the ECG, the cardiologist focuses his or her attention on several points of the trace, seeking signs of disease. It seems obvious, but is not often considered, that some segments of the signal are more important for a doctor than the remaining parts. Depending on a doctor's habits and experience, the interpretation starts from the most severe or most suspected abnormality or from the most unusual signal component. The order of the ECG inspection is based on the investigation strategy and is determined by irregular distribution of medical information in the ECG. These assumptions have already been explored with regard to speech or audio signals, resulting in numerous successful applications, such as the MP3 compression algorithm.

Three alternative approaches to the investigation of standard medical information distribution in ECG signals are presented in detail. The first approach is the local spectrum of the signal as a common 'technical' strategy to the temporal data-stream variability. This approach is simplified as much as possible, thus it defines the statistically expected bandwidth neglecting medical aspects of the heart cycle. Several methods, including Short Term Fourier Transform and wavelets, were used to estimate the local spectrum of the ECG. The literature review and original authors' research results are presented in this chapter with highlights of their advantages and drawbacks.

The second approach to the ECG data-stream assessment is output oriented and based on ECG diagnostic parameters. The parameters set is weighted according to parameters importance, and the resulting measure is used to correlate the diagnostic result deviation with the frequency and occurrence time of local bandwidth reduction. The main advantage of such an approach is the assessment of instantaneous transmission channel requirements, based on the measurements of the accuracy of diagnostic parameters that are derived automatically. Therefore, all differences resulting from bandwidth limitation are not expressed as a signal distortion (e.g., PRD), but directly as a deviation of diagnostic parameters.

Finally, the conceptual approach to the informative contents of the ECG signal assumes an analysis of observer gaze points during the manual inspection of the trace. The study yielded several general rules on how the cardiology expert perceives the electrocardiogram and revealed important steps in human reasoning. The results of this research are used to estimate the ECG signal features from on a background of medical findings and measurements of the waveforms. This approach is the one-dimensional analogy to the 'region of interest' commonly used to define special areas in images.

INVESTIGATION OF THE LOCAL SPECTRUM

Introductory Remarks

In the storage and transmission of an electrocardiographic signal (and for other sequences of samples), a full informative capacity (bandwidth) transmitting channel is usually used (Bailey et al., 1990). However, in the case of the ECG, the occurrence of particular signal components is limited by the physiology of intra-cardiac stimulus propagation. Additionally, the phases of a cardiac cycle are defined by cellular actions in tissues of different conduction speed, limiting their own variability and consequently the local bandwidth of the representing signal (Macfarlane & Lawrie, 1989). Moreover, the automatic recognition of the heart cycle phases, developed 40 years ago for medical purposes, is commonly used as a P, QRS, and T wave delimitation algorithm and nowadays yields results of acceptable reliability (Willems et al., 1985a, 1985b, 1987). These facts suggest that the electrocardiogram is a far more predictable signal than speech or audio signals, even in the case of pathologies. Therefore, the use of typical ECG pre-processing strategies (i.e., automatic wave recognition procedures) seems to be appropriate as background for the correct adaptation of the transmission channel instantaneous bandwidth to the local density of information. The first issue is to determine statistically the typical bandwidth or density of information and its variance for all ECG components. Different wave morphologies, for the QRS-complex in particular, should be considered. The work presented in this section is aimed at determining the indispensable minimum of parameters that the pre-processor should deliver for optimum bandwidth adjustment for the transmission or storage of records. The adjustment method is not taken under consideration here because it is constrained by technical aspects of implementation.

The Experimental Setup

A well-known source of annotated ECG beats of different morphology is the CSE-Multilead Database (Willems, 1990) (sampling parameters: 500 Hz, 16 bit), which provides the exact start- and endpoints of the P, QRS, and T waves. Knowing these points for each signal allows retrieval of their closest references in the time-frequency (t-f) representation of an ECG.

The differences in ECG waves lengths must be suppressed by the means of the time-normalized inter-signal averaging. Corresponding sections of all ECG records were expanded or contacted in order to fit a standard number of samples. For this purpose, having wave borders as signal section delimiters, we first calculated the average target sample count for each wave type and took the nearest integer value of the form 2^k for the convenient usage of wavelet transforms. A cubic spline interpolation technique was next used to calculate the waves representation of each signal with regard to their target length. The original ECG signal section of native length $N_j(\{n, v(n)\})$ was first interpolated (Aldroubi & Feichtinger, 1998) by a continuous cubic polynomial function:

$$S_i(x) = a_i + b_i(x - x_i) + c_i(x - x_i)^2 + d_i(x - x_i)^3 \tag{6.1}$$

$x \in [x_i, x_{i+1}]$, $i \in \{0, 1, ...n\text{-}1\}$ best fitted to the time series N_j.

The interpolation yielded a representation for each section by sampling the $S_i(x)$ at the desired time points m corresponding to target representation samples:

$$N'_j(m) = \sum_m S_i(x) \cdot \delta(x - mT) \tag{6.2}$$

These signals represent the electrocardiogram sections of the length unified through all signals for averaging and decomposition without further necessity of length adjustment (e.g., zero padding, etc.).

Two trials of time-scale decomposition were performed: one using a standard pyramidal decomposition (i.e., wavelets) and the second using an optimized tree decomposition (i.e., wavelet packets; Bradie, 1996).

Although many time-frequency transforms are widely known, for this particular task the transform is expected to meet the following criteria:

- the condition of losslessness, needed to control all signal properties in the t-f domain and guaranteeing that every change in the output signal results from the manipulations done in the t-f domain; and
- the use of filters with compact and relatively short support.

For the wavelet decomposition, we used a Mallat QMF-based wavelet (Mallat, 1989) that provides sufficient frequency-band separation and time accuracy, as well as the 5th order Daubechies (1992) wavelet transform. The use of 5th order filters is a compromise between the support length and frequency bands separation. The decomposition using the pyramid decimation scheme is executed down to level 3. That extracts three high-frequency octaves and the coarse approximation signal. The effective sampling frequency for the coarse approximation signal is equal to ⅛ of the original sampling frequency (64 Hz).

The wavelet-packet decomposition has adjustable resolution in both the time and frequency domains, as far as the surface of the time-frequency representation atom complies with the uncertainty rule. However, the flexibility of the decomposition tree increases computational complexity and requires the output data-stream to be completed by the tree structure description. Since the decomposition in the leaves consists of a few samples (four for P and QRS, and eight for T waves), the simple bi-orthogonal filter of order 1.1 was used for a better temporal resolution with regard to the cost of inferior band separation. The decomposition was performed for the first four levels and yielded 16 frequency bands. The temporal size of the atoms was 32 ms and the frequency band was 16 Hz, which defines the resolution grid for a time-frequency representation (Hilton, 1997).

To minimize the edge-effect distortion, all signals were prepared for the t-f transformation by subtracting a constant value and slope, and then standardized in length to a value of 2^k. The lengths were 32 ms (16 samples) for the baseline, 128 ms for the P and QRS waves, and 256 ms for the T waves. These values determine the lowest frequency band for each wave: 32 Hz for the baseline, 8 Hz for the P and QRS waves, and 4 Hz for the T wave. As suggested in the CSE comments (CSE Working Party, 1985), the true positions of the waves for a particular signal were assumed to be equal in all leads. The t-f representation for each wave was related to the baseline content of the same signal in the same lead in order to assess the significance of the particular t-f items. The baseline (i.e., the P-end to QRS-start section) is commonly considered as a representation of a non-cardiac electrical activity period and thus widely used as a reference. Due to the very short baseline (1...4 t-f samples depending on the frequency band), a simple threshold method was used for the assessment instead of a statistical non-parametric significance test (Tadeusiewicz, Izworski, & Majewski, 1993).

Signal Preprocessing

Assuming the extra-cardiac signal (noise or other phenomena) to be stationary and not correlated to the ECG, the average energy E and its variance δE were measured at the baseline for each frequency band (6.3). The t-f representation of every wave was thresholded with the t-f values (6.4) representing the noise level in all frequency bands and in all leads: I, II, III, aVR, aVL, aVF, V1, V2, V3, V4, V5, V6, X, Y, Z.

$$th_f = E_f + \delta E_f \tag{6.3}$$

$$S_{t,f} = \begin{cases} S_{t,f} & \text{when } S_{t,f} > th_f \\ 0 & \text{otherwise} \end{cases} \tag{6.4}$$

The thresholded t-f representations were then averaged through all leads available and normalized in energy in order to eliminate the influence of amplitude variations on the results of intra-signal averaging. That resulted in three sets of wave-specific normalized averaged thresholded t-f representations: NATTF-P, NATTF-QRS, and NATTF-T. All these representations were next averaged through all signals represented in the database, excluding the pacemaker stimulated waves and some signals of extremely low quality.

The effective count of the averaged t-f representations was: 99 for the P wave, 123 for the QRS-complex, and 103 for the T wave. For the QRS-complex, averaging of t-f representations was additionally made separately for the ventricular V (non-P wave) and the supra-ventricular SV morphology in order to maintain the differences in their t-f content.

The effective bandwidth of the ECG was initially set to 16 Hz (the lowest frequency represented on the baseline). It may be lower in some circumstances, but the use of the baseline as a reference is questionable in that case. For sections where P, QRS, and T waves were detected, the effective bandwidth was expanded to a value corresponding to 95% of the energy throughput. Temporal variability of that value inside the wave is referred to as 'instantaneous bandwidth'. At the application stage, depending on the adjustment method's properties, a compromise between time and frequency precision should be made. The instantaneous bandwidth is expressed in information density units and then is compared to the full bandwidth.

The comparison of the NATTF-QRS-V subset (11 elements) with the NATTF-QRS-SV subset (111 elements) was done with the use of the non-parametric Kolmogorow-Smirnoff significance test ($p < 0.05$). This comparison is expected to confirm or deny the application of a morphology detector in the pre-processing phase.

Results

The experiment yielded three kinds of results:

- the definition of the *electrocardiogram instantaneous bandwidth function* (EIBF) for an assumed tolerance for distortions;
- an estimation of the number of essential t-f samples carrying the ECG information found below the electrocardiogram instantaneous bandwidth function for an assumed value of tolerance for distortions, and an expected compression ratio for each decomposition type; and
- a comparison of the decompositions of two basic ECG morphologies (supraventricular and ventricular) as a background for the use of morphology detectors.

Figure 6.1 displays the EIBF for an average P-QRS-T segment representing the wavelet time-frequency plane, and Figure 6.2 indicates the EIBF for an average P-QRS-T segment representing the wavelet packet time-frequency plane.

Figure 6.1 presents the averaged NATTF-P, NATTF-QRS, and NATTF-T planes. The horizontal axis is time in sample numbers (sampling frequency equals 500 Hz), and the vertical axis is time in octave numbers: octave 1 corresponds to frequency band 125...250 Hz, octave 2: 62.5...125 Hz, and so on.

The average lengths of each ECG component are summarized in Table 6.1.

The black line in Figures 6.1 and 6.2 separates above it coefficients representing less than 5% of instantaneous energy and thus determines the instantaneous bandwidth of the signal. All samples on and above this line could be cancelled (set to zero or not transmitted) without disturbing the signal more than 5%. The assumed distortion level can be set to another value that directly influences the EIBF.

Estimated from a sufficient number of representative signals, the borderline between essential and non-essential atoms in time-frequency ECG representation may be considered as a source of *a priori* knowledge about the expected nature of the ECG. Therefore, we call it the *standard local bandwidth* (SLB) of the ECG. The main advantage of the wavelet-based local bandwidth function is its definition in

Figure 6.1. Normalized averaged thresholded time-frequency (NATTF) planes (wavelets) of the main components of the heart cycle along with multilead signals in time domain; black lines separate coefficients representing less than of 5% instantaneous energy

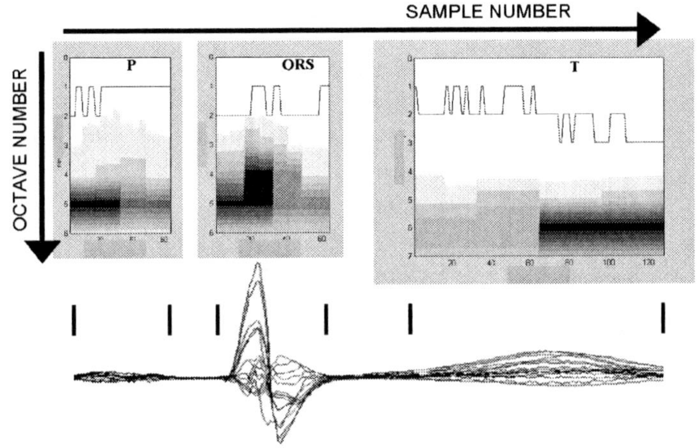

Figure 6.2. NATTF planes (wavelet packets) of main components of heart cycle along with multilead signals in time domain; black lines separate coefficients representing less than 5% of the instantaneous energy

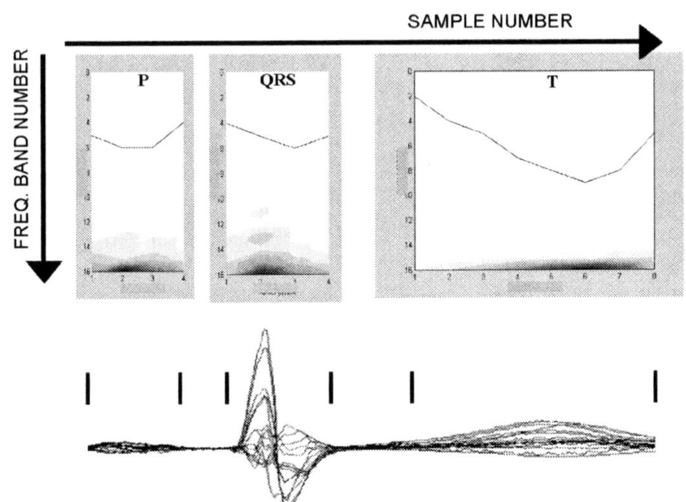

Table 6.1. Average lengths of ECG components (in samples, each representing 2 ms)

	RR	P	QRS	T
average	443.62	55.61	54.75	146.27
st. dev.	106.35	6.49	11.56	18.17
% of RR	100	12.5	12.3	24.0

Table 6.2. Wavelet decomposition, the number of essential samples for P, QRS, and T waves

samples	P	QRS	T	izoline	entire RR
original normalized	64	64	128	187	443
essential	29	20	26	11	86
% of original	45.3	31.3	20.3	5.8	19.4

Table 6.3. Wavelet packet decomposition, the number of essential samples for P, QRS, and T waves

samples	P	QRS	T	izoline	entire RR
original normalized	64	64	128	187	443
essential	35	36	64	11	146
% of original	54.7	56.3	50.0	5.8	33.0

the time-frequency domain, while the concurrent local susceptibility function (see Equation 6.3) is defined in time domain.

The averaged t-f plane allows us to calculate the number of samples that are essential to maintain the signal's properties. Similar t-f planes were computed for P and T waves and for QRS-SV and QSR-V morphologies separately (Figure 6.3). Table 6.2 summarizes the number of essential samples for each wave out of the cut-off level of 5%.

When comparing wavelet-based to wavelet packet-based $EIBF_{5\%}$, we stated that in the case of wavelet decomposition, thanks to exponential frequency scales, the number of time-frequency plane coefficients essential for the correct reconstruction of the signal is much lower. That results directly in higher compression ratios, of the order of 5 obtained with wavelets and only 3 with wavelet packets.

With regard to the question about the use of morphology detectors in local bandwidth estimations, we compared time-frequency signal representations averaged separately for supra-ventricular and ventricular heartbeats. Using the Kolmonogorov-Smirnoff non-parametric test, we put a zero hypothesis about significant differences between time-frequency coefficients in both groups. The result is a time-frequency plane of binary coefficients equaling zero (white on central t-f plane in Figure 6.3) whenever the hypothesis does not hold at a confidence level of 0.01%, and one (black on central t-f plane in Figure 6.3) when differences are found significant. Figure 6.3 displays the result of this comparison.

Discussion

A compression factor of 5 can easily be achieved when using the instantaneous bandwidth-based coding of an electrocardiogram. The length normalization of waves verifies on average their real lengths (P and QRS are overestimated and T is underestimated). The use of a non-parametric test showed no significant difference between corresponding samples of NATTF-QRS-V and NATTF-QRS-SV planes outside of the intersection of their bandwidths. That means that the use of morphology recognition algorithm does not improve the compression efficacy. The wavelength processing algorithm does not need to be very precise—the sample length at the second octave equals 8 ms.

The difference between two basic QRS morphologies does not justify the use of additional morphology detectors. This result is slightly surprising since the smooth-

Figure 6.3. Comparing average time frequency places for supra-ventricular (SV) and ventricular (V) QRS-morphologies

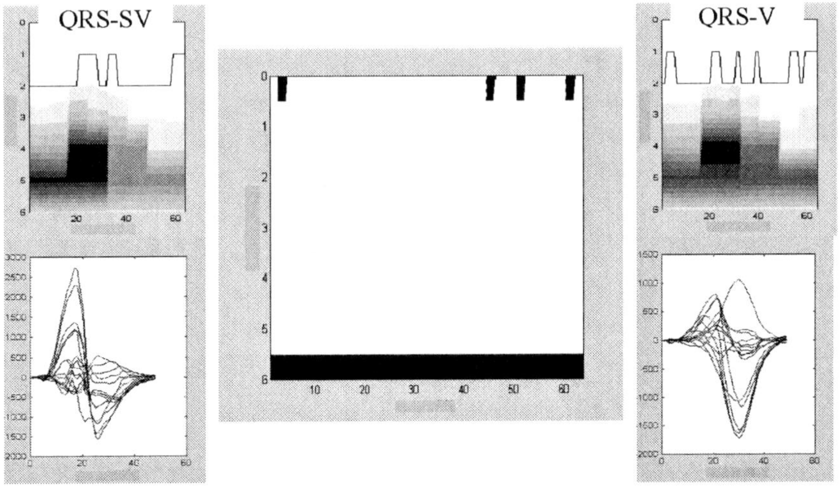

ness of the ventricular QRS wave is visually distinctive. Nevertheless, from the compression viewpoint, the ventricular QRS wave could be interesting because of its origin. Since the stimulus is triggered in ventricles, no atrial action is recorded. The lack of P waves allows up to 25 samples (out of total 443, see Table 6.2) to be discarded in order to increase the compression factor to the value of 7.25 in the case of wavelet decomposition.

The Application of the EIBF

The ECG signal recorded in unstable conditions (e.g., ambulatory or home care) suffers from the influence of extra-cardiac bioelectrical phenomena. Due to the simultaneous activity of adjacent muscles, this influence can hardly be avoided using technical means. Classical noise removal techniques assume noise stability, however this requirement is not fulfilled because in home care recordings the broadband noise contribution varies in energy. The need for an intelligent noise discrimination method comes from the common use of wearable devices and telemedicine. In these applications, the recorder is expected to yield a signal suitable for automated interpretation, even if it is operated by an untrained user.

The documented electrical inactivity of the heart during the slow conduction of the stimulus in the atrio-ventricular node is the foundation for the commonly performed measurement of the noise level in the PR section of the ECG (Nikolaev, Gotchev, Egiazarian, & Nikolov, 2001; Nikolaev & Gotchev, 1998, 2000; Nikolaev, Nikolov, Gotchev, & Egiazarian, 2000; Paul, Reddy, & Kumar, 2000). This requirement is met thanks to the central position of the AV Node close to the electrical center of the heart. Consequently, the baseline level is a widely recognized reference point in the electrocardiogram. Unfortunately, this approach has important limitations in real applications of ECG recordings: short durations of the baseline limiting the bandwidth and rare, irregular occurrences of the baseline.

The background activity, despite its unavoidable character, is limited by the laws of electro-physiology and thus predictable to a considerable extent. The main idea of our proposal is to discriminate the cardiac-originated components and the background electrophysiological signs into a time-frequency plane. The domain allows for the setting of a maximum number of noise measurement points, and only a few gaps must be filled using interpolation or extrapolation techniques in order to obtain a quasi-continuous noise model. Finally, the noise model is subtracted from the original signal, yielding rectified ECG records. This approach considers local variability of background activity, variability of the heart rate, and favors measured over estimated noise information (Augustyniak, 2003).

The heuristic function of the local bandwidth expected at the time point n is expressed by the discrete function $f(n)$:

$$f : \forall n \in \{0,1,...N\} \rightarrow f(n) \in [0;0.5) \quad (6.5)$$

representing the local relative cut-off frequency. This function, using $k_1 ...k_5 \in \{0, 1, ...N\}$ as the representation of the standard positions of wave borders, is projected to the local position of current heartbeat wave borders $h_1 ...h_5 \in \{0, 1, ...M\}$ for each point $i = 1...5$ (Figure 6.4):

$$\forall n \in [k_i, k_{i+1}], \forall m \in [h_i, h_{i+1}] \quad f'(m) = P^{S_i}(f(n)) \quad (6.6)$$

with a projection scale of S_i varying from section to section:

$$S_i = \frac{h_{i+1} - h_i}{k_{i+1} - k_i} \quad (6.7)$$

The time-frequency atoms of raw ECG representations are categorized as cardiac components only for scale j and time point m satisfying: $f'(m) > 2^{-j-1}$. Otherwise they are considered as extra-cardiac components (noise representations).

In separate octaves N_j, $j \in \{1...3\}$, noise measurement points are considered as non-uniformly sampled time series $N_j(\{n, v(n)\})$ and projected to the regular space (Aldroubi & Feichtinger, 1998) according to Equations 6.1 and 6.2 (Figure 6.5a): As the scale number increases, the contribution of cardiac representation grows. Below 32 Hz ($j > 3$), a reliable measurement of noise is never possible because the bandwidth is entirely occupied by the representation of cardiac activity. Instead of measurement, a noise extrapolation based on the first three scale coefficients is used to estimate the noise print in lower frequencies. This extrapolation uses sec-

Figure 6.4. (a) The example heartbeat (solid) and the adapted bandwidth variability function (dashed); (b) Corresponding time-frequency signal representations divided in the noise measurement region (above the local cut-off frequency) and the cardiac representation region (below)

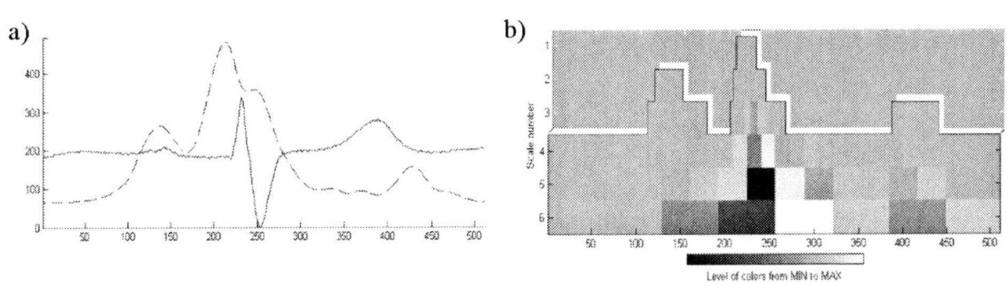

ond-order polynomials generated by all of the atoms of embedded trees originating from the considered coefficient. Therefore, the estimation of the noise level at a given time point k on scale j is based on the three average values $M_j(k, i)$ cumulating all the corresponding time-frequency atoms $s(n, i)$ on each of the first three scales (Figure 6.5b).

The time-frequency ECG background activity model contains partially measured and partially computed atoms of noise N' matching exactly the time-frequency plane of the raw signal. At this point, the time domain noise pattern may easily be recovered; however, with respect to noise discrimination, it is interesting to continue the calculations in the time-frequency domain. The values of time-frequency atoms in the noise model $N'(j, m)$ are subtracted from the values of the corresponding atoms in the representation of the raw signal $R(j, m)$:

$$D(j,m) = R(j,m) - N'(j,m) \tag{6.8}$$

This operation yields a modified time-frequency plane representing the distilled cardiac signal $D(j, m)$. This plane is then fed to the inverse wavelet transform, which produces time-domain ECG signal with removed noises.

The ECG-dedicated adaptive wavelet discrimination of muscular noise was tested with CSE Multilead Database signals accompanied by reference segmentation points and with synthesized noise-free ECGs. Both kinds of signals were mixed with real recordings from the MIT-BIH Noise Stress Database (resampled from 360 Hz), normalized with respect to the ECG signal to four test levels 50%, 20%, 10%, and 5% (corresponding to -3dB, -7dB, -10dB, and -13 dB SNR) and with another mathematically synthesized noise representing three patterns:

- poor electrode contact (abrupt baseline changes),
- electromagnetic interference (sinus wave, 60 Hz), and
- muscle fibrillation (high-frequency noise).

Figure 6.5. (a) Distribution of noise measurement and interpolation samples in the first three scales; (b) Extrapolation of noise values to low-frequency bands with averaging of the noise print in the time domain—missing values 'o' are estimated from adjacent measured values 'x'

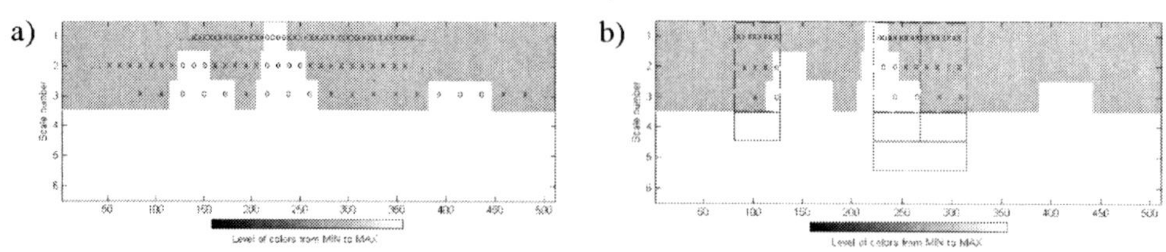

The measure of noise discrimination efficiency was the PRD ratio representing how far the noise-contaminated test signal and distilled signal approximates the original. Tests with artificial noise patterns provide a proper estimate of noise discrimination efficiency (Table 10).

The dynamics of the noise model adaptation was also tested with the use of sinus-modulated noise. In order to avoid any correlation with the ECG, the modulating function uses frequencies constantly increasing from 1 to 10 Hz.

The noise discrimination efficiency for static and sinus-modulated signals were 95.4% (11.6 dB) and 92.6% (11.1 dB), respectively. The time-frequency noise model is quasi-continuous, and it adapts to physiological changes in muscular activity.

CORRELATIONS OF SIGNAL DISTORTIONS AND DEVIATIONS OF DIAGNOSTIC PARAMETERS

Introduction

The idea of non-equal density of medical information in the electrocardiogram is of particular importance when designing signal compression systems. The distortions of reconstructed signals, considered to be an unavoidable consequence of data reduction in other traditional systems, are now subject to control. The temporal distribution of distortions, within the confines of a heart evolution, may be designed as signal-feature dependent, application-dependent, or even controlled by the human operator. Being similar in technical aspects, the resulting compression algorithms differ in favoring a particular zone in the signal according to physiological expectations. The compression ratio, which is a principal estimate of compression efficiency, gives priority to the signal quality that is indisputably essential for electrodiagnostic applications. Controlling the temporal distribution of the distortions is achieved in time-frequency domains by means of a 'function of interest', a one-dimensional

Table 6.4. The average difference of denoised and original synthesized signals for patterns of static and sinus-modulated noises; the values represent the percentage of remaining noise

Noise Pattern	PRD (%) Static Noise				Modulated Noise			
	50	20	10	5	50	20	10	5
poor electrode contact	46	11	4.3	2.1	47	13	4.5	2.4
electromagnetic interference	17	4.3	1.3	0.95	17	4.4	1.4	1.1
muscle fibrillation	10	1.4	0.71	0.33	11	1.6	0.78	0.37

equivalent of the 'region of interest' (ROI) in images. This function represents information about the local diagnostic importance of the ECG.

The attention received by ECG-compression methods in the scientific world is proven by a dozen reports (Karlsson, 1967; Cox, Nolle, Fouzzard, & Oliver, 1968; Pahlm, Börjesson, & Werner, 1979; Ruttiman & Pipberger, 1979; Peden, 1982; Ishijiama, Shin, Hostetter, & Sklansky, 1983; Kuklinski, 1983; Lee, Chang, & Thakor, 1987; Furth & Perez, 1988; Lamberti & Coccia, 1988; Hsia, 1989; Iwata, Nagasaka, & Suzumura, 1990; Jalaleddine & Hutchens, 1990; Jalaleddine, Hutchens, Strattan, & Coberly, 1990; Hamilton & Tompkins, 1991; Tai, 1991, 1992; Hamilton, 1993; Ishijiama, 1993; Nave & Cohen, 1993; Takahashi, Takeuchi, & Ohsawa, 1993; Uchiyama, Akazawa, & Sasamori, 1993; Hamilton, Thomson, & Sandham, 1995; Reddy & Murthy, 1996; Ramakrishnan & Supratim, 1997; Zigel, Cohen, Abu-Ful, Wagshal, & Katz, 1997; Chen & Itoh, 1998; Cohen & Zigel, 1998; Zigel & Cohen, 1998, 1999, 2000; Kuzume & Niijima, 2000; Lu, Kim, & Pearlman, 2000; Duda, Turcza, & Zieliński, 2001; Nygaard, Melnikov, & Katsaggelos, 2001; Reza, Moghaddam, & Nayebi, 2001; Miaou & Lin, 2002; Bilgin, Marcellin, & Altbach, 2003; Miaou, Chen, & Chao, 2005; Tai, Sun, & Yan, 2005). Detailed studies of some of the proposed compression methods, particularly those using time-frequency signal representations (Bradie, 1996; Hilton, 1997) led to the formulation of the following general remarks:

- *Lossy and Lossless Methods*—Existing methods are usually described as lossy or lossless, or strictly speaking: *bit-accurate*. The bit-accurate methods guarantee the identity of digital representations for original signals and their reconstructed copy. Despite the common belief, the bit-accurate compression methods represent the continuous real signal only as close as it results from the digitizing parameters. The bit-accurate compression is featured at a cost of considerably lower compression efficiency, and in many countries is the only legal way for storing medical data.
- *Medical Interpretation of Distortion*—Compression efficiency is usually the main feature in compression assessments. For lossy compression methods, the distortion coefficient is seen as a necessary evil because of the monotone function of the compression ratio. The commonly used distortion estimators (like Percent Root-mean-square Difference PRD) do not reflect the time-domain variability of signal importance in medical examinations, thus such a technical parameter is hardly interpretable in terms of medical diagnosis.
- *Signal-Specific or General-Purpose Algorithms*—The cyclic behavior of heart muscles represented in the structure of the ECG offers a rare opportunity to relate the local density of diagnostic information to easily detectable points on the ECG curve. Some epochs in the heart's cycle (e.g., the ventricle's contrac-

tion) are diagnostically more important to the human expert than the other parts. Consequently, the corresponding sections in the ECG must be handled with special care, while the others may be simplified without altering the medical interpretation of the data. Because of the lack of medical knowledge about local ECG signal importance, this time function is to be assumed in an application-specific way.

Considering all the remarks above, it seemed reasonable to propose new design guidelines favorable to the signal quality and to the maximum reproducibility of medical data. Such a system would prompt the doctor to manage temporal distribution of distortions. Consequently, distortions concentrate on the zones indicated as less important, while the zones of particular interest remain unaffected. Our method joins the advantage of high efficiency typical to lossy compressions (it is a lossy compression indeed) and the control of the medical aspects of the signal. Additionally, with regard to the medical aspect, local distortions tolerance borders or local signal importance functions are easier to interpret and manage than a global distortions estimate.

A Revised Approach Local Signal Quality Estimator

The medical knowledge about the importance of particular sections in the ECG signal is not easy to express. Despite the lack of guidelines, we carry out experiments and poll doctors in our investigations of the electrocardiogram process. Although every doctor looks at ECG traces differently, there are some similarities:

- A huge percentage of ECG examinations are made to answer a particular question or verify a hypothesis, and only a few are 'general-purpose' recordings with no presumptions. ECG interpretation depends on *a priori* knowledge about the patient's health. Consequently, the importance of ECG information is patient specific.
- In accordance with the medical goal of an examination, specialized recording equipment is used. Stress-test systems, long-term Holter recorders, and bedside cardiomonitors are expected to satisfy different requirements and to issue different kinds of information from the ECG. The local importance of an ECG depends in some way on the specific purpose of the application.
- In spite of tendencies for 'normalization', the doctors' experience still plays an important role in interpretation of ECG traces. Cardiologists, after a certain period of time, become more or less specialized in the diagnosis and treatment of particular heart disease. In that respect, ECG usage is also doctor specific.

The above-mentioned findings suggest that a unified approach to local data density in the interpretation of ECG should not be expected soon. Instead, the custom-defined importance function ought to be applied.

Vulnerability of Diagnostic Parameters to the Signal Distortion

To estimate the importance of the diagnostic parameters issued by a 12-lead recorder, we first studied their vulnerability to distortions. Table 6.5 indicates the precision of the segmentation points positioning as an appropriate background for *global estimator of ECG diagnostic parameters quality* (GEQ) since it influences the precision of computation of all temporal relationships between the cardiac events. On the other hand, this parameter is particularly sensitive to bandwidth limitation, which typically originates from compression-caused distortion.

The GEQ is based on values that are important with regard to electrodiagnostic aspects and that are monotonically less precise when the datastream decreases. It seems most reasonable that the positioning of P-onset, P-end, QRS-onset, QRS-end, and T-end segmentation points are selected to contribute to the global estimator value. They are medically very meaningful, because they represent the stimulus conduction function and are not fully recoverable by mathematical tools if lost as a result of simplification of the ECG signal.

To compute the individual contributions of each positioning difference to the GEQ, we processed the CSE guidelines for the expected precision of the segmentation positioning points given in Table 6.6, according to Equation 6.9.

$$w_i = \frac{\frac{1}{dl_i}}{\sum_{i=1}^{5} \frac{1}{dl_i}} \tag{6.9}$$

The thresholds difference recommended by CSE dl_i and the contribution coefficients of each point are summarized in Table 6.6. The formulae (6.10) defines the GEQ [ms] as:

$$GEQ = d_{P-onset} \cdot w_1 + d_{P-end} \cdot w_2 + d_{QRS-onset} \cdot w_3 + d_{QRS-end} \cdot w_4 + d_{T-end} \cdot w_5 \tag{6.10}$$

The principal assumption of the proposed quality estimator is that the parameters' quality is expected to monotonically decrease with a decrease of data rate. We tested the signal quality for a set of 125 signals from the 12-lead CSE Multilead Database

Table 6.5. Discussion about the vulnerability of ECG diagnostic parameters to signal distortions

Parameter	Diagnostic Meaning	Vulnerability to the Signal Quality
precision of the R wave peak positioning	The fundamental parameter for heart rate (HR) and heart rate variability (HRV) computations. Commonly used also for arrhythmia, premature beat detection, and many other diseases.	The correct position of the R wave peak may result from the parabola fitting to the sparse data. The loss of data can be compensated with a precision greater than the sampling interval.
precision of the segmentation points positioning	Basic parameters for the computation of all temporal relationships between cardiac events. Precise segmentation is the key to assessing the correctness of the functionality of the heart conducting system.	With regard to the complexity of the phenomena, wave border mathematical models are not precise enough for diagnostic purposes, hence data loss cannot be recovered with use of mathematical tools.
measure of ventricular late potentials (VLPs)	Ventricular late potentials represent the susceptibility of ventricular muscle fibrils with regard to spontaneous contractions that are out of the control of the heart-conductive system. Life-critical if not detected.	Limiting the signal bandwidth below a value of 250 Hz makes VLP detection impossible.
measurement of the level and the slope of ST segment (ischemia)	Depressions or elevations of the ST segment, exceeding given limits, are considered as symptoms of ischemia. Ischemia is the most frequent disease of the cardiovascular system, with mortality rates being the highest in the developed countries. Risk factors are stress, physical overload, overweight, and bad diet.	The correct assessment of the ST segment change is conditioned by the acquisition of low-frequency components of the ECG signal. Data reduction in the high-frequency range does not affect the performance of ST segment measurements.

(Willems, 1990). The ECG segmentation procedure designed for 500 Hz/12bit signals was obtained as an executable file from a commercial ECG software manufacturer. The segmentation was performed for a whole set of signals and compared with the reference points provided by the database. In the subsequent trials, the signal bandwidth was truncated with a low pass filter (FIR, 12 dB/oct) to 200, 150, 100, and 50 Hz. For each simplified version of the signal, the segmentation was performed by the same subroutine and the results were compared with the reference. Figure 6.6 displays the mean inaccuracy of P-onset, P-end, QRS-onset, QRS-end, and T-end segmentation points positioning for the original and restricted-bandwidth data. The value of the GEQ is displayed as well.

The results of testing the GEQ with the restricted bandwidth signal set support the further use of GEQ as a reliable representation of data quality. An additional test verified the correlation (r-Pearson) between GEQ and the bandwidth. The value of 91.7 % indicates the close relation of GEQ and the bit rate.

Calculating the Importance Function Based on the Diagnostic Parameters Quality Loss

A numerical experiment was designed and carried out to estimate the local ECG relevance function. The experiment was expected to prove that removing a specified amount of information causes different results with regard to the diagnostic parameters' quality, depending on the part of the heart's cycle that is subjected to the removal. Additionally, moving the data modification window along the time in the heart cycle indicates the zones in the ECG signal where the resulting diagnostic parameters are particularly susceptible to distortion.

For the application of ECG signal compression, the idea is to maintain the diagnostic parameters as little affected as possible by means of keeping the GEQ value as low as possible. Hence the importance function should have values proportional to the local signal vulnerability. The data reduction will then be subtler on the zones described as particularly vulnerable.

Like in the tests for the GEQ (see Equation 6.10), a set of 125 signals from the 12-lead CSE Multilead Database (Willems, 1990) were used to test the average local vulnerability to distortions. Thirty-seven signals containing ventricular, pacemaker stimulations, and low heart rate beats were discarded from the test signal set. The segmentation was performed by the previously described external procedure for a whole set of signals and compared with the reference points provided by the database.

Table 6.6 CSE recommendations concerning the precision of the P-QRS-T segmentation and the calculated weight coefficients (Morlet, 1986)

i	**1** **P-onset**	**2** **P-end**	**3** **QRS-onset**	**4** **QRS-end**	**5** **T-end**
maximum accepted difference [ms] dl_i	8.0	7.8	4.4	5.8	15.6
calculated weight coefficient w_i	0.174	0.179	0.317	0.240	0.090

Figure 6.6. Mean inaccuracy of segmentation points positioning for the original and restricted-bandwidth data and the corresponding value of global diagnostic parameters' quality GEQ

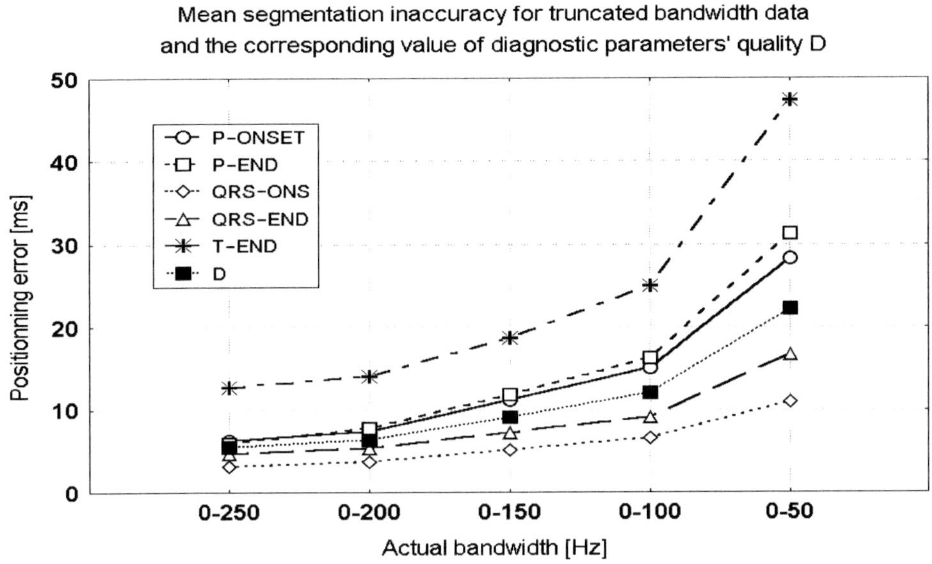

In each trial were modified six randomly selected t-f coefficients out of 14 in octaves 1-3 (32...250 Hz) in the window spanning for 32 ms. Five trials of removal were performed for each of 89 signals and for each of 27 positions of sliding window.

To represent the ECG signal equivalently in the time and the time-frequency domains, the Daubechies (1992) 5th order compactly supported wavelet transform was selected. It satisfies the following features:

- the perfect reconstruction property, in order to guarantee that every change in the time domain signal is due to coefficient removal in the time-frequency domain;
- the compact and relatively short support, to represent the heartbeat components in a temporal selective way; and
- good separation of adjacent frequency octaves to minimize frequency band cross-talk.

The main part of the experiment consisted of eliminating time-frequency coefficients in the sliding window. The altered signal is then reconstructed and processed for segmentation. The values of the difference for the P-onset, P-end, QRS-onset, QRS-end, and T-end are calculated with respect to the references from the database.

Finally, the GEQ was computed according to Equation 6.10. For each particular time-frequency window position, the GEQ value was averaged over the five trials of random modification, with a total of 89 test signals and 12 traces in each signal.

The experiment was repeated for 27 subsequent time positions of the window covering the average length of a heartbeat of 864 ms (Figure 6.7). Each experiment resulted in the average GEQ estimator value specific for the window's position with reference to the segmentation points. Despite the fact that the amount of information lost is always the same (six time-frequency samples), the global quality of medical data, expressed by the value of GEQ, changes with the position of time zone where the removal was performed (Figure 6.8). That proves the temporal non-uniform vulnerability of medical data to ECG signal distortion. Additionally, the function GEQ(t) quantitatively assesses the extent to which the diagnostic parameters' quality is affected with regard to each position of the modification window.

Figure 6.7. The principle of canceling the time-frequency coefficients randomly selected in a moving window: octave 1-3 (32...250 Hz), time span 32 ms

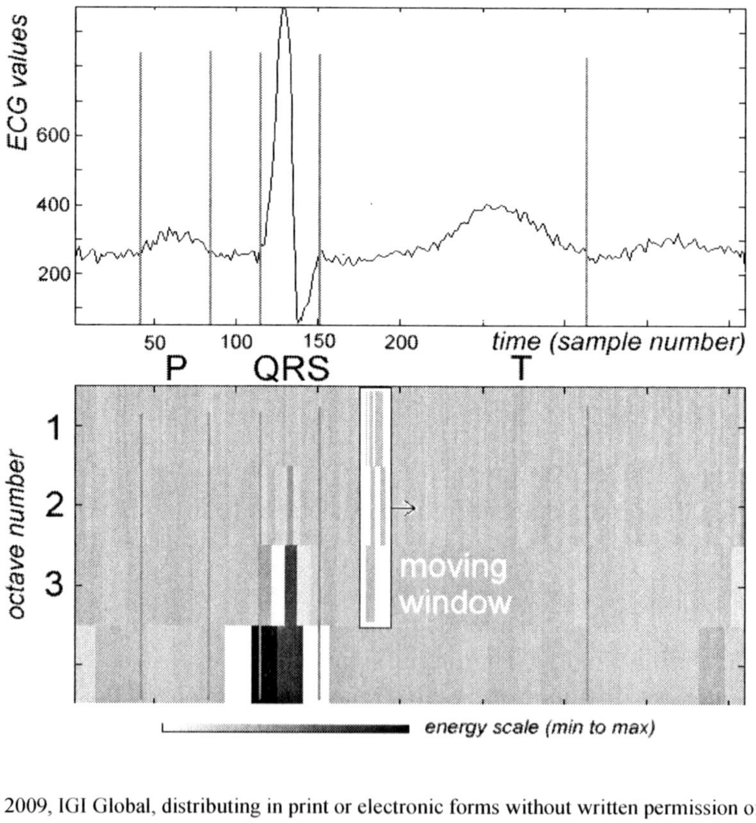

Discussion

The main goal of the research was to explore the possibility of controlling the time-domain distortion distribution in the wavelet packed-based ECG signal compression. Distortions, being unavoidable in lossy but efficient compression algorithms, no longer appear as a phenomena of unknown behavior described with use of a meaningless global parameter such as PRD (see Equation 6.14). From now on, the distortions may be removed from the most important zones of the ECG according to user-defined rules.

In principle, the future user is practically unrestricted in defining his own importance function related to the heart cycle time. Suppressing distortions in a particular section causes a proportional increase in distortions in the neighboring parts of the signal, so the overall distortion level remains unchanged. The local distortion level may be suppressed to very low values; and with use of lifting wavelet transform (Unser & Zerubia, 1998), even a segmentary bit-accurate compression is possible.

Designing an Application-Dependent Compression Algorithm

When aiming at a best result for the compression, there is an interest in finding the optimal representation that best preserves the features contained in the signal. For

Figure 6.8 The function of diagnostic parameters' susceptibility to distortion caused by the local random canceling of time-frequency coefficients; additionally, average wave borders are marked

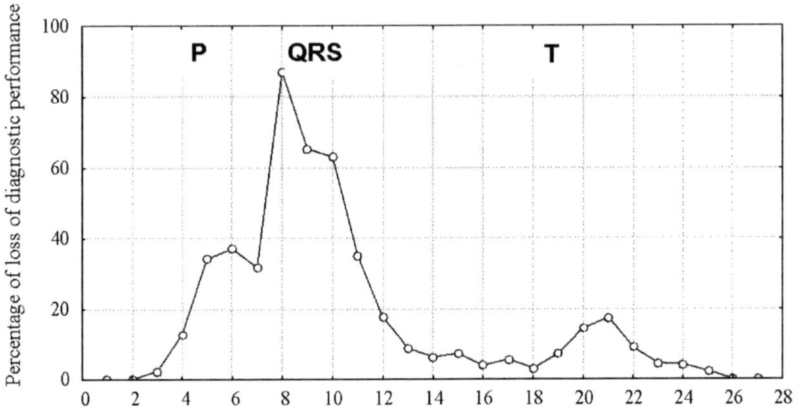

this purpose, we used wavelet packets (Mallat, 1996), which are an extension of the wavelet concept. The orthogonal decomposition of the time-domain signal splits its bandwidth into two half-band components: the step-down signal approximation and the detail signal. At each node of the decomposition tree, a decision must be made whether band splitting is interesting. For efficient searching of the binary-tree structure, entropy-like cost functions are commonly used. The compression is achieved by minimizing the value of the cost function at each node. Consequently, some branches of the binary tree are pruned, and the remaining irregular structure, which is adapted to the time-frequency properties of the analyzed signal, is called the "best tree." It contains the most relevant time-frequency atoms of the signal, but some information is lost during the optimization, hence the compression is lossy. In keeping with the previous experiment, we used Daubechies (1992) 5th order compactly supported wavelet.

All the cost functions reported in the literature, in particular in papers on wavelet-packet-based ECG compression (Bradie, 1996; Hilton, 1997), use s_i, the value of the wavelet packet coefficient, to compute the cost function E:

$$E = \sum_i P(s_i) \tag{6.11}$$

where P is a functional operator like a logarithm, square, absolute value, and so forth. The computation of the cost function is carried out in the same way for all of the coefficients, not taking into account their temporal position.

Modulating the local compression parameters and, as a result, controlling the temporal distortion's distribution are the main novelties of our approach. In our application the previously derived importance function was used as a source of modulation, since we found it reasonable for a stand-alone 12-lead recorder. It ought to be mentioned, however, that any other modulating sequence relative to the time of a heart cycle may be applied alternatively.

Modulating the compression parameters consists of modifying the cost function computation rules, with the use of weighting coefficients provided by the importance function. Time-frequency representation contains true values that may be used for decompression without any additional modifiers. The cost function, used for the best tree lookup, must respect the temporal position i expressed by the weighting coefficient w_i (6.12).

$$E = \sum_i P(s_i \cdot w_i) \tag{6.12}$$

A vector of consecutive values of w_i is computed for the segmented heartbeat signal. For the convenience of the dyadic wavelet decomposition, its length is expected to be an integer power of 2. For the lack of assumptions about the importance of function sampling, it is necessary to calculate each w_i value with respect to its temporal distance to the nearest segmentation points. The interpolation must consider the temporal variability of each section in the heartbeat. The temporal re-scaling of each section length in the importance function to the actual section length in the segmented signal is used to fit all the wave start- and endpoints.

The weighting coefficient's vector, computed for the first decomposition level, must be adapted for the use at the lower nodes of the decomposition tree. Using the dyadic scheme wavelet decomposition simplifies this adaptation—the only necessary processing is the successive decimation of the weighting coefficient vectors.

For testing purposes, the segmentation procedure is not necessary, since all wave start- and endpoints are provided in the CSE Multilead Database. All the traces belonging to the same recording were processed as separate single-channel records, but because they have common segmentation points, the importance function and weighting coefficient vectors are calculated once per recording. Two recordings containing pacemaker stimulated beats and five recordings with low heart rates were excluded from the test signal set. The remaining 118 beats are of supra-ventricular and ventricular origin.

The algorithm starts directly with the temporal rescaling of the importance function. For each interval in the heart evolution (i.e., P, P-Q, QRS, etc.), the length expressed in importance function samples is compared with the actual interval length. The importance function is then resampled in segments using the appropriate higher number of sampling points. For computational simplicity, linear interpolation was used. The last operation is the normalization of values in the weighting coefficient vectors, so the average of all the coefficients equals 1.

The wavelet packet decomposition uses the Daubechies 5th order compactly supported wavelet, and the pursuit for the best tree is performed using the modified logarithm function of the energy entropy:

$$E = \sum_i \log(s_i^2 \cdot w_i) \qquad (6.13)$$

where w_i are elements of weighting coefficient vectors.

All the nodes at the given wavelet-packet decomposition level use the same version of weighting coefficient vectors. When proceeding to a lower level, all the signal representations are decimated since they contain one-half of the previous bandwidth. In order to maintain temporal compatibility, decimation is applied to the weighting coefficient vectors as well.

The essential components of the compressed signal are:

- best tree values,
- position parameters of the best tree components, and
- synchronization and scale parameters.

Following the guidelines given in Bradie (1996), the positioning of the best tree nodes is encoded in a 16-bit value. The values of the decomposition components are expressed in floating-point format as a consequence of applying a real-valued wavelet transform and weighting coefficients. These values are subject to quantization, and similarly to the original signals, are represented in 12-bit integers. The quantization is a source of additional data loss, but considering that the prevalence of the local signal energy is represented in the best tree values, the estimated error is comparable with the quantization error during the analog-to-digital conversion. Thanks to additional amplitude normalization, the best tree coefficients always use the full dynamic range of 12-bit coding.

The decompression procedure is very straightforward. The signal samples are retrieved from the best tree values at the node position coordinates with the use of inverse wavelet transform. Amplitude rescaling and temporal synchronization of the heartbeat end the decompression.

Compression ratio results and global distortion estimates (percent root-mean-square difference, PRD, according to Equation 6.14) are presented in Table 6.7, as averaged over all traces in each CSE recording.

$$PRD = \sqrt{\frac{\sum_{k=1}^{N}\left(s_{k,i} - s_{k,j}\right)^2}{\sum_{k=1}^{N}\left(s_{k,i}\right)^2}} \cdot 100\% \qquad (6.14)$$

The compression efficiency, as a global estimate coherent within the result achieved above, is not the most important parameter of our approach because it does not reflect the distortion's distribution strategy. The distortion's distribution is a time-domain function that is expected to show a correlation with the ECG segmentation points. For each signal, however, the segmentation points are set individually with respect to the detected signal features. In order to collect the corresponding information on error distribution from various signals, the appropriate segmentary resampling of individual difference functions must be used to match the positions of the segmentation points. Additionally, there is no solution suitable for the ventricular beats without the P wave.

Although all the traces are considered as separate ECG signals for processing, the 12 components of a particular recording have common segmentation points. Consequently, the temporal distortions' distribution may be displayed individually for each recording as the average absolute difference of the original and decom-

Table 6.7. General results of application dependent upon the compression algorithm for CSE database files

CSE-ID	Compression Ratio	Total Distortion PRD (%)
1	4.6390	6.4871
2	7.9102	3.5952
3	6.3116	4.6818
4	5.0881	6.1332
123	6.5532	5.0970
124	4.9714	5.8661
125	5.8650	4.7592
mean value	**5.9006**	**5.1711**

pressed signal. The distribution plots were studied for all 118 files, but because of a lack of space, only two examples are given here (Figure 6.9).

Segmentary values of PRD are summarized in Table 6.8. The additional parameter is the correlation coefficient (*r*-Pearson) of the distortion percentage and the values of the weighting coefficient vector at zero level. The data in Table 6.8 are also averaged over all 12 traces in each file.

The efficiency test compression ratio result of 5.9 is not outstanding compared to other published methods. Some of them show significantly higher values of compression ratios, particularly when a superposition of transforms is used. The global PRD (5.17%) is fairly low, but even for this order of distortion level, significant alterations of medical findings are reported by other authors (Bradie, 1996; Zigel, Cohen, & Katz, 1996). The global distortion coefficient does not reflect the temporal distortion concentration, so it is not appropriate to make judgment about the main advantage of our algorithm.

Particularly interesting are results for the distortion's distribution. A visual inspection of Figure 6.9 sheds some light on the local distortion's concentration with respect to the medical events detected in the electrocardiogram. The zones defined as more important—that is, P, QRS, and T waves—are less affected than the remaining part of the signal. The results of the segmentary PRD value (Table 6.8), which is the quantitative comparison for the distortion level, also yield similar conclusions. Another very meaningful parameter is the correlation of the values of the weighting coefficient's vector at the zero level with the local distortion's amplitude. The value of the correlation expresses the extent to which the temporal distortion's distribution matches the local vulnerability of diagnostic parameters.

The average value of -0.86 means that the local distortion level is almost inversely proportional to the signal importance. As expected, the distortions are concentrated in less important sections of the signal.

The algorithm was not optimized for speed or computing efficiency. Despite the use of floating-point representation and the Fourier Transform, real-time application was prototyped with the use of a modern DSP chip (Kowacki & Augustyniak, 2007).

INVESTIGATION OF FOCUS ATTENTION DISTRIBUTION DURING VISUAL ECG INSPECTION

Introduction to the Visual Task Methodology

The control of adaptive biosignals and data transmission in distributed monitoring networks is an emerging area of prospective applications for the general rules describing datastream variability in relation to the medical content of the signal to its expected statistical parameters. Searching for signal meaning beyond its technical parameters (e.g., spectrum) and the involvement of medical knowledge would not be feasible without the cooperation of experienced people. In this case, however, results are very sensitive to human factors: prejudging, verbalization, and other ones (Hitch & Baddeley, 1976; Baddeley, 1986). Making use of expert surveys usually involves the statistical processing of their outcomes, very effective in reducing inter-subject variability, but inadequate for limiting systematic errors.

Figure 6.9. Temporal distortion distributions averaged for all 12 traces of selected files along with the lead V2 original (the top-first) and reconstructed (the top-second) traces: (a) supra-ventricular beat CSE Mo001, (b) ventricular beat CSE Mo045; note that the vertical axes' values apply to distortion plots only

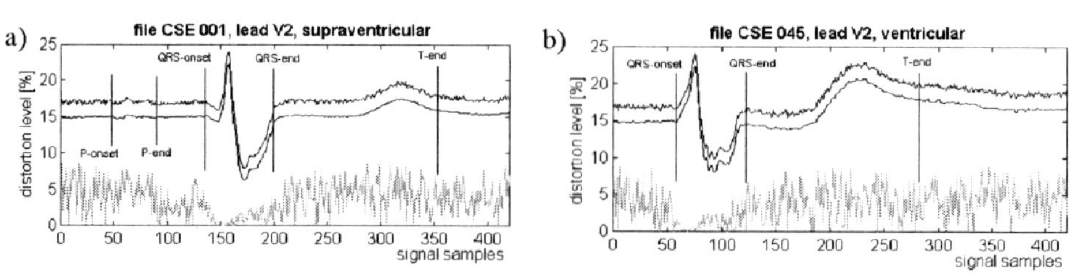

An original alternative to a standard questionnaire is a visual experiment performed on cardiology experts aimed at capturing and investigating local variations of the ECG trace conspicuity. Assuming proper engagement of an observer in the trace inspection, the gaze is controlled instinctively. Consequently, the eyeglobe movements objectively represent the information gathering sequence. An analysis of expert eye-globe trajectories carried out during the visual interpretation not only reveals regions of particular importance in the signal trace, but also reconstructs the human reasoning involved in the interpretation process. Therefore, except for our main interest in the prediction of required parameters of the transmission channel from the automatic rough estimation of medical contents, the eye-track features captured during the visual inspection of biosignals may be applicable in the:

- implementation of human reasoning and non-verbalized rules in machine interpretation algorithms,
- objective assessment of cardiologist interpretation skills,
- teaching visual interpretation using the guided repetition method during scan-paths, and
- application of human reasoning and non-verbalized rules in machine interpretation algorithms.

Perceptual models (PMs) of various scenes have been recently recognized as valuable tools for improving human interaction with sophisticated devices (Dick, 1980; Salvucci & Anderson, 2001; Ober et al., 2002). The PM of the ECG is an outcome of the statistical processing of the scan-paths, analyzed within the context of background visual information. The eye fixation time and gaze order correspond to the amount of data visually gathered by the observer and represent the diagnostic importance of particular regions in the scene (Boccignone, 2001). In the case of the ECG, the waves' positions represent subsequent events in the cardiac cycle, and in this context the concentration of foveation time along the horizontal axis expresses the local density of medical data.

The scan-path features are representative of the quantitative measurement of the datastream gathered from a particular point in the visual scene only when considering the physiology of human perception and the oculomotoric system (Pelz & Canosa, 2001). Three groups of issues were identified as affecting the visual perception time:

- the randomness of observation start and finish moments,
- the dynamics of seeking new targets and the accuracy of eyeball positioning, and
- the ambiguity of binocular perception.

Table 6.8. Local distortion results of the application-dependent compression algorithm for CSE database files (distortions PRD in %)

CSE-ID	compression ratio	total distortions	P wave distortions	QRS wave distortions	T wave distortions	extra wave distortions	correlation *r*
1	4.6390	6.4871	0.8756	0.2335	0.9770	4.4010	-0.78
2	7.9102	3.5952	0.7901	0.2195	0.7317	1.8539	-0.84
45	5.9507	5.2612	-	0.3144	0.9810	3.9658	-0.81
124	4.9714	5.8661	1.0644	0.4177	0.8760	3.5080	-0.91
125	5.8650	4.7592	0.9817	0.2914	0.8426	2.6435	-0.86

Automatic extraction of local conspicuity estimate from recorded polygonal curves requires proper detection of all the phenomena mentioned above and correction of foveation time for each section of the electrocardiogram. For this purpose, we developed a heuristic-driven pre-processing algorithm correcting these observer-dependant issues obscuring the relationship of gaze time and localization of the observer's interest.

The aim of our research was the analysis of expert eyeball trajectories captured during the visual ECG interpretation in the following three aspects:

- the identification of the particularly important regions in the signal trace in the context of represented medical information,
- the examining and generalization of visual information pursuit strategies, and
- selecting the eye-track parameters that discriminate the experienced and the untrained observer.

Since traditional ECG interpretation is considered to be a purely visual process, research on the perceptual model of the electrocardiogram was based on a series of visual experiments. Two effects determined the range of foveation time in which the attention-to-foveation time relation is expected to be linear:

- The resolving power of the retina is limited outside the central zone of the fovea (Pelz & Canosa, 2001). Therefore, all of the information in the corresponding zone of the scene is captured in about 500 ms. Even if the gaze remains longer at one point, no additional detail can be extracted.
- Very short presentations (0.01-60 ms) are 'memorized' on the surface of the fovea and are later analyzed by the human visual system. Thanks to this feature, the sequence of images is perceived as a continuous motion picture, if only the presentation rate is high enough.

Within the range specified above, the correlation between foveation and attention was the goal of the visual experiment carried out in our laboratory. Thirty random sequences of characters (length 3 to 10) were presented to 13 observers (all male, age 18-35) in limited time: 100-800 ms. Immediately after each presentation, the observer was expected to speak out the sequence and the completeness of the information was scored. Apart from interpersonal differences, for each observer the scores were better for shorter sequences and for longer presentation time. This result, evidenced also in everyday life, justifies the use of fixation point densities as an estimate of the local relevance of the image.

Each experiment was carried out using a human volunteer sequentially performing a set of visual tasks. Before each visual task, the observer underwent a calibration procedure resulting in an individual scan-path transposition matrix. The matrix is calculated from the differences between the coordinates of the standard calibration rectangle and the corresponding scan-path trace, and is used in the correction of the geometrical issues as long as the eyeball acquisition conditions are maintained. Each visual task consisted of three stages:

1. The observer received a standardized initial message and was motivated to complete the information from the scene.
2. The observer scrutinized the scene in an unrestricted manner, however only eight initial seconds of scan-path signal were analyzed.
3. The observer announced the completion of the task.

At each stage, the scan-path may be influenced by unexpected observer behavior or other human factors, so a high degree of cooperation is essential.

Eye-Tracking Devices

In the visual experiments, we used the infrared reflection-based eye-tracker OBER-2 (Ober et al., 1997). The goggles illuminate each eye-globe with four adjacent spots for a total power of 5 mW/cm^2 in infrared pulses (wavelength 940nm) lasting for 80μs repeated at the sampling frequency. Four IR sensors per eye work in a pair-wise space-differential configuration and capture two-dimensional traces of each eye at the speed of 750 samples per second during the ECG presentation lasting for 8s. Since the sensor captures the visual light as well, a double sampling time-differential measurement is used for sidelight discrimination. This specific method relates the actual infrared reflection readout to the sidelight background captured about 80μs before the LEDs become active. This eliminates the influence of all common light sources and allows the eyetracker to achieve an angular resolution of 0.02 degrees. This value is equivalent to an ECG time interval of 30 ms if a standard chart plot (25mm/s) is viewed from a typical reading distance (40 cm). The position of both eyes was recorded simultaneously, however only the dominant eye was used to determine the scene conspicuity. Figure 6.10 displays the physical background of the differential infrared reflection-based eye-track acquisition.

Processing the Scan-Path Signal

Each visual experiment yields a four-column matrix representing raw eye-globe coordinates at the evenly spaced time points (Salvucci & Anderson, 2001). All signal processing routines were developed in Matlab as a customary toolbox with regard to the aims of the visual experiments. The main stages of this calculation include:

- detecting the true confines of visual perception in the scan-path, including the end of the initial idle time and the interpretation task completion time;
- qualifying each foveation point in the scan-path as corresponding to the particular ECG section (i.e., P, QRS, and T) with the use of a set of reference wave borders provided in the CSE database (Willems, 1990);
- averaging the number and duration describing the foveation regions, separately for each ECG section in all of the ECG displays; and
- referring the contribution of each section's conspicuity to the total time qualified as the active perception.

Since the foveation points are not directly referred to the ECG temporal coordinate, intrinsic wave length variability does not influence the result.

Apart from the wave conspicuity statistics, the duration and order describing foveation regions reveal the perceptual strategy related to the main stages of the ECG interpretation process. The strategy description is based on identification of the most attractive coordinate points and their gaze order aimed at relating the foveation regions to the ECG events and displayed ECG leads.

Reference ECG Traces and Observer Population

Visual targets in the experiment were ECG strips randomly selected from CSE records (Willems, 1990). The reference wave borders were not displayed but provided the cardio-physiological background for scan-path signal processing. Considering the borders of the electrocardiogram waves in the scan-path analysis was a key point in finding the relationship between a cardiac event and the amount of information its representation contributes to a final diagnosis.

Each observer was asked to interpret eight traces. Each trace from Dataset 3 appeared two to four times (2.43 on average). Pacemaker-stimulated recording numbers 67 and 70 were excluded because of the lack of waveform measurement points in the database.

Waveforms were presented on a computer display, simulating a typical 12-lead paper recording. The reading distance was set to 40 centimeters and was controlled with the use of a chin support. Each presentation of the ECG trace was interlaced with a fixation point in the middle of the display.

The recordings of the scan-paths were made in similar laboratory conditions with volunteers during the manual interpretation of ECG traces. Seventeen experts (12 +/- 4 years of experience) accepted the invitation for the visual experiment. We

Figure 6.10. (a) Physical principles and (b) technical details of the infrared reflection-based eye-tracker OBER-2

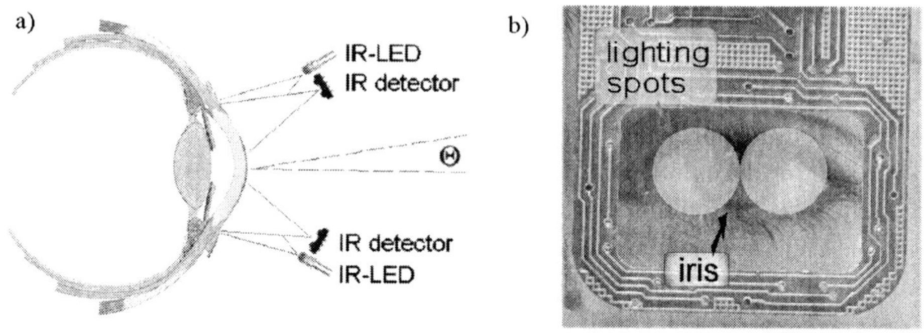

Figure 6.11. Scan-path signal processing diagram

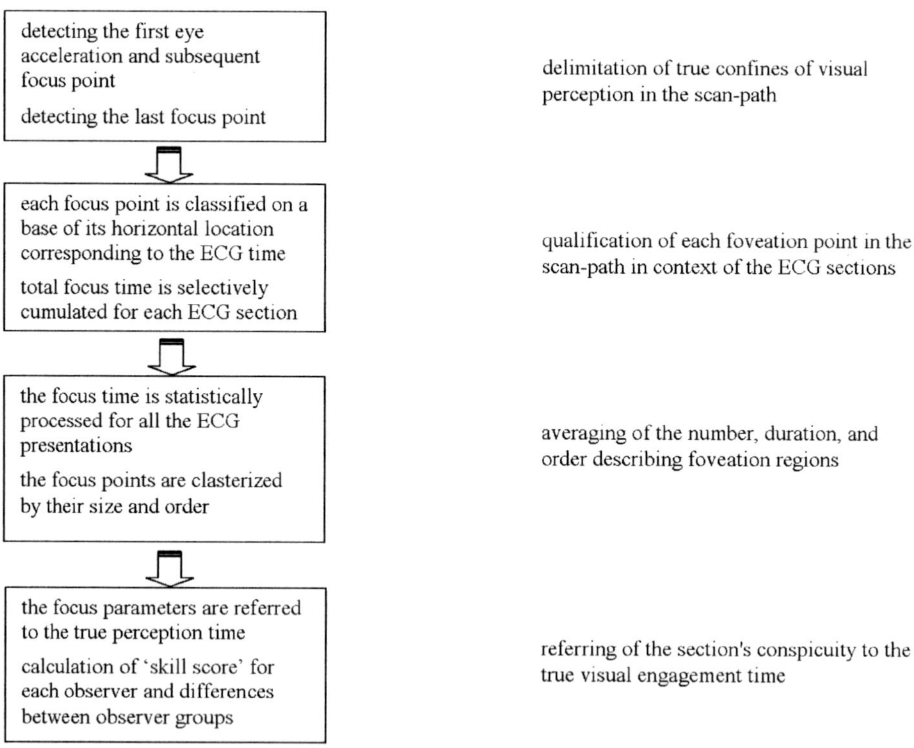

included also 21 student volunteers having only basic knowledge of ECG (Figure 6.12). Before attempting the visual task, all observers completed a questionnaire specifying their professional specialization, experience, and skills in ECG interpretation, as well as describing their eyesight defects. Because most of the experts wore glasses, we had to determine their impact on the scan-paths. We found no significant difference in traces, but only if the positions of the glasses and of the eye-tracker goggles remain unchanged from the calibration to the measurement phase.

Quantitative Results Concerning the Description of the Medical Data Distribution

Statistically processed results of all visual experiments are summarized in Table 6.9. Figures 6.13 and 6.14 display examples of the eye-globe trajectory over a 12-lead ECG plot and the corresponding bar graph of the attention density that is representative of two groups of observers: experts and students.

Figure 6.12. An expert volunteer performing the visual task of ECG inspection

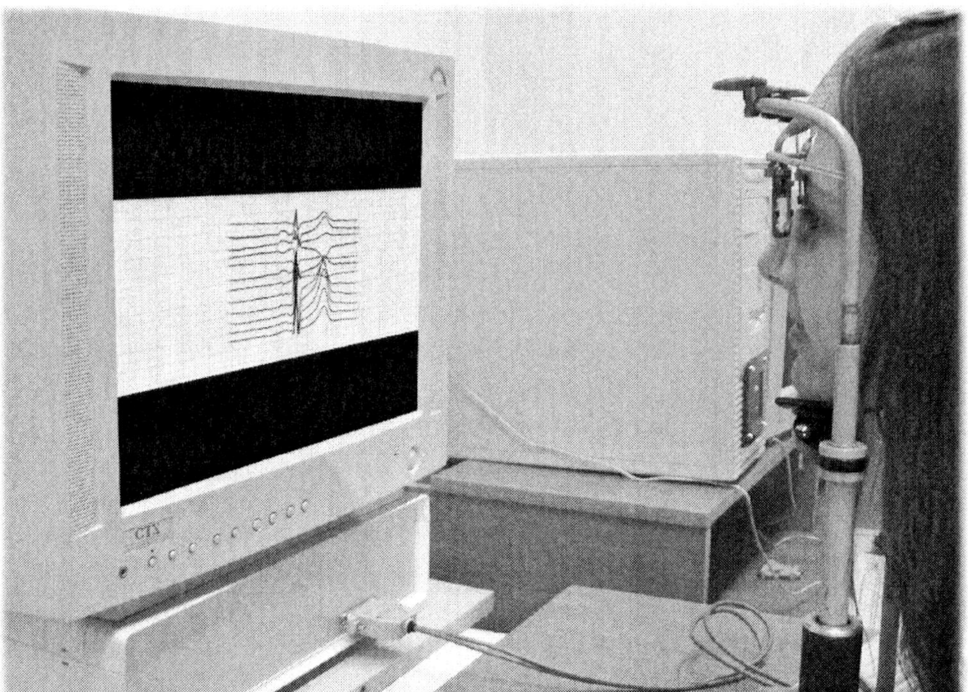

Assuming that the student volunteers are untrained observers, the only reason for the difference in the attention density variations between the two groups are expert perceptual habits developed over years of practice. Therefore, highlighting the attention density variations is of particular interest in objective skills assessment. The local difference in attention density between two groups is particularly high within the QRS wave borders, indicating the information represented in the QRS shape as important for diagnostic decisions.

The Results of the Visual Interpretation Strategy

The second group of results were derived from the analysis of the perceptual strategy. The strategy is attributed by the focus points coordinates and time, and by the gaze order. Figures 6.15 and 6.16 display examples of the strategy over a 12-lead ECG plot. The focus point origins are represented by the circle centers and focus time—by their diameters. Small flashes represent gaze movements to the next focus point and help to follow the observer's gaze order. Table 6.10 summarizes the corresponding strategy description parameters.

Studies of the scan-path examples given in Figures 6.15 and 6.16 reveal the main principles of perceptual strategy typical for both groups:

- Experts (Figure 6.15) scan purposely selected traces for expected waveforms:
  - first circle is the main focus point and represents 31% of the total focus attention, and
  - subsequent points order may be justified by: (2) rhythm detection, (3) QRS-verification, (4) rhythm verification, or (5) T segment assessment.
- Students (Figure 6.16) scan every trace for anything interesting:
  - chaotic or ineffective systematic scan,
  - seventh circle is detected as the main focus point (perhaps because it is a turning point),
  - main focus point represents 17% of the total focus attention, and
  - subsequent points order corresponds to the trace order.

For the additional studies, which were aimed at perceptual strategy repeatability, we selected electrocardiogram images interpreted by at least two observers from the same group. By comparing the positions and gaze order of the five most important foveation points in the scan-paths, we found that the similarity between two experts is much more probable (37%) than between two students (17%). Because students are untrained observers applying general conspicuity rules to the ECG plot,

Table 6.9. Quantitative results of the ECG inspection scan-path analysis

Parameter		Unit	Observers Experts	 Students
observers population			17	21
idle time		ms	73 ± 55	88 ± 105
interpretation time		s	5.5 ± 1.5	6.2 ± 1.7
local foveation	within P wave	%	23 ± 12	17 ± 12
	within PQ section	%	7 ± 5	11 ± 10
	within QRS wave	%	38 ± 15	26 ± 19
	within T wave	%	18 ± 10	21 ± 10
	within TP section	%	14 ± 5	25 ± 14
attention density [1]	maximum	s/s	21.0	16.0
	minimum	s/s	1.9	3.9

[1] *Attention density represents the time the eye-globe spends over a time unit in the ECG plot (recorded typically at 25mm/s) and thus is expressed in seconds per second ([s/s]). It should be noted that although scan-path and ECG time are both temporal variables given in seconds, the eyesight and the ECG record are not simultaneous processes.*

Figure 6.13. (a) An example expert eye-globe trajectory over a 12-lead ECG plot (CSE-Mo-001); (b) corresponding bar graph of the attention density

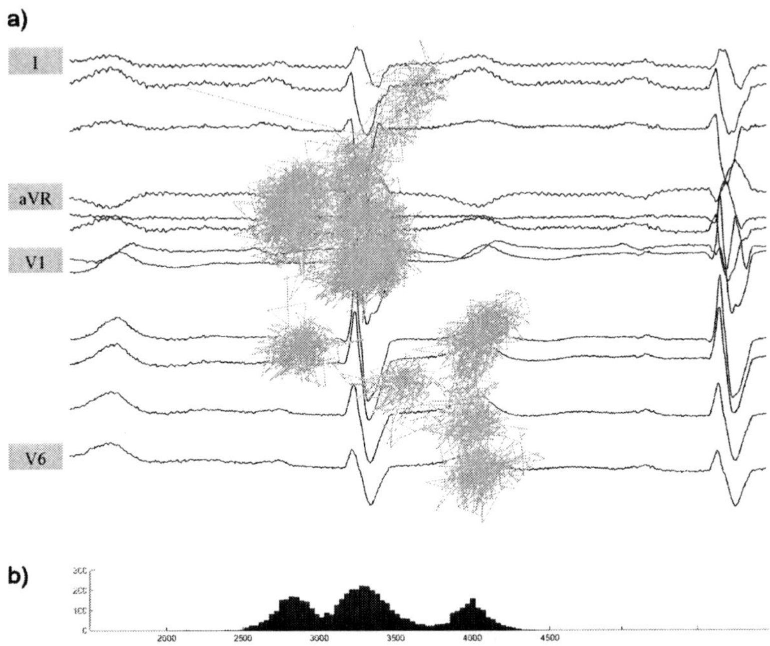

Figure 6.14. (a) An example of a student 's eye-globe trajectory over a 12-lead ECG plot (CSE-Mo-021); (b) corresponding bar graph of the attention density

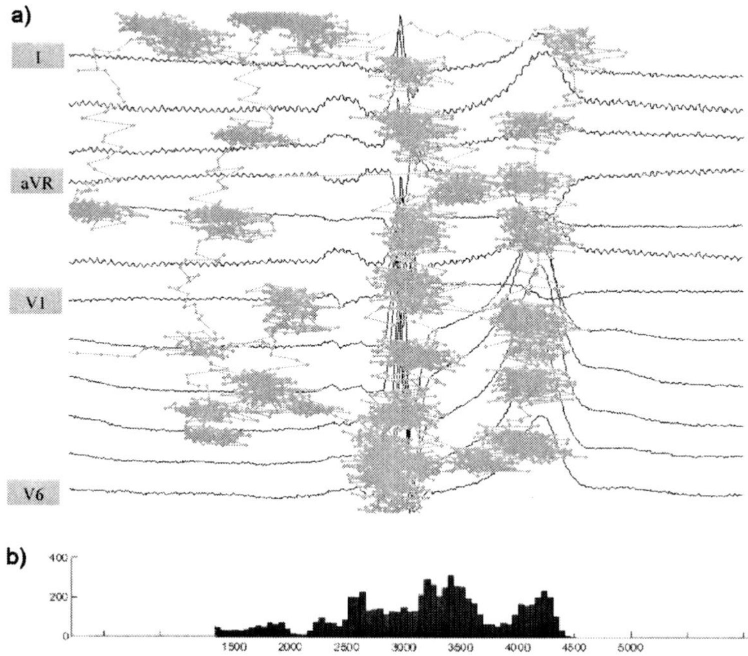

their perceptual strategy is chaotic and thus their reliability is weak. The experts apply medically justified conspicuity rules and scrutinize the ECG scene in more consistent way, so the probability of similar scan-paths increases. This result is an accurate representation of the ECG interpretation process and personal skills of the observers in the visual strategy process.

The eye tracks gathered during the visual experiments need additional research and contextual analysis with regard to the CSE database records and the medical significance of the data. An example of an unexplored area is the correctness of medical diagnoses based on visually inspected traces.

Discussion

Scan-path analysis is reported as a useful tool for investigation of human mental processes, surrounding perception and interaction, as well as man-machine interfacing (Yarbus, 1967; Noton & Stark, 1971; Levine, 1985; Aloimonos, Weiss, &

Table 6.10. Quantitative descriptions of the perceptual strategy

Parameter	Unit	Observers Experts	Students
observer population		17	21
relative foveation time for the main focus point	%	31 ± 12	17 ± 10
number of foveation points [a]		6.1 ± 1.7	9.2 ± 3.9
distance of adjacent foveation point	deg.	5.7 ± 2.4	3.1 ± 1.2
scan-path length to the last foveation point [b]	deg.	34.7 ± 5.1	28.5 ± 6.6
scan-path duration to the last foveation point [a]	s	3.6 ± 1.3	5.7 ± 1.5

[a] *Including first points having at least 5% of relative foveation time*

[b] *From the beginning to the last point having at least 5% of relative foveation time*

Bandyodaphyay, 1987; Bajcsy, 1987; Carpenter, 1988; Becker, 1989, 1991; Kowler. 1990; Irwin, 1991; Skavenski, 1990; Viviani, 1990; Swain, Kahn, & Ballard, 1992; Pashler, Carrier, & Hoffman, 1993; Ballard, Hayhoe, & Pelz, 1995). Visual experiments provide a quantitative description of trace conspicuity in the context of cardiac events represented in the signal.

Although very informative, the scan-path is very sensitive to voluntary observer cooperation during the visual tasks and thus has to be carefully interpreted. Some parameters show high inter-observer variability of unexplained origin. Being aware of the difficulties and familiar with other visual experiments, we eliminated 18% of the scan-path records because of poor cooperation or a misunderstanding of the visual task rules. Unfortunately, the result is still influenced by psycho-physiological factors during the visual experiment which are beyond our control:

- observer-dependent features varying from one person to another which include eyesight impairments, variations in anatomy, perceptual and motor skills, sex, race, and so forth; and
- observer status-dependent properties for each particular person varying from one day to another which include psycho-physiological status, drug, climate influence, and so forth.

The identification of basic phenomena interfering with the relationship between scan-paths and visual perception information flow took three years and needed the analysis of various results of visual experiments. Another challenge was the development of scan-path pre-processing software requiring minimum operator assistance in recognition of desired trace features.

Figure 6.15. Example of an expert perceptual strategy over a 12-lead ECG plot (CSE-Mo-001); the circle diameter represents the foveation time

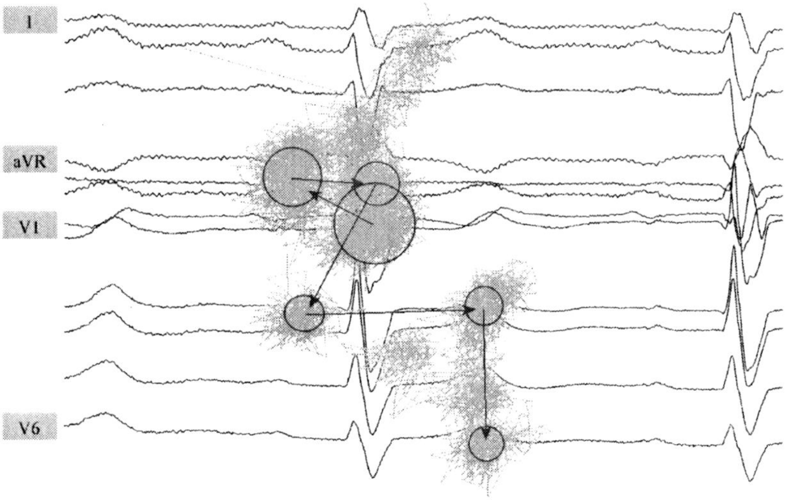

Figure 6.16. Example of a student perceptual strategy over a 12-lead ECG plot (CSE-Mo-021); the circle diameter represents the foveation time

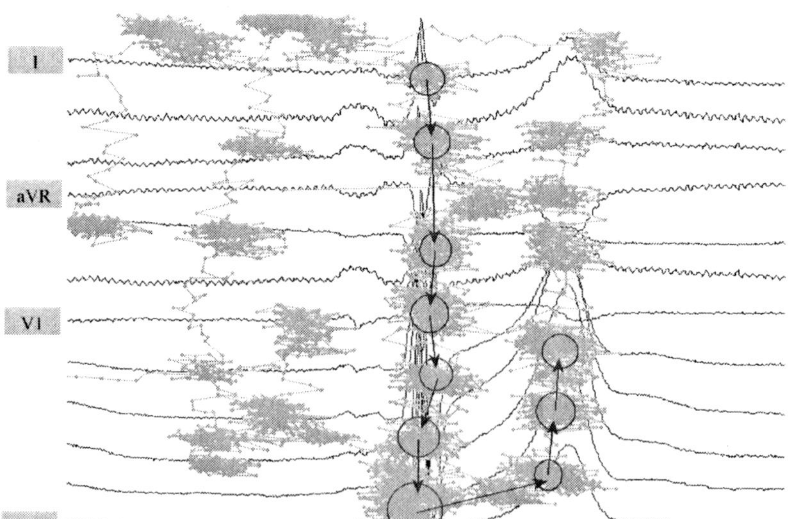

The scan-path-dedicated signal processing, interpretation, and statistics revealed many differences between cardiology experts and untrained observers concerning ECG inspection methods and perceptual strategies. The most discriminative parameters of the scan-path are as follows:

- Attention density is a significantly higher variability in the expert group.
- The number of foveation points is lower in the expert group, which is similar to the results we obtained with the 'fast reading' people in one of our previous research studies (Augustyniak, 2006).
- The distance between the foveation points is higher in the experts group.
- Total scan-path duration with reference to the last significant foveation point is shorter, indicating that the expert is first searching for the most important.

All these parameters indicate a very precise and consistent way of searching information with regard to the experts. Moreover, the high variation of focus time and distance for the first foveation points suggests hierarchical information gathering which reflects the parallel decisive process.

This experiment demonstrates that the common belief about irregular medical data distributions is fully justified with regard to electrocardiograms. With the use of scan-path analysis, local data distribution can be effectively measured and expressed as attention density.

Applications: The Objective Assessment of Personal Interpretation Skills

The objective assessment of personal interpretation skills for a given class of scenes is a very promising field of scan-path application. A comparison of certain parameters of scan-paths significantly discriminates the expert and student groups, highlights experience-justified differences, and provides a quantitative measure of observation skills. When using this approach to interpret the ECG, differences in fixation time (expressed as a percentage of the total observation time) were found within the QRS wave (38% with experts, 26% with students) and within the T-P section (14% with experts, 25% with students). Both groups showed irregularity in the fixation time per ECG plot time unit, however with regard to the experts it varies in range from 21 s/s at the QRS to 1.9 s/s at the baseline, and in students only from 16 s/s to 3.9 s/s, respectively.

With reference to the perception of a typical image by an untrained observer, some features in the scene are particularly conspicuous. The example given in Tadeusiewicz and Ogiela (2004) shows the edges as elements attracting much attention. In the electrocardiogram, although the QRS complex having the highest contribution of high-frequency components is at the same time the most conspicuous for both groups of observers, the P wave is hardly distinguishable from the baseline and the very smooth T wave is lower, but not far from the QRS result. For these waves, the information is more difficult to extract and visual pursuit requires more time.

For the untrained group of students in front of the ECG plot, we found some typical relationships for the scan-path and the local quantitative features of the scene (e.g., the frequency). Similar relationships are significantly weaker within the group of experts. The difference in perception between students and experts can only be explained by perceptual and oculo-motoric habits developed during years of practice. A particular difference was in the QRS wave foveation time, which was up to 50% longer by experts than by students. This indicates that the information represented in the QRS shape is important for a diagnostic decision.

Scan-path analysis provides us not only with an image-assessment tool, but also observer-assessment one. Expert and student eyeball trajectories, captured during the visual inspection of the record, provide reliable quantitative measures of observer interpretation skills. Similar visual experiment-based methods may be applicable to other signals and images.

REFERENCES

Akay, M. (1995). Wavelets in biomedical engineering. *Annals of Biomedical Engineering, 23,* 531-542.

Aldroubi, H., & Feichtinger, J. (1998). Exact iterative reconstruction algorithm for multivariate irregularly sampled functions in spline-like spaces: The Lp theory. *Proceedings of the American Mathematical Society, 126*(9), 2677–2686.

Aloimonos, Y., Weiss, I., & Bandyodaphyay, A. (1987). Active vision. *Proceedings of the 1st ICCV* (pp. 35-54), London.

Augustyniak, P. (2003). Time-frequency modelling and discrimination of noise in the electrocardiogram. *Physiological Measurement, 24*(3), 753-767.

Augustyniak, P. (2006). Scanpath analysis in objective evaluation of reading skills. *Proceedings of the Symposium on Medical Informatics and Technologies* (pp. 261-266).

Baddeley, A. (1986). *Working memory.* Oxford: Clarendon Press.

Bailey, J. J., Berson, A. S., Garson, A. et al. (1990). Recommendations for standardization and specifications in automated electrocardiography: Bandwidth and digital signal processing. *Circulation, 81,* 730-739.

Bajcsy, R. (1988). Active perception. *Proceedings of IEEE 76* (pp. 996-1005).

Ballard, D. H., Hayhoe, M. M., & Pelz, J. B. (1995). Memory representations in natural tasks. *Journal of Cognitive Neuroscience, 7*(1), 68-82.

Becker, W. (1989). Metrics. In M. E. Goldburg & R. H. Wurtz (Eds.), *The neurobiology of saccadic eye movements.* Englewood Cliffs, NJ: Elsevier Science.

Becker, W. (1991). Saccades. In R.H.S. Carpenter (Ed.), *Vision and visual dysfunction* vol. 8: *Eye movements.* Boca Raton, FL: CRC Press.

Bilgin, A., Marcellin, M. W., & Altbach, M. I. (2003). Compression of electrocardiogram signals using JPEG2000. *IEEE Transactions on Biomedical Engineering, 50*(4), 833-840.

Boccignone, G. (2001). An information-theory approach to active vision. *Proceedings of the 11th International Conference on Image Analysis and Processing.*

Bradie, B. (1996). Wavelet packet-based compression of single lead ECG. *IEEE Transactions on Biomedical Engineering, 43,* 493-501.

Calderbank, A. R., Daubechies, I., Sweldens, W., & Yeo, B. L. (1997). Lossless image compression using integer to integer wavelet transforms *Proceedings of the IEEE International Conference of Image Processing* (vol. 1, pp. 596599).

Carpenter, R. H. S. (1988). *Movements of the eye.* London: Pion Press.

Chen, J., & Itoh, S. (1998). A wavelet transform-based ECG compression method guaranteeing desired signal quality *IEEE Transactions on BME, 45,* 1414-1419.

Cohen, A., & Zigel, Y. (1998). Compression of multichannel ECG through multichannel long-term prediction. *IEEE Engineering in Medicine and Biology, 17*(1), 109-115.

Cox, J. R., Nolle, F. M., Fozzard, H. A., & Oliver, G. G. (1968). AZTEC, a preprocessing program for real-time ECG rhythm analysis. *IEEE Transactions on Biomedical Engineering, 15,* 128-129.

CSE Working Party. (1985). Recommendations for measurement standards in quantitative electrocardiography. *European Heart Journal, 6,* 815-825.

Daubechies, I. (1992). *Ten lectures on wavelets.* CBMS-NSF Conference Series in Applied Mathematics.

Dick, A. O. (1980). *Instrument scanning and controlling: Using eye-movement data to understand pilot behavior and strategies.* NASA CR 3306.

Duda, K., Turcza, P., & Zieliński, T. P. (2001). Lossless ECG compression with lifting wavelet transform. *Proceedings of the IEEE Instrumentation and Measurement Technology Conference* (pp. 640-644).

Furth, B., & Perez, A. (1988). An adaptive real-time ECG compression algorithm with variable threshold. *IEEE Transactions on Biomedical Engineering, 35*(6), 489-494.

Hamilton, D. J., Thomson, D. C., & Sandham, W. A. (1995). ANN compression of morphologically similar ECG complexes. *Medical and Biological Engineering and Computing, 33,* 841-843.

Hamilton, P. S. (1993). Adaptive compression of the ambulatory electrocardiogram. *Biomedical Instrumentation & Technology,* vol. 27 No. 1 (January), 56-63

Hamilton, P. S., & Tompkins, W. J. (1991). Compression of the ambulatory ECG by average beat subtraction and residual differencing. *IEEE Transactions on Biomedical Engineering, 38,* 253-259.

Hilton, M. (1997). Wavelet and wavelet packet compression of electrocardiograms. *IEEE Transactions on Biomedical Engineering, 44,* 394-402.

Hitch, G. J., & Baddeley, A. (1976). Verbal reasoning and working memory. *Quarterly Journal of Experimental Psychology, 28,* 603-621.

Hsia, P. W. (1989). Electrocardiographic data compression using precoding consecutive QRS information. *IEEE Transactions on Biomedical Engineering, 36,* 465-468.

Irwin, D. E. (1991). Information integration across saccadic eye movements. *Cognitive Psychology, 23,* 420-456.

Irwin, D. E. (1992). Visual memory within and across fixations. In K. Raynor (Ed.), *Eye movements and visual cognition; scene perception and reading.* New York: Springer-Verlag.

Ishijiama, M. (1993). Fundamentals of the decision of optimum factors in the ECG data compression. *IEICE Transactions Information and Systems, E76-D*(12), 1398-1403.

Ishijiama, M., Shin, S., Hostetter, G., & Sklansky, J. (1983). Scan-along polygonal approximation for data compression of electrocardiograms. *IEEE Transactions on Biomedical Engineering, 30*(11), 723-729.

Iwata, A., Nagasaka, Y., & Suzumura, N. (1990). Data compression of ECG using neural network for digital Holter monitor. *IEEE Engineering in Medicine and Biology Magazine*, (September), 53-57.

Jalaleddine, S. M., & Hutchens, C. G. (1990). SAIES—a new ECG data compression algorithm. *Journal of Clinical Engineering, 15*(1), 45-51.

Jalaleddine, S. M., Hutchens, C. G., Strattan, R. D., & Coberly, W. A. (1990). ECG data compression techniques—a unified approach. *IEEE Transactions on Biomedical Engineering, 37*(4), 329-343.

Jayant, N. S., & Noll, P. (1984). *Digital coding of waveforms.* Englewood Cliffs, NJ: Prentice Hall.

Karlsson, S. (1967). Representation of ECG records by Karhunen-Loève expansions. *Proceedings of the 7th International Conference on Medical and Biological Engineering* (p. 105).

Kowacki, L., & Augustyniak, P. (2007). Implementation of wavelet compression of the electrocariogram in signal processor. *Journal of Medical Informatics and Technologies.*vol. 11 pp. 147–153

Kowler, E. (1990). The role of visual and cognitive processes in the control of eye movement. In K. Kowler (Ed.), *Eye movements and their role in visual and cognitive processes.* Englewood Cliffs, NJ: Elsevier Science.

Kuklinski, W. S. (1983). Fast Walsh transform data-compression algorithm: ECG application. *Medical and Biological Engineering and Computing, 21,* 465-472.

Kuzume, K., & Niijima, K. (2000). Design of optimal lifting wavelet filters for data compression. *Proceedings of the IEEE, 88*(11).

Lamberti, C., & Coccia, P. (1988). ECG data compression for ambulatory device. *Computers in Cardiology, 15,* 171-178.

Lee, H., Cheng, Q., & Thakor, N. (1987). ECG waveform analysis by significant point extraction. *Computers and Biomedical Research, 20,* 410-427.

Levine, M. D. (1985). *Vision in man and machine.* New York: McGraw-Hill.

Lu, Z., Kim, D. Y., & Pearlman, W. A. (2000). Wavelet compression of ECG signals by the set partitioning in hierarchical trees algorithm. *IEEE Transactions on Biomedical Engineering, 47*(7), 849-856.

Macfarlane, P. W., & Lawrie, T. D. V. (Eds.). (1989). *Comprehensive electrocardiology. Theory and practice in health and disease.* Oxford: Pergamon Press.

Mallat, S. G. (1989). A theory for multiresolution signal decomposition: The wavelet representation. *IEEE Transactions on Pattern Analysis and Machine Intelligence, 11*(7).

Mallat, S. G. (1996). *A wavelet tour of signal processing.* New York: Academic Press.

Miaou, S.-G., Chen, S.-T., & Chao, S.-N. (2005). Wavelet-based lossy-to-lossless ECG compression in a unified vector quantization framework. *IEEE Transactions on Biomedical Engineering, 52*(3), 539-545.

Miaou, S.-G., & Lin, C.-L. (2002). A quality-on-demand algorithm for wavelet-based compression of electrocardiogram signals. *IEEE Transactions on Biomedical Engineering, 49*(3), 233-239.

Morlet, D. (1986). *Contribution a l'analyse automatique des electrocardiogrammes—algorithmes de localisation, classification et delimitation precise des ondes dans le systeme de Lyon.* PhD thesis, INSA-Lyon, France.

Nave, G., & Cohen, A. (1993). ECG compression using long term prediction. *IEEE Transactions on Biomedical Engineering, 40,* 877-885.

Nikolaev, N., & Gotchev, A. (1998). De-noising of ECG signals using wavelet shrinkage with time-frequency dependant threshold. *Proceedings of the European Signal Processing Conference* (pp. 2449-2453), Island of Rhodes, Greece.

Nikolaev, N., & Gotchev, A. (2000). ECG signal denoising using wavelet domain Wiener filtering. *Proceedings of the European Signal Processing Conference* (pp. 51-54), Tampere, Finland.

Nikolaev, N., Gotchev, A., Egiazarian, K., & Nikolov, Z. (2001). Suppression of electromyogram interference on the electrocardiogram by transform domain denoising. *Medical and Biological Engineering and Computing, 39,* 649-655.

Nikolaev, N., Nikolov, Z., Gotchev, A., & Egiazarian, K. (2000). Wavelet domain Wiener filtering for ECG denoising using an improved signal estimate. *Proceedings of the International Conference on Acoustics, Speech, and Signal Processing* (pp. 2210-2213), Istanbul, Turkey.

Noton, D., & Stark, L. (1971). Eye movements and visual perception. *Scientific American, 224,* 34-43.

Nygaard, R., Melnikov, G., & Katsaggelos, A. K. (2001). A rate distortion optimal ECG coding algorithm *IEEE Transactions on Biomedical Engineering, 48*(1), 28-40.

Ober, J. K., Ober, J. J., Malawski, M., Skibniewski, W., Przedpelska-Ober, E., & Hryniewiecki, J. (2002). Monitoring pilot eye movements during the combat flights□the white box. *Biocybernetics and Biomedical Engineering, 22*(2-3), 241-264.

Pahlm, O., Börjesson, P., & Werner, O. (1979). Compact digital storage of ECGs. *Computer Programs in Biomedicine, 9,* 293-300.

Pashler, H., Carrier, M., & Hoffman, J. (1993). Saccadic eye movements and dual-task interference. *Quarterly Journal of Experimental Psychology, 46A*(1), 51-82.

Paul, J., Reddy, M., & Kumar, V. (2000). A transform domain SVD filter for suppression of muscle noise artifacts in exercise ECGs. *IEEE Transactions on Biomedical Engineering, 47,* 654-662.

Peden, J. (1982). ECG data compression: Some practical considerations. In J. Paul, M. Jordan, M. Ferguson-Pell, & B. Andrews (Eds.), *Computing in Medicine.* Macmillan, London.

Pelz, J. B., & Canosa, R. (2001). Oculomotor behavior and perceptual strategies in complex tasks. *Vision Research, 41,* 3587-3596.

Ramakrishnan, A.G., & Supratim, S. (1997). ECG coding by wavelet-based linear prediction. *IEEE Transactions on BME, 44*(12).

Reddy, B. R. S., & Murthy, I. S. N. (1986). ECG data compression using Fourier descriptors. *IEEE Transactions on Biomedical Engineering, 33,* 428-434.

Reza, A., Moghaddam, A., & Nayebi, K. (2001). A two dimensional wavelet packet approach for ECG compression. *Proceedings of the International Symposium on Signal Processing Application* (pp. 226-229).

Ruttiman, U. E., & Pipberger, H. V. (1979). Compression of the ECG by prediction or interpolation and entropy encoding. *IEEE Transactions on Biomedical Engineering, 26,* 613-623.

Salvucci, D. D., & Anderson, J. R. (2001). Automated eye-movement protocol analysis. *Human-Computer Interaction, 16*, 39-86.

Skavenski, A. A. (1990). Eye movement and visual localization of objects in space. In E. Kowler (Ed.), *Eye movements and their role in visual and cognitive processes.* Englewood Cliffs, NJ: Elsevier.

Swain, M. J., Kahn, R. E., & Ballard, D. H. (1992). Low resolution cues for guiding saccadic eye movements. *Proceedings of the Computer Vision and Pattern Recognition Conference,* Urbana, IL.

Tadeusiewicz, R., Izworski, A., & Majewski, J. (1993). *Biometry.* Kraków: AGH.

Tadeusiewicz, R., & Ogiela, M. R. (2004). Medical image understanding technology. *Studies in Fuzziness and Soft Computing,* 156. Berlin: Springer-Verlag.

Tai, S. C. (1991). SLOPE—a real time ECG data compression. *Medical and Biological Engineering and Computing, 29,* 175-179.

Tai, S. C. (1992). ECG data compression by corner detection. *Medical and Biological Engineering and Computing, 30,* 584-590.

Tai, S.-C., Sun, C.-C., & Yan, W.-C. (2005). A 2-D ECG compression method based on wavelet transform and modified SPIHT. *IEEE Transactions on Biomedical Engineering, 52*(6), 999-1008.

Takahashi, K., Takeuchi, S., & Ohsawa, N. (1993). Performance evaluation of ECG compression algorithms by reconstruction error and diagnostic response. *IEICE Transactions on Information and Systems, E76-D*(12), 1404-1410.

Uchiyama, T., Akazawa, K., & Sasamori, A. (1993). Data compression of ambulatory ECG by using multi-template matching and residual coding. *IEICE Transactions on Information and Systems, E76-D*(12), 1419-1424.

Unser, M., & Zerubia, J. A. (1998). Generalized sampling theory without bandlimiting constraints. *Transactions on Circuits and Systems–II: Analog and Digital Signal Processing, 45*(8), 959-969.

Viviani, P. (1990). Eye movements in visual search: Cognitive, perceptual, and motor control aspects. In E. Kowler (Ed.), *Eye movements and their role in visual and cognitive processes. Reviews of oculomotor research V4* (pp. 353-383). Englewood Cliffs, NJ: Elsevier.

Willems, J. L. (1990). *Common standards for quantitative electrocardiography: 10th CSE progress report.* Leuven, Belgium: ACCO.

Willems, J. L., Arnaud, P., van Bemmel, J. H. et al. (1985a). Assessment of the performance of electrocardiographic computer programs with the use of a reference database. *Circulation, 71,* 523-534.

Willems, J. L., Arnaud, P., van Bemmel, J. H. et al. (1985b). Establishment of a reference library for evaluating computer ECG measurement programs. *Computers and Biomedical Research, 18,* 439-457.

Willems, J. L., Zywietz, C., Arnaud, P. et al. (1987). Influence of noise on wave boundary recognition by ECG measurement programs. Recommendations for preprocessing. *Computers and Biomedical Research, 20,* 543-562.

Yarbus, A. F. (1967). *Eye movements and vision.* New York: Plenum Press.

Zigel, Y. (1998, August). *ECG signal compression.* MSc thesis, Ben-Gurion University, Beer-Sheva, Israel. Retrieved from http://www.ee.bgu.ac.il/~spl/publication

Zigel, Y., & Cohen, A. (1998). ECG signal compression using analysis by synthesis coding and diagnostic distortion. *IEEE Transactions on Biomedical Engineering, 47*(10), 1308-1316.

Zigel, Y., & Cohen, A. (1999). On the optimal distortion measure for ECG compression. *Proceedings of the European Medical and Biological Engineering Conference.*

Zigel, Y., & Cohen, A. (2000). ECG signal compression using analysis by synthesis coding and diagnostic distortion. *IEEE Transactions on Biomedical Engineering, 47*(10), 1308-1316.

Zigel, Y., Cohen, A., Abu-Ful, A., Wagshal, A., & Katz, A. (1997). Analysis by synthesis ECG signal compression. *Computers in Cardiology, 24,* 279-282.

Zigel, Y., Cohen, A., & Katz, A. (1996). A diagnostic meaningful distortion measure for ECG compression. *Proceedings of the 19th Convention of Electrical & Electronic Engineering in Israel* (pp. 117-120).

Chapter VII
Optimization of ECG Procedures Chain for Reliability and Data Reduction

This chapter deals with various aspects of improvements in the typical ECG processing chain. Particular procedures designed for the computation of specified diagnostic results are usually developed in long research projects and rarely disclosed as a source code. Without challenging well-established calculation methods, we aimed at optimizing the data flow and minimizing the propagation of computational errors. These issues are of particular importance in telemedical applications because the ECG interpretation process is distributed in the network and partly unsupervised.

The ECG signal contains some cardiac-independent components and represents heart activity with limited reliability. The process is based on many heuristics, expected signal features, and general knowledge, and thus it implies an additional uncertainty factor. In this chapter we present the analysis of global uncertainty of the ECG diagnostic result and its dependence on the configuration of procedures in the processing chain. We also reveal sources of errors and discuss selected methods, aiming at minimizing their influence.

The ECG interpretation is investigated with reference to data volume at particular stages of the processing chain. In this respect, the interpretation is similar to the data compression, but specific enough to reduce the raw record to a few bytes of patient status description. The data volume is always reduced to a considerable extent from the recorded signal to the final diagnostic decision. However, in distributed systems sharing the interpretation tasks between distant devices, it is interesting to reduce the data volume as much as possible at the beginning of the processing. This chapter summarizes the error propagation and data reduction analyses performed for many possible configurations of the processing chain. An optimal solution is proposed as a result of the authors' original research.

ESTIMATION OF THE RELIABILITY OF PARTICULAR ECG PROCEDURES AND ERROR PROPAGATION IN THE INTERPRETATION CHAIN

Dependencies in the ECG Interpretation Chain

Various implementations of automatic ECG interpretation are currently widespread in many devices, ranging from large servers to small wearable cardiomonitors. The appearance of autonomous recorders for real-time monitoring and interpretation, communicating over a wireless digital link (Chiarugi et al., 2003; Pinna, Maestri, Gobbi, La Rovere, & Scanferlato, 2003; Banitsas, Georgiadis, Tachakra, & Cavouras, 2004), necessitated new prerequisites for the interpretive software architecture. For this purpose we studied several example ECG processing chains to highlight and catalog the main dependencies between the procedures, and to become aware of the scale of the error propagation problem (Table 7.1).

The above qualitative survey demonstrates the complexity of the information flow and approaches mutual dependencies within the processing chain. These relations helped us to follow not only the information but also the error propagation pathways.

The Measurement of Diagnostic Procedure Uncertainty

The first aspect to be considered with respect to the uncertainty is whether diagnostic reliability is directly affecting interpretation autonomy and the need for external supervision. The second aspect is the local data reduction ratio, which is the main condition for maintaining the communication service expenses within the margins of acceptance.

Despite studies based on algorithms from various manufacturers (IBM, 1974; HP, 1994; DRG, 1995; Nihon Kohden, 2001; Cardiosoft, 2005), all the investigated applications follow a very similar software architecture originating from their version histories or the upgradeable modules concept. This functional-growth architecture is very convenient for manufacturers tailoring software for diverse users from the

Table 7.1. Error propagation and the mutual influences of result quality between principal ECG interpretation procedures

Signal Quality Assessment	The purpose of signal quality assessment is twofold: • In systems with flexible contributions of ECG channels in subsequent interpretation procedures, the ranking of individual channel quality estimates is a background for channel weighting. • In all systems, the average quality estimate of best channels is used for the assessment of the overall quality of diagnostic results. In the case of very poor signals, most systems assume that no ECG input is present, inhibiting the procedure's ability to adapt and disable the output. This quality assessment procedure uses common features of the ECG signal like global-to-local amplitude ratio, slope of power spectrum decay, percentage of monotonic sections, number of isolated signal accelerations and decelerations, and so forth. These parameters have poor discriminative value if used separately, but the aggregated decision is usually reliable enough to identify the ECGs correctly. The main disadvantage of this approach is high correlation of reliability and computational complexity resulting in processing huge amounts of raw data. Therefore, the implementation of precise signal quality assessment procedures are limited to stationary powerful systems. A solution for mobile interpretive systems, which partly overcomes the problem, is the feedback from the QRS detector and classifier confirming the amplitude and temporal position of a heartbeat representation in the signal. The reliability of the signal quality assessment is still poor in the presence of some rare, but important cardiac abnormalities: • *Atrial Flutter or Fibrillation*—Continuous P wave-like trains of small amplitude may easily be confused with noise originating from muscles. • *Ventricular Fibrillation*—Continuous sine wave-like signals without acceleration, which is characteristic for a spontaneous synchronized ventricle action with the addition of noise caused by patient motion, may be confused with poor electrode contact.

continued on following page

Table 7.1. continued

Pacemaker Pulse Detection	The number of remotely monitored pacemaker users has recently increased to a considerable amount of 10% of all Holter recordings. Long-term monitoring has been found useful for supervising pacemaker functionality with regard to both hardware and software levels. Concerning those patients, it is estimated that on average only during about 10% of the monitoring time, heart activity is driven by the pacemaker; nevertheless pacemaker pulse detection is very important for the correct identification of the heart rhythm and the appropriate diagnostic description of the patient. Unlike the endogenous rhythm, the pacemaker pulse is artificially generated and surprisingly causes several technical problems caused mainly by the lack of direct connection between the implanted device and the recording system. The pacemaker pulse is very short (30-500 μs) and the amplitude adapts to the electrical sensitivity of the heart muscle tissue. Two solutions are commonly used in advanced recorders to correctly capture the pacing spike: • signal over-sampling up to 100kHz followed by time-amplitude discrimination of pacemaker pulses and the decimation of all the remaining signals like muscle-originated responses or endogenous electrical discharge; and • hardware detection latch circuits triggered by the fast rising slope of the pacemaker pulse and insensitive to all the other components recorded from the leads; their status is checked and reset together with the signal sampling sequence. Similarly, the uncertainty of pacemaker pulse detection from surface ECGs may also be caused by external electromagnetic interferences (like power switching electronics). These misinterpretations may be partly limited by the use of additional pacemaker recording channels with electrodes positioned individually according to the pacing lead of the pacemaker. The consequence of a missed pacemaker pulse is the false-positive report of pacemaker failure (Failure to Pace or Failure to Capture) and the erroneous classification of the resultant heartbeat as endogenous. Usually a cluster of these false paced beats can easily be identified (manually and by automation) due to very high beat-to-beat similarity. In the case of extra detection of non-existent pacemaker pulse, the system reports oversensitivity of the pacemaker and non-effective pacing. The false pacemaker can easily be detected by the absence of consequences in the recorded action potential.

continued on following page

Table 7.1. continued

Heartbeat Detection	The heartbeat detection procedure is the first step in each automated ECG interpretation. Heartbeat detection accuracy determines the quality of the whole process, since missing or extra heartbeats influence rhythm and contour analysis and all principal diagnostic parameters. The heartbeat is usually detected by the presence of the highest essential electrical phenomenon in the record—the QRS complex representing the ventricles contraction. The algorithms in use favor features that are common to the signal: • high acceleration and deceleration, • specific frequency ranges, and • expected time intervals, to transform the single or weighted multi-channel ECG record to a time function (referred to as a detection function), quantitatively representing the selected features. Such functions are expected to have: • irrelevant values when no heartbeat is present, and • a single significant maximum within the confines of the QRS complex. The detection function is a background for further processing aimed at a final binary result, which is related to the time coordinate of a sample when the QRS complex is present. This coordinate is the first approach of the fiducial point; however due to detector's flexibility, the accuracy of its final position is influenced by the content of preceding record strips. In the course of further processing, the precision of the detection point position may be significantly improved with use of approximation techniques. To compensate for heart rate and signal amplitude variations, rhythm type diversity, and so forth, the calculation of the detection function and the thresholding of its values contains a history of adaptive factors. These variables aim at maintaining a balance between artifact-immunity based on the expected similarity of consecutive heartbeats and the responsiveness to sudden changes in the cardiac action.

continued on following page

Table 7.1. continued

Baseline Estimation	Baseline level is a voltage reference value for all amplitude-based measurements in the electrocardiogram, in particular for ST segment evaluations. The commonly accepted rule defines the baseline as a PQ segment representing the stimulus transmitted through the atrio-ventricular (AV) node; however, definitions based on T-P segments are also in use. The advantage of the first approach is the reduced speed of stimulus conduction in the AV node and its close location to the geometrical center of the heart. The PQ segment is rarely a true iso-electric section because of noise and accompanying bio-electric phenomena. Its length may vary on a beat-to-beat basis due to atrio-ventricular desynchronization or it may be absent in the case of the ventricular rhythm. Fortunately, these cardiac abnormalities also exclude ST segment evaluations, performed usually only in the sections of normal sinus rhythm. With regard to other diagnostic parameters, the imprecise estimation of the baseline is well compensated by the algorithms (e.g., wave border delimitations) and the local baseline is computed instead (e.g., QT dispersions) or no baseline information is needed at all (e.g., rhythm classification).
Heart Rate Estimation	The basic frequency of heartbeats, referred to as the heart rate, is the first diagnostic parameter usually computed even by the simplest interpretation algorithm. The value is immune to signal quality variation as far as QRS detection is correctly made. To avoid the influence of false detections, the output value is usually averaged from seven consecutive RR intervals, excluding the longest and the two shortest of them. The heart rate is in turn one of the principal inputs for other diagnostic procedures like rhythm classification, arrhythmia detection, and the analysis of heart rate variability (HRV).

continued on following page

Table 7.1. continued

Heartbeat Classification	The sections of the signal representing the ventricle contraction are classified according to their shape. The classification aims at determining the number of internal stimulating centers and their contribution to the rhythm statistic. With regard to the rhythm analysis, the main borderline separates the atrial beats, all having one dominant shape, triggered by the sino-atrial (SA) node, and ventricular beats having multiple shapes corresponding to the trigger centers, which in frequent cases are distributed in various locations in the ventricles. The heartbeat classification is prone to input noise and artifacts because the correlation of the cluster representation and the classified beat is used as a membership condition. Variations in the baseline level are compensated by removing the mean value of the selection. Possible inaccuracy in fiducial point positioning is corrected with the use of the multiple time-shifted correlation attempts. Classification errors have severe consequences only if heartbeats that are different with respect to their physiological background are merged in one cluster. This causes missing their differences as potential carriers of information about abnormalities. Conversely, multiplying clusters of similar background only influences the general complexity of the processing.
Wave Measurement	Waves P, QRS, and T are representative of the heart cycle event. Because the diagnostic meaning of time dependencies is fundamental for the assessment of heart activity based on the surface electrical recordings, the precise delimitation of wave borders is a key point in the overall diagnosis. These parameters, usually represented by five variables—P-onset, P-end, QRS-onset, QRS-end, and T-end—are referenced in databases for diagnostic quality assessment (such as CSE; Willems, 1990; Laguna, Jané, & Caminal, 1994), and the maximum acceptable differences in the corresponding intervals are specified by the IEC standard for interpretive software (see Chapter II, IEC60601-2-51). Wave measurement reliability is limited by signal quality. Instability and high noise, low-signal amplitude, abrupt changes of the baseline level, and so forth imply rough errors of wave border computation, while various shapes of the waves usually cause small differences. Wave measurement precision influences rhythm classification, ST segment assessment, and contour analysis—the principal diagnostic procedures typical for a 12-lead ECG interpretation.

continued on following page

Table 7.1. continued

Axis Determination	Determination of the main electrical axis of the heart is usually interpreted as the heart's position and significantly varies with physical training or during delivery. Short-term variability of the atrial depolarization axes (the P wave) and the relative P and QRS axes is one of the factors determining normal sinus rhythm, various atrial rhythms, and the conducting volume of the heart ventricles (QRS complex). The re-polarization axis variability (T wave) is often used to assess the influence of the drugs on the electric tissue at the cellular level. A significant correlation with the ventricular tachycardia is used to predict the VT from the T wave alternans. Axis determination is highly dependent on the signal quality, and the influence of muscular noise may be eliminated by the interpolation of expected wave shapes in the 2D or 3D space at the cost of computation complexity. Artifacts or baseline wandering are the reasons for errors in determining the maximum time-point in the heart vector module, and consequently bad orientation of the estimated axis. The other factor is the accurate placement of electrodes, because the axis determining algorithms uses assumptions from the standard Einthoven triangle.
Dominant Rhythm Detection	To classify the rhythm as a normal sinus rhythm (i.e., sino-atrial rhythm), four essential conditions must be satisfied: (1) the presence of a single P wave within given temporal confines, (2) stable P-R interval lengths, (3) a stable P wave axis, and (4) stable differences in the P and QRS axis. Any departure from these conditions is interpreted as a sign of abnormality. Whether the first two conditions are satisfied, the rhythm is classified as supraventricular or ventricular otherwise. These two rhythm origins are essential for arrhythmia detection, and misinterpretation of any single beat results in erroneous arrhythmia detection. The unstable length of the P-R interval is a sign of probable atrio-ventricular de-synchronization, which means two independent stimulus sources for atries and ventricles contraction. Further signal processing aimed at a detailed localization of a stimulus source with the use of P and QRS axis variations is performed only in the most sophisticated interpretive systems.

continued on following page

Table 7.1. continued

Arrhythmia Detection	Arrhythmias are detected as predefined patterns of stimulus sequences with given conditions for the RR interval. They are representative of mutual influence of stimulus sources active in the heart. The presence and frequency of arrhythmia provides us with information as to the extent of the electrical conduction abnormalities in the heart and determines patient diagnosis. Arrhythmia detection is based on logical operations of selective heartbeat counting and thus is a very accurate procedure. However, it is significantly influenced by heartbeat detection accuracy, P wave and QRS-complex borders detection, and the determination of the electrical axes of these waves. Moreover, the priority of particular arrhythmia types is undefined. Because some of them are mutually exclusive, computer programs may behave differently (e.g., a sequence SVSVSVV could be interpreted as a bigeminy or as a ventricular couplet).

same bricks (Bonner & Schwetman, 1968; Balda, Diller, Deardorff, Doue, & Hsieh, 1977; Abenstien, 1978; Tompkins, 1980; Abenstein & Thakor, 1981; Tompkins, Tompkins, & Weisner, 1983; Daskalov, Dotsinsky, & Christov, 1998; Paoletti & Marchesi, 2004). Nevertheless, that approach neither optimizes the diagnostic reliability nor effectively reduces the datastream.

Our research investigates the existing interpretive software for electrocardiographs and generalizes rules concerning the optimal architecture for satisfying both previously mentioned criteria: a high data reduction ratio and high immunity to errors at the subsequent stages of the processing chain.

Over the course of the research, we expected to identify the areas for improvement of wearable ECG recorder performance brought to light by the structural rearrangement of the interpretive software. Therefore, we consider diagnostic subroutines as black boxes and never attempt to modify the interpretive algorithms or their mathematical foundations. In the experimental part of the research, we used standard ECG databases—MIT-BIH (Moody, 1993) and CSE (Willems, 1990)—recommended for testing of the software performance and a standard interpretive software designed to be embedded in a stand-alone ECG machine. In order to estimate the probability of each function call, we assumed that particular heart diseases are proportionally represented in the database.

In Figure 7.1, a typical data flow diagram is presented for the basic ECG interpretation process, with many references to the raw signal. Certainly, the software architecture rearrangements are constrained by the logical flow of ECG diagnostic procedures. In some rare cases the data processing chain must follow a specified order, first providing general information (e.g., a heartbeat was detected) and then more precise details (e.g., morphology types or wave lengths). Within these constraints the reduction-effective and frequently used procedures were identified in the first experiment.

The aim of the first experiment was to estimate values of two statistical parameters for each interpretive procedure:

δ—outcome relative inaccuracy (%), and
ε—probability of false outcome (%).

In order to favor more frequent, more accurate, and more reduction-effective functions in access to the datastreams, each procedure was attributed a priority level derived from estimated statistical parameters (Table 7.2).

Figure 7.1. Typical data flow diagram for the basic ECG interpretation process

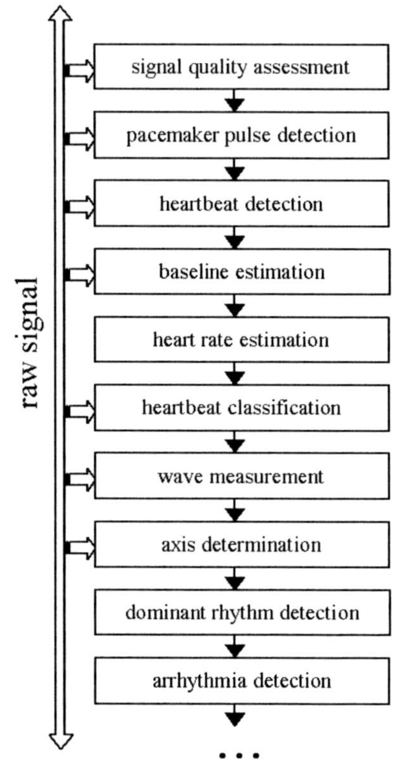

Figure 7.2. An excerpt of the ECG processing chain block diagram with a statistical description of the procedure and signal quality

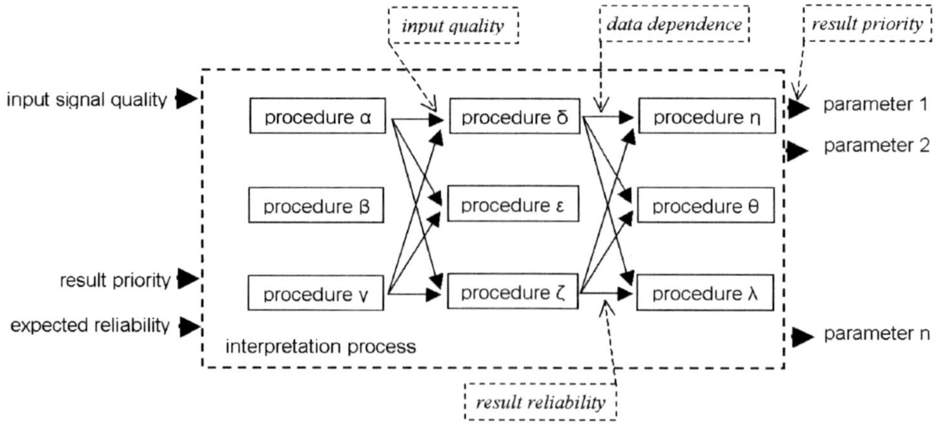

Table 7.2. Basic ECG interpretation procedures, their statistical parameters, and attributed priority levels

Procedure Name	Statistical Parameters		Priority Level
	δ	ε	
signal quality assessment	10	3,3	1
pacemaker pulse detection	<1	8,3	4
heartbeat detection	1,5	2,5	2
baseline estimation	3	<1	3
heart rate estimation	<1	<1	1
heartbeat classification	10	3	1
wave measurement	3	5	2
axis determination	3	5	3
dominant rhythm detection	0	8,5	1
arrhythmia detection	0	10	2
...			

ESTIMATION OF EXPECTED DATAFLOW IN THE CONTEXT OF DISEASE PROBABILITY

The expected dataflow may be estimated by two principal factors:

1. the standard data flow characteristic to each procedure, and
2. the estimated usage frequency corresponding to the probability of the supported disease.

An Example of a Data Flow Characteristic

The first step in the investigation concerned the example ECG interpretation source code and was aimed at approaching the standard dataflow in the inputs and outputs of each procedure in the context of the procedure calls in the interpretation tree (Figure 7.3, Table 7.3).

The comparison of the input and output sizes yields the theoretical datastream compression ratio for each procedure single call. Two remarks are worthy of mention as implied by the analysis of data in Table 7.3.:

Figure 7.3 Root of the example ECG interpretation tree

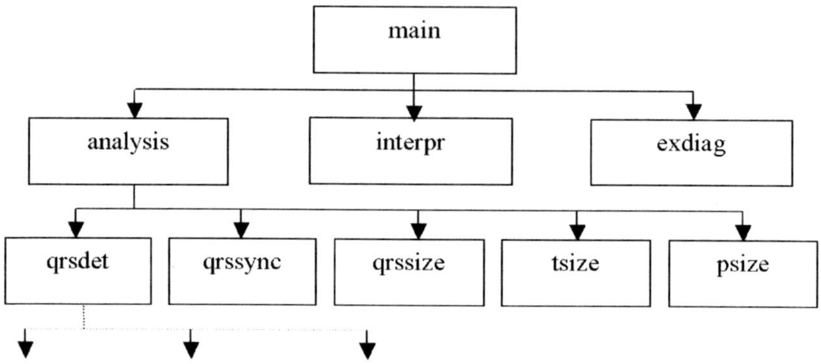

1. For some procedures the value of the compression ratio is quite high.
2. The resulting compression ratio needs to consider mandatory and conditional procedures separately or to include procedure usage probability as a weighting coefficient.

A set of statistical parameters for each interpretive procedure has been completed for two additional variables:

r—the data reduction ratio, and
p—probability usage (%) (depending on the frequency of related disease occurrence).

Estimation of the Procedure Usage Probability

The probability usage for each diagnostic procedure is difficult to estimate, so the problem is often neglected by assuming a flat distribution of procedure usage.

Establishing a general estimate of the procedure's usage contribution in a final diagnosis seems to be inadequate because the values refer to the disease probability, which in turn is highly dependent upon factors like patient history, drugs, sex, race, lifestyle, diet, and so forth. Nevertheless, being conscious of the limitations of the result, we modified the example 12-lead interpretive system used in a general practitioner office by adding procedure execution marks. During the automated

Table 7.3. Example datastreams and calling sequence in the real 12-leads ECG interpretation software

Call Level	Procedure Name	Called By	Calls	Input	Size	Output	Size
0	main	-	init_cfg init_analiza analiza interpr exdiag	ECG signal configuration structure	8000*16 bps 20 bytes	diagnostic code QRS equivalent representation	10 bytes 300 bytes
1	analysis	main	ampli_chk qrsdet qrssync qrsasize qrssize tsize psize QRS->qrsvmax QRS->qrssubs QRS->qrsclass P->qrsvmax P->qrssubs P->qrsclass p_qrs_t_axis	ECG signal configuration structure	8000*16 bps 20 bytes	measurement point descriptors without ST	200 bytes/qrs
1	interpr	main	rh_anal cnt_anal st_anal	ECG signal configuration structure measurement point descriptors without ST	8000*16 bps 20 bytes 200 bytes/qrs	measurement point descriptors diagnostic code	300 bytes/qrs 10 bytes

continued on following page

Table 7.3. continued

Call Level	Procedure Name	Called By	Calls	Input	Size	Output	Size
1	exdiag	main	qtd_anal vlp_anal twa_anal	ECG signal configuration structure measurement point descriptors	8000*16 bps 20 bytes 300 bytes/qrs	dispersion descriptors diagnosti code	10 bytes/qrs 10 bytes
2	qrsdet	analysis	HiPass LoPass Deriv4 MovInt ProgDet	single-channel ECG signal	1000*16 bps	detection points	2 bytes/qrs
2	ampli_chk	analysis		eight-channel ECG signals	8000*16 bps	quality estimate	2 bytes
2	qrssync	analysis		single-channel ECG signal	1000*16 bps	synchronization points	2 bytes/qrs
2	qrsasize	analysis		single-channel ECG signal	1000*16 bps	approximate QRS start/end points	2 bytes/qrs
2	qrssize	analysis	as2_asc as2_dsc mod_one	twelve-channel buffered ECG signal	12x 1200 bytes/qrs	QRS border error code	6 bytes/qrs 1 byte/qrs

continued on following page

Table 7.3. continued

Call Level	Procedure Name	Called By	Calls	Input	Size	Output	Size
2	tsize	analysis	FDPBuff izol_one ss2_asc recal ChkIntRange as2_asc mod_one as2_dsc mod_one	twelve-channel buffered ECG signal	12x 1200 bytes/ qrs	T wave borders error code	4 bytes/ qrs 1 byte/ qrs
2	psize	analysis	izol_one ss2_asc recal ChkIntRange as2_asc mod_one as2_dsc mod_one	twelve-channel buffered ECG signal	12x 1200 baytes/ qrs	P wave borders error code	4 bytes/ qrs 1 byte/ qrs
2	SetPtsAvg	analysis		twelve-channel result structure	12x 20 bytes/qrs	result structure (averaged)	20 bytes/ qrs
2	qrsvmax	analysis		single-channel ECG signal	1000*16 bps	signal velocity value	2 bytes/ qrs
2	qrssubs	analysis		single-channel ECG signal	1000*16 bps	QRS equivalent representation	103 bytes/qrs

continued on following page

Table 7.3. continued

Call Level	Procedure Name	Called By	Calls	Input	Size	Output	Size
2	qrsclass	analysis	set_class verify_class center_class merge_class count_class	QRS-equivalent representation	105 bytes/qrs	class number pattern reference	1 byte/ qrs 1 byte/ qrs
2	p_qrs_t_axis	analysis	maxmod FHanMax f_ang	three-channel ECG signal result structure (averaged)	3000*16 bps 20 bytes/qrs	angular values	6 bytes/ qrs

continued on following page

Table 7.4. Basic ECG interpretation procedures: statistical parameters and attributed priority levels

Procedure Name	Data Reduction Ratio *r*	Probability of Use *p*	Priority Level
signal quality assessment	20	97	1
pacemaker pulse detection	70	3	4
heartbeat detection	70	100	2
baseline estimation	20	97	3
heart rate estimation	1	100	1
heartbeat classification	50	88	1
wave measurement	100	85	2
axis determination	300	85	3
dominant rhythm detection	1,5	100	1
arrhythmia detection	1,3	80	2
...			

ECG analysis, each subroutine call increments the value of a respective marker. For each patient, once the interpretation was completed, the doctor selected the relevant part of the diagnostic report. After the doctor's choice was made, we followed the interpretation tree in backward direction to identify procedures making no impact on the final report and cancel their usage mark. Remaining values were related to the total number of interpretation attempts (Table 7.4).

When considering the purchase of specialized medical equipment like interpretive electrocardiographs, the user projects future diagnostic cases from his or her experience. The cost of the device usually depends upon its interpretation capability, allowing the user a flexible choice of target-optimized performance at a minimum cost. However, payment is required before the first usage, and not related to the actual number of patients nor to the actual contribution of the particular subroutines in the final diagnosis. That justifies the statement that the price covers the potential capability of the equipment, the upper estimate of which is sometimes far above the actual needs.

Optimization of Internal Data Flow

Each heuristic subroutine in the ECG interpretation chain shows a non-zero probability of inappropriate processing and incorrect outcome. Despite the application of very thorough testing procedures, no software engineer is able to foresee all possible signal recording conditions combined with all possible heart diseases. In a typical processing chain, subsequent procedures use results based on previous ones, thus misinterpretations and inaccuracies may compensate or accumulate (Straszecka & Straszecka, 2004; Clifford, 2006). Unfortunately, the error-accumulative scenario is much more probable, because statistically speaking the correct and accurate result is a singularity in a cloud of all possible outcomes. Three approaches aimed at the reduction of overall error probability may be applied, separately or in combination:

- reducing the processing chain length,
- using the most accurate procedures at the front of the processing chain, and
- applying the auto-assessment functions.

The first two methods were the subject of our studies because the auto-assessment functions are often already implemented as a part of the diagnostic subroutines. Moreover, the application of first two methods in a real system do not require additional computation power.

Data Reduction Efficiency Investigations

Each interpretive subroutine transforms the input data to its output. Since the whole interpretation process begins from a collection of signal samples (sometimes of diverse nature) to a final diagnostic outcome, from a statistical viewpoint it is a sort of data reduction task. For each specialized subroutine, the information stream reduction ratio can be quantitatively measured by comparing the expected throughput of the outputs with reference to the inputs. Effective data reduction at the beginning of the process, postulated by wearable recorder implementation, can be achieved by putting either the most reduction-effective procedures or the most frequently used procedures in front of the processing chain. The particular challenge is the consolidation of all functions having access to the raw signal at their inputs. Unfortunately, the meaning of many signal-derived parameters depends on advanced calculations within long processing chains.

A second, complementary approach to the interpretive software optimization is based on a concept of data busses. These inter-procedure information channels are sorted by the value of expected throughput (Figure 7.4). Procedures are arranged on each data bus by their priority level, also reflecting the degree of signal processing advancement and the dependence on previously calculated parameters. Each data flow was assigned a throughput level combining statistical parameters of the data:

- average datastream used,
- frequency of usage (depending on the data refresh rate), and
- probability of usage (depending on the frequency of related disease occurrence).

The concept of data busses limits access to unprocessed data representation to subroutines of high peak throughput and high usage frequency. Consequently, several such procedures may need redesigning in order to access a common and very reliable data interface. With regard to wave measurement and axis determination procedures, highly dependent on previous computation results, two solutions were considered:

1. a continuous direct connection to the raw signal bus and an approximate estimation of calculation starting points, and
2. an occasional connection to a buffer caching a copy of raw signal dependent on the detection point position.

Figure 7.4. Data bus concept combined with interpretation procedure priority levels

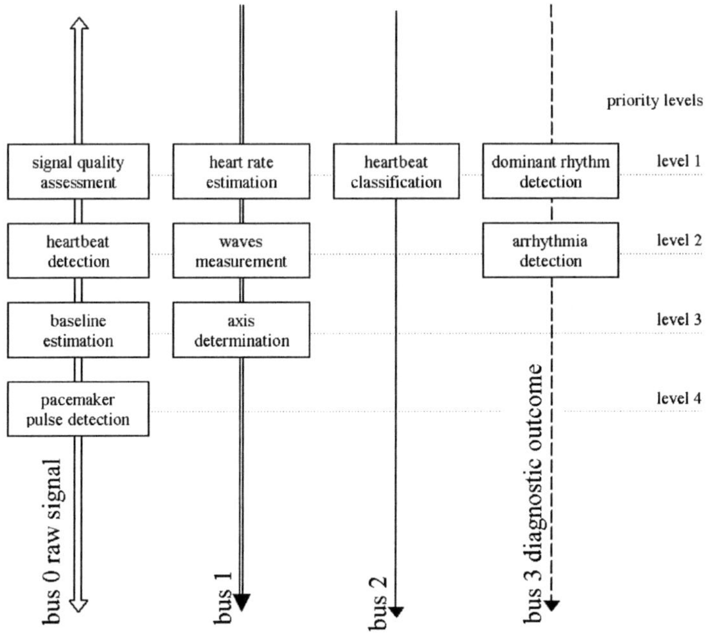

Since wave measurement and axis determination performance dramatically drops with the use of estimate instead of accurate detection points, the second method was chosen.

REDESIGN OF THE ARCHITECTURE OF THE ECG INTERPRETATION CHAIN CONSIDERING OPTIMAL RELIABILITY AND DATA REDUCTION

The Optimized Architecture Proposal

The final architecture of ECG interpretation software is optimized for reliability and early datastream reduction (Figure 7.5). It contains three raw signal access points:

1. common interface for signal quality estimation, baseline estimation, and pacemaker detection procedures;

Figure 7.5. The final architecture of ECG interpretation software optimized for reliability and early datastream reduction

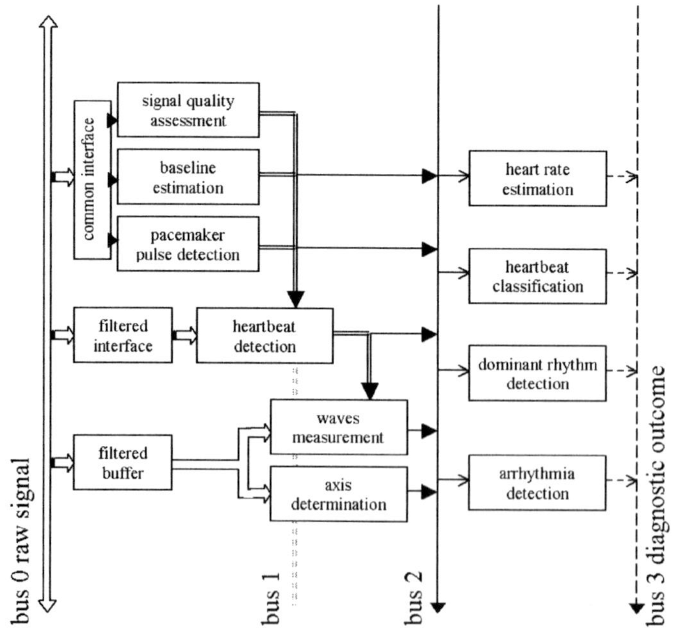

2. heartbeat detection filtered real-time input; and
3. wave measurement and axis determination filtered off-line buffer (provided also for ST measurement and P-averaging not considered here).

The group of functions accessing the raw signal issues a complete description of a heartbeat (bus 2), which is not the diagnostic outcome, but contains all the metadata necessary for further processing and thus the raw signal is no longer necessary. These data appear occasionally, once per heart cycle, but even for as high a heart rate as 180 bps, the datastream is 8.2 times lower than for a 12-lead 500 sps raw signal. If a remote ECG interpretation has to be transferred to a central node, this point is a convenient opportunity.

Experimental Results

The architecture optimization was performed on standard ECG interpretation software provided by a regional manufacturer. The structured source code was written in C++ programming language. The original target application was the interpretive bedside ECG recorder, and the purpose of the optimization was the manufacturer's interest in migrating to a wearable computer platform. Two factors were assessed separately for the original and the modified architectures:

1. the average reduction of the data rate at subsequent processing stages, and
2. the average inaccuracy and probability of error for selected diagnostic parameters.

Because of architecture optimization, the processing stages could not be set up in a similar way for the original and modified software. Therefore, with regard to the identical testing conditions, we used processing time as an estimation of the interpretation progress. The control stages were set up at every 20% of the total interpretation time. The reason for this relative approach was twofold:

1. particular ECG files vary in processing time; and
2. although not intended as a main goal, the software redesign reduced the average processing time.

Table 7.5 compares the average data reduction ratio during the subsequent stages of the interpretation process. The right column highlights the differences between the original and the optimized architectures, and proves that significant data reduction was achieved as a result of the modified architecture in the early stages of the interpretation process.

Table 7.5. The average data reduction ratio (%) in the subsequent stages of interpretation process

Interpretation Progress (% of total processing time)	**Data Reduction Related to Raw Signals (%)**		**Data Reduction Gain (%)**
	Original Architecture	Optimized Architecture	
0	100	100	0
20	78	47	31
40	54	31	23
60	32	22	10
80	14	12	2
100	8	8	0

Table 7.6. Diagnostic parameter quality achieved by the original and the optimized architectures; the meaning of δ and ε are explained further on in the text

Procedure Name	**Statistical Parameters**			
	Original Architecture		Optimized Architecture	
	δ	ε	δ	ε
pacemaker pulse detection	2.8	9.3	1.5	9.0
heartbeat detection	2.5	3.5	1.7	2.9
baseline estimation	4.3	1.3	4.3	1.3
heart rate estimation	1.0	1.2	1.0	1.2
heartbeat classification	14	7.1	12	4
wave measurement	5.1	7.5	3.3	5.3
axis determination	6.3	7.8	3.7	5.1
dominant rhythm detection	0	10.5	0	8.8
arrhythmia detection	0	13	0	11.8

The second aspect of architecture optimization, the result accuracy, was tested according to international standards (IEC 60601-2-51 2003). The quantitative results for both architectures are summarized in Table 7.6. The comparison of the diagnostic reliability for isolated procedures (Table 7.3) with the corresponding results of the whole processing chain (Table 7.6) leads to the conclusion that in the case of the optimized architecture, the overall reliability of each parameter is much less affected by the remaining procedures of the ECG interpretation chain.

This improvement is achieved mainly by shortening the processing chains. Consequently, dependence upon subsequent function input data and the results of previous processing stages is looser and no longer favors cumulative error propagation.

Discussion

The work presented in this chapter was motivated by recent changes in cardiac monitoring techniques, taking into account the applications of modern digital communication technology. The classical approach to the ECG interpretation processing chain was revised, and important software architecture modifications were proposed to overcome two principal drawbacks:

1. the necessity of raw signal access in the advanced processing stages, and
2. cumulative error propagation resulting from data dependencies in the processing chain.

Both aspects were thoroughly studied and the findings were applied to the real interpretive software, in close cooperation with the ECG equipment manufacturer. The modular software was modified only at the subroutine interconnection level without changes or adjustment to the mathematical foundations. The main result is the relative improvement of diagnostic outcome accuracy and datastream reduction, rather than their absolute values. Therefore, any manufacturer may check his software for concordance with the guidelines issued herein.

The aim of our research was fully achieved. We proved that software architecture optimization is suitable for improved interpretation in the following areas:

- in moving reduction-effective functions to the beginning of the processing chain and consequently reducing the inter-procedure data flows, thus lowering communication costs with regard to prospective distributed implementation of the ECG interpretation process;
- in reducing cumulative error propagation by the parallel use of multiple short processing chains instead of one long chain; and
- in reducing interpretation processing time and the required computational power, thus extending the wearable device longevity.

Even more promising results could be expected if the particular processing parameters were fully independent. However, in this case many processing steps must be repeated in the same signal. Nevertheless, as a future consideration we propose to completely rewrite each interpretive function to minimize the use of parameters computed at preceding stages of signal processing.

REFERENCES

Abenstein, J. P. (1978). Algorithms for real-time ambulatory ECG monitoring. *Biomedical Sciences Instrumentation*. Vol. 14 . pp.73-77.

Abenstein, J. P., & Thakor, N. V. (1981). A detailed design example—ambulatory ECG monitoring. In W. J. Tompkins & J. G. Webster (Eds.), *Design of microcomputer-based medical instrumentation*. Englewood Cliffs, NJ: Prentice Hall.

Balda, R. A., Diller, G., Deardorff, E., Doue, J., & Hsieh, P. (1977). The HP ECG analysis program. In J. H. van Bemmel & J. L. Willems (Eds.), *Trends in computer-processed electrocardiograms* (pp. 197-205). Amsterdam: North Holland.

Banitsas, K. A., Georgiadis, P., Tachakra, S., & Cavouras, D. (2004). Using handheld devices for real-time wireless tele-consultation. *Proceedings of the 26th Annual International Conference of the IEEE EMBS* (pp. 3105-3108).

Bonner, R. E., & Schwetman, H. D. (1968). Computer diagnosis of the electrocardiogram II. *Computers and Biomedical Research, 1,* 366.

CardioSoft. (2005). *Version 6.0 operator's manual.* Milwaukee, WI: GE Medical Systems Information Technologies.

Chiarugi, F. et al. (2003). Continuous ECG monitoring in the management of pre-hospital health emergencies. *Computers in Cardiology, 30,* 205-208.

Clifford, G. D. (2006). ECG statistics, noise, artifacts and missing data. In G. D. Clifford, F. Azuaje, & P. E. McSharry (Eds.), *Advanced methods and tools for ECG data analysis* (pp. 55-99). Boston, Artech House.

Daskalov, I. K., Dotsinsky, I. A., & Christov, I. I. (1998). Developments in ECG acquisition, preprocessing, parameter measurement and recording. *IEEE Engineering in Medicine and Biology Magazine, 17,* 50-58.

DRG. (1995). *MediArc premier IV operator's manual* (version 2.2.).

Friesen, G. M., Jannett T. C. et al. (1990). A comparison of the noise sensitivity of nine QRS detection algorithms. *IEEE Transactions on Biomedical Engineering, 37*(1), 85-98.

HP. (1994). *M1700A interpretive cardiograph physician's guide* (4th ed.). Hewlett-Packard.

IBM. (1974). *Electrocardiogram analysis program physician's guide* (5736-H15; 2nd ed.).

IEC 60601-2-51. (2003). Medical electrical equipment: Particular requirements for the safety, including essential performance, of ambulatory electrocardiographic systems. First edition 2003-02, International Electrotechnical Commission, Geneva,

Laguna, P., Jané, R., & Caminal, P. (1994). Automatic detection of wave boundaries in multilead ECG signals: Validation with the CSE database. *Computers and Biomedical Research, 27*(1), 45-60.

Moody, G. (1993). *MIT/BIH arrhythmia database distribution.* Cambridge, MA: MIT Division of Health Science and Technology.

Nihon Kohden. (2001). *ECAPS-12C user guide: Interpretation standard* (revision A).

Paoletti, M., & Marchesi, C. (2004). Low computational cost algorithms for portable ECG monitoring units *IFMBE Proceedings of Medicon 2004* (paper 231).

Pinna, G. D., Maestri, R., Gobbi, E., La Rovere, M. T., & Scanferlato, J. L. (2003). Home tele-monitoring of chronic heart failure patients: Novel system architecture of the home or hospital in heart failure study. *Computers in Cardiology, 30,* 105-108.

Straszecka, E., & Straszecka, J. (2004). Uncertainty and imprecision representation in medical diagnostic rules. *IFMBE Proceedings of Medicon 2004* (paper 172).

Tompkins, W. J. (1980). Modular design of microcomputer-based medical instruments. *Medical Instrumentation , 14,* 315-318.

Tompkins, W. J., Tompkins, B. M., & Weisner, S. J. (1983). Microprocessor-based device for real-time ECG processing in the operating room. *Proceedings of AAMI.*

Willems, J. L. (1990). *Common standards for quantitative electrocardiography: 10th CSE progress report.* Leuven, Belgium: ACCO.

Chapter VIII
Interpretation of the ECG as a Web-Based Subscriber Service

This chapter is about the idea of medical information interchange networks providing signal and possibly image interpretation services. Technically, the issue is similar to Web-accessible services: document conversion, searching the Web, photo development, video on demand, electronic booking of hotels or airline ticketing. Various services use state-of-the-art Internet technology for commerce and entertainment purposes. Unfortunately, medical applications are rarely represented in that form.

In the first part we present a software manufacturer viewpoint resulting from a typical consideration of costs vs. benefits. The important point here is that simple basic procedures are commonly and more frequently used than sophisticated and specialized subroutines. The development of newly introduced diagnostic procedures or calculations of diagnostic parameters recently proposed by cardiologists is very expensive, and the resultant products are unknown, so they are rarely purchased, which makes them more costly.

Such conclusion and past experience discourage manufacturers from implementing new methods in devices designated for average customers. These also discourage customers from paying for the potential, but rarely used possibility of performing very uncommon diagnoses. The alternative solution is limiting hardware-embedded procedures at a certain level and creating worldwide-accessible, highly specialized interpretation centers to deal with rare cases automatically or with occasional supervision from human experts.

The idea of distributed interpretation services challenges the current definition of telemedicine because the software, instead of the human, is supposed to be the main agent in the network. The doctor's role is shifted to resolving uniquely unusual cases or to the occasional verification of system performance. His or her work will require greater expertise and responsibility. Clients of medical subscriber services will be human cardiologists, but also the software implemented in wearable devices. Such a multi-modal monitoring system is able to measure vital signs without the patient's intervention, send the digital data for interpretation, and initiate emergency procedures when necessary.

The remote interpretation as a subscriber service needs two areas of data security to be considered: (1) patient privacy and the consistency of raw data and returned reports; and (2) server security and immunity to erroneous signals, network violation acts, or attempts at unauthorized access.

The prototype Internet service for diagnosis based on T wave dispersions was set up and provided the authors with an opportunity to meet several technical constraints for this idea. This chapter is about small-scale network experimental results. This experimental service is aimed at revealing and testing emerging problems, and is also a test bed for similar applications.

THE CONCEPT OF KNOWLEDGE SPACE

Introduction

The importance of recordings or sketches has never been neglected in the medical sciences, and even the oldest surgical manuals contain descriptions of reference cases. For many years collections of ECG recordings were only on paper, except for long-term recordings stored on magnetic tapes. Nowadays, digital storage remains the only practical data carrier, and we often wonder how we could ever manage without it.

Since the first issue of the American Heart Association Standard for the ECG (AHA, 1967), databases played several roles in electrocardiology, including these most important ones:

- as references for interpreting (manual or automatic) medical signals,
- to impose standards on data storage and transmission formats, and
- as starting points for new challenges in the of signal content exploration.

Databases have two principal aspects in cardiology: to provide specific raw records and an exemplary knowledge explaining the interpretation. Considering that knowledge is on a continuum, increasing the number of examples leads to better knowledge representation.

Data Formatting and Medical Knowledge

The data format is an inherent part of the database, although it is usually specified by a separate document. The description of physiological parameters contains data of various origin (time sequences, text, still images, movies, and audio) and the format must support such diverse data. Despite the need for a general format, the recording-specific formats are in common use (e.g., SCP ECG Protocol for the 12-lead ECG and VCG; Willems, 1991). The existence of well-established common formats is of paramount importance to patients because examinations are no longer limited to health centers or by manufacturers of medical equipment.

Joint representation of signals along with the accompanying medical information was the principal area of applications for early databases. The examples recognized worldwide are the MIT-BIH Arrhythmia Database (Moody & Mark, 1993) and the CSE Multilead Database (Willems, 1990). Many other databases were a result of clinical trials performed in leading research centers, and some of them are freely available from Physionet (www.physionet.org). At the moment, these databases are used for training cardiology students as well as for tuning and validating software. Apart from problem-oriented databases, few recent data collections (e.g., ICU-Database) describe the simultaneous vital signs that provide researchers with an opportunity to study correlations between the activities of different human organs.

Clinical practice is under continuous development, and the data format must provide support for currently unknown vital signs and annotations. The most frequent disadvantage of the current formats is their poor flexibility as new parameters emerge and old ones die out. The format extensibility may partially be achieved in a combination of DICOM Waveform Interchange (or HL7 level 3.0) standards and XML-structured reporting forms.

Wedding Data and Methods

During medical research, various experiments must be completed resulting in unusual recordings made in atypical conditions (e.g., tele-ECG in rats). These data often require specialized processing, approximating clinical conditions. Software engineers usually develop procedures for this purpose on demand, but very often they copy other people's work. Such software needs to be evaluated over a long period of time before being used. This is costly because computation errors may lead to the misinterpretation of results and erroneous conclusions.

The proposed extension of the database is the knowledge space (KS), which integrates the signal with medical annotations as well as the information technology-based methods of data interpretation. The KS is accessible to a wide range of medical researchers over the Internet. As a conventional database, the KS service contains downloadable reference ECG data, however its main advantage is the offer of a choice of the most recent interpretation methods too. The server interface is able not only to demonstrate the ability of a particular method to solve a given problem, but also to perform the requested computation on the uploaded user data and to return the result. The source code is ready to use in multiple asynchronous threads remotely launched and controlled by the user via a limited set of options. User interface software is not required because modern graphic-based Web browsers support user file transfer, method selection and options, and the presentation of results. The transfer of computation results in separate files also under consideration, allowing for the support of text interface-based terminals. The graphics may then be reconstructed from the file in the vector format more suitable for the purpose of publishing in unlimited quality.

The user manual and knowledge guide are provided in HTML format and contain links to the original papers. Although the medical library is not the main function of the KS server, the collection of publications provides the medical researcher with the most appropriate knowledge facilitating the preparation of an experiment and the right choice of data processing method and options.

Knowledge Representation and Exchange

The idea of knowledge space follows the example of software engineering, which in the early 1970s defined computer programs as an aggregate of data and methods (Wirth, 1976). However, the notion of data and particularly the notion of methods are much extended in the case of knowledge space for cardiology (Figure 8.1).

Figure 8.1. Block diagram of knowledge space components

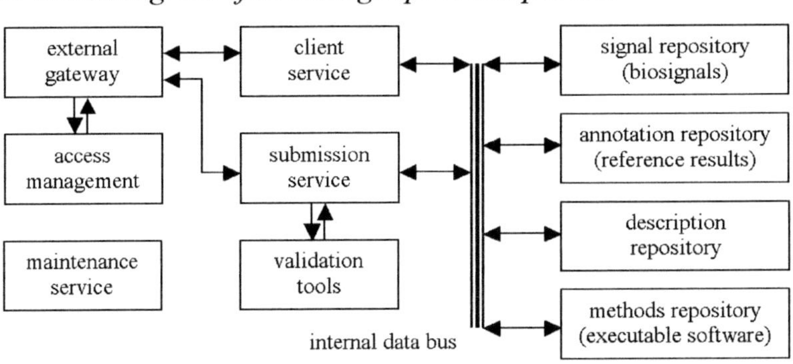

In a regular expert system based on a database, data is compared for similarity, correlation, and covariance, thus no knowledge about calculation methods is used. For a given input data vector, the most similar data vector is searched in the database and the corresponding result is reproduced as output. The data are generally understood as one or more of the following forms:

- *Raw signal,* which is the unprocessed digital representation of electrical measurements of the surface ECG and synchronous other phenomena (respiration, blood pressure, patient motion, oxygen saturation, acoustic, and many others). Various data-types follow their proper technical specification of measurement (sampling frequency, amplitude scale, etc.). Although not typical for electrocardiography, some applications like polysomnography may include static or motion pictures as raw signal as well. Despite some processing performed, the conditioned signal or ECG with the baseline removed also falls into the raw signal category. The raw signal is characterized by huge data flow and storage requirements.
- *Metadata,* which are all intermediate results yielded by the interpretation procedures. Except for the values, the complete data description is composed of attributes indicating the processing result or identifying the source procedure and the reliability. Metadata may be scalar values or symbols, vectors of various sampling frequency, and images. They may represent numerical values and semantic descriptions of the ECG contents. Metadata are characterized by free data forms, depended only upon the requirements of the interfaced procedures, limited reliability, and average dataflow and volume. Metadata are usually not readable by humans. However, metadata compatibility is the key point for the distributed processing or Web-based subscriber interpretation service.
- *Diagnostic data,* which are all the numerical values and string constants describing the final findings about patient status. Their form usually conforms to human habits and standardization rules. Diagnostic data reliability is reduced by all the quality compromises in the processing chain; however, at the moment the uncertainty level is determined by a doctor's guess or suspicions rather than a quantitative assessment. Diagnostic data have the most concise form. The final decision—however rarely made automatically—is usually a binary choice.

The methods, being novel but essential components of the knowledge space, are technically very similar to the data and represent knowledge about the derivation of results from the data. They represent 'thinking and reasoning' rather than the 'searching' process. Several methods may coexist in the knowledge space in a common application area. They have a standardized interface, and they will be externally characterized only by computational complexity and result accuracy. Software manufacturers usually develop various methods for key procedures in the interpretation chain in order to have the flexibility to tailor any final product. The methods also have various forms in the knowledge space, depending on their origin and intended application:

- The scientific paper is the principal form of a message identifying the problem and methods, and proposing a solution. Despite its widespread use in all the sciences, the scientific paper is not directly applicable to automatic signal processing. Its value is mainly informative, and usually this is the only form disclosing the methodological background of selected interpretation aspects.
- The reference is an essential part of data processing and redirection management. This category includes all forms of electronic recipient identification messages like hypertext links for cross-referencing data within the knowledge space itself, Internet addresses for automatic messaging within the network, and phone numbers for voice and data messaging. Each time a diagnostic problem is submitted to the knowledge space, the reference system automatically searches for similar problems and their solutions within the database, propagates the automatic interpretation query in the network, and searches for the most suitable cardiology expert on duty.
- The algorithm is the main engine of the automatic interpretation service providing effective data processing towards a diagnostic outcome. Details of technological and numerical methods are not important and may be kept confidential. Nevertheless, the algorithm is subject to assessment of accuracy and medical correctness performed by human experts during the development stage and continued into the maintenance stage. For reasons of applicability, the algorithms cooperating within the knowledge space or in the network must be designed with respect to common interfacing rules. These rules and the quality assessment protocol must be normalized and published in the future in the interest of network development.

The Scientific Impact of Knowledge Spaces

The dynamic structure of the KS is supported by experts in bio-signal interpretation and supervised by the International Scientific Committee, which validates new proposals in order to guarantee state-of-the-art representation procedures. The KS is supposed to soon receive wide recognition in centers of medical research because of the impact it has on the development and standardization of electrocardiology.

Thanks to this independent validation, the contribution of KS may be recognized in academic societies as equal to a submission of a scientific paper.

The idea of providing a computational service in cardiology closes the gap between high-quality but closed commercial applications and public domain subroutines of poor reliability. Because the source code of methods is not published at any stage, the user is not bored by technical issues like compilation, and the range of methods may include high-quality patented algorithms or special versions of software typically embedded in interpretive ECG recorders. Commercial ECG equipment manufacturers are also welcome to submit their contributions and manifest their authorship using their company name or visual identification system, and to profit from the software usage.

THE IDEA OF INTERPRETATION AS A WEB-AVAILABLE SUBSCRIBER SERVICE

Procedure Complexity vs. Probability of Usage

Computerized ECG interpretation is currently a clinical standard in basic diagnostic procedures. Unfortunately, for software manufacturers, the most sophisticated interpretation algorithms have a limited demand, so research expenditures are not rewarded. With regard to clinical practice, the specialized functions that increase the price of sophisticated equipment are rarely justified because the corresponding medical cases are relatively infrequent. Moreover, some methods invented recently are fully or partially patented, causing the work-repetitive development of custom solutions by competitive companies. Consequently, instead of interoperability, new constraints are created with regard to the standardization of the ECG interpretation procedures.

Our proposal is motivated by the studies on human relations between cardiologists and has procedure-use statistics as a background. Following the human network of specialization in cardiology, we found it interesting that common universal skills reach a certain level, from which upward only a very particular domain is practiced and reaches the maximum. On a national scale, every cardiologist is able to interpret a certain range of most common cases, whereas with infrequent diseases, regional or national specialists must usually be involved. This limits the costs that must be borne to train every doctor in all aspects of cardiology without impacting upon quality. The specialists are then treating pre-selected cases matching their interest. The above-mentioned principles are particularly useful because they are based on years of clinical practice.

The stand-alone interpretive software was conceived as a model of reasoning of an individual cardiologist. In a similar way, distributed healthcare networks may be modeled with some constraint in a computer network (Tadeusiewicz, 2004). General-purpose patient-side recorders play the role of basic-skilled cardiologists and report every unusual case as unresolved to the specialized center. The centers play the role of regional or national specialists and are realized as Unix-based multitask and multi-user servers scaled to the estimated demand for particular interpretation tasks. We make no assumption on the number of the centers; in particular, each heart disease may be supported by several physical interpretation nodes using independent interpretation methods and located in different parts of the world (Augustyniak, 2003). The interpretation of difficult diseases needs the transmission of a considerable amount of data over the network, however this affects the overall performance only slightly due to the rare occurrence of these cases.

Some of the commercial advantages of Web-based ECG interpretation services are worth mentioning:

- The recorder is marketed as a low-cost general-purpose device; the potential ability of specialized interpretation does not increase its price and the client only pays for the actual number of interpretations.
- The inventor of a specialized interpretation method may be rewarded for the service in proportion to its usage and quality.

Figure 8.2. Worldwide accessibility of ECG-specialized interpretive services

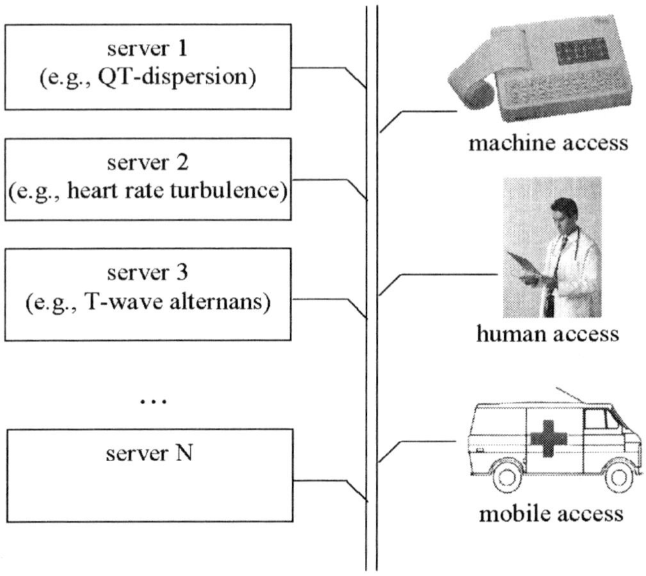

- The inventor's intellectual property rights are well protected because the distribution of the software source code or executable file is no longer required.
- The interpretation method is widely standardized and does not depend on recorder manufacturer or the physical location of the patient.

Another advantage of our proposal is no involvement of changes in the bedside interpretive ECG recorders in use today. The only modification consists of extending the connectivity, used only for electronic patient records, by a procedure that is in accordance with multiple method-specialized remote interpretation services. The service could be organized independently and managed by the inventor of a particular diagnostic method or another healthcare provider.

The purpose of our research is to implement a well-known diagnostic procedure as a Web-accessible service. This new technical solution may be proposed for the implementation of any existing highly specialized procedure as well as of new algorithms that will appear in the future. The service, under consideration, is designed and developed for QT dispersion interpretation, and the principle of this experiment presented earlier was rather to face and solve a range of technical issues than to open a healthcare center. Other medical signal processing-based services, not limited to cardiology, may follow this solution considering the advantages of the service:

- high reliability of interpretation and protection of inventors intellectual rights,
- worldwide standardization of procedures and interoperability, and
- low cost.

Future Web-based ECG interpretation service investigations should precisely identify the interpretation tasks for the recorder and for the center, however shared methods are still interesting. Various aspects should be considered in the design of ECG machine families for a Web-based service. The most important are:

- interpretation feasibility in constrained remote resources,
- manufacturing costs,
- frequency of disease occurrence, and
- medical severity and urgency of parameters out of 'normal' range.

DATA SECURITY AND AUTHORIZATION ISSUES IN DISTRIBUTED INTERPRETATION NETWORKS

Signal Quality Verification

The purpose of signal quality verification is the correct estimation of diagnostic outcome reliability. In the case of weak amplitude, noisy signals, spikes in the T-end area, or baseline wander, the analysis may end with incorrect results. The signal is analyzed but not altered in any way before diagnostic processing starts. Suspicious input signals are identified, and a warning message is issued together with the diagnostic outcome. When the result does not satisfy the recipient, a client-side filtered version or another, distortion-free signal section may be re-submitted for interpretation. Signal quality is estimated by the computation of several parameters: the slope of the power spectrum decay, the percentage of monotonic sections, the number of isolated signal accelerations and decelerations, and so forth. With regard to this aspect, signal quality is not a precise term, and its definition is dependent on the procedure in use—some parameters are vulnerable to certain distortion types.

Multi-Threading and Human Assistance

The diagnostic subroutines of service software were designed to be launched as multiple asynchronous remotely controlled threads (Figure 8.3) assigned by the system to clients in login order. The clients have regular user privileges, with access limited to their thread and parent directory. Two methods of supervision are designed for the service: server administration and medical expert assistance. Help from a qualified cardiologist is crucial at this point, because he or she not only resolves conflicts or misinterpretations, but also gathers and qualifies information on errors. Consequently, these remarks are considered as a background for future versions of the interpretive software.

There are several aspects of human assistance that are expected at the specialized interpretation server:

- supervising the adequacy of basic case interpretation performed remotely,
- controlling and correcting the task assignment,
- supervising and improving the specialized interpretation procedure,
- using the knowledge base and extra-cardiac information, and
- authorizing the output diagnosis.

Figure 8.3. Interpretation request processing chain

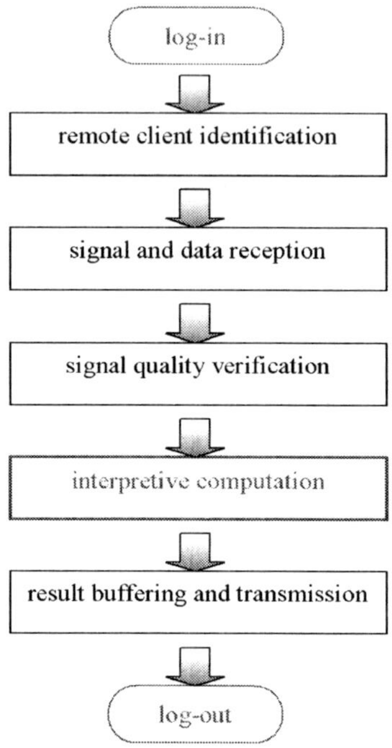

Improving the automated diagnosis quality will reduce the supervisory tasks expected from the human expert, increasing his or her efficiency and limiting his or her duties to the manual interpretation of very rare cases currently not supported by the software.

Remote Access and Client Identification

Our target approach was only designed for machine access. However at the testing stage, we had to consider the human access as well because we found it useful in some circumstances.

The general-purpose ECG recorder provides the acquired signal for the network, requests the interpretation service, and receives the diagnostic outcome. Although the service in its experimental stage is accessed by a closed group of remote clients recognized by their IP addresses, the remote client identification procedure was implemented for the future system expansion. The purpose of this procedure is twofold:

- assignment of the diagnostic outcome to the appropriate client request, and
- identification of service subscriber status and prevention from unauthorized or multiple task requests.

The client identification procedure is used as a substantial tool for the service usage statistic. These procedures are expandable when the subscription will be payable. This solution may be considered a first approach to the service's financial support. The subscribers must pay for the number of interpretation tasks requested over a given period and not for the potential ability of the analysis like it is in the case of recorder-embedded ECG interpretation software.

The human access is maintained in the final version of the service (e.g., for medical researchers). The server interface is able to perform the requested computation on the uploaded user data and to return the result without disclosure of the software code. The service can be manually launched and controlled by the client with use of a limited set of parameters. Any modern graphic-based Web browser is suitable as a user interface. The only requirements are the support of user file transfer, the selection of options, and the results presentation. The transfer of computation results as a file is also under consideration to allow for the use of text interface-based terminals.

THE EXPERIMENTAL DESIGN OF INTERPRETATION SERVICES

QT Interval Durations in the Stratification of Re-Polarization Abnormalities

As an implementation example, throughout this book we present principal technical problems encountered during the design and development of the example QT dispersion service and discuss alternative solutions. Only the signal processing algorithm is process-specific, while all other issues are common for any ECG interpretation routine designed as a Web service. The QT dispersion, derived from inter-lead comparisons of QT interval duration in several leads of standard ECGs, is one of the most significant predictive factors of re-polarization abnormalities (Figure 8.4). Extensive research (Algra, Le Brunand, & Zeelenberg, 1987; Benhorin et al., 1990; Merri et al., 1992; Coumel et al., 1995; Maison-Blanche, Catuli, Fayn, & Coumel, 1996; Sosnowski, Czyz, Leski, Petelenz, & Tendera, 1996; Berger et al., 1997; Marciano, Cuomo, Migaux, & Vetrano, 1998; Daskalov & Christov, 1999; Extramiana et al., 1999; Malik & Batchvarov, 2000; Zareba, 2001; Murabayashi et al., 2002; Strumillo, 2002; Berger, 2003; Kardys et al., 2003; Lang, Neilson, & Flapan, 2004;

Figure 8.4. A pre-cordial lead representation of an example heartbeat: (a) normal; (b) high QT dispersion (long QT syndrome)

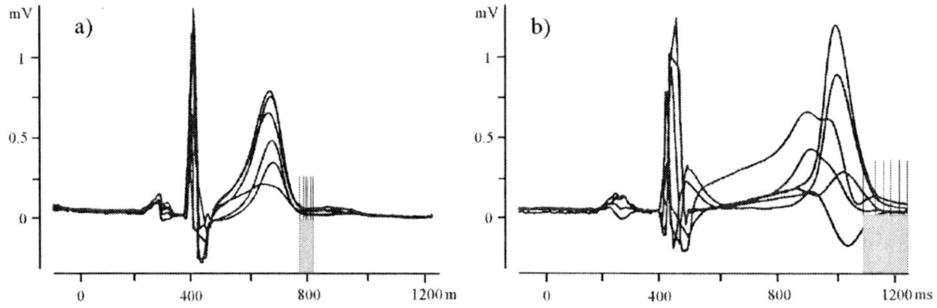

Jensen et al., 2005; Pueyo, Malik, & Laguna, 2005; Christov et al., 2006) shows that the heterogeneity of refractoriness in myocardial tissues contribute to increased vulnerability in the ventricular tachyarrhythmias. Increased QT dispersions are associated with cardiac death in non-ischemic patients, and with ventricular fibrillation and sustained tachycardia and other severe heart failures. This parameter is also used to identify high-risk patients awaiting heart transplants.

THE QT DISPERSION COMPUTATION ALGORITHM

Studies of QT dispersion algorithms in various manufacturers' products (HP, 1994; Nihon Kohden, 2001; CardioSoft, 2005) reveal that AHA guidelines are implemented in different ways and that the software yield significantly diverse results from the same test signal. The most problematic issue is the correct delimitation of T-end points independently for each ECG lead. As sources of differences we found:

- various approximation techniques to be responsible for the differences; and
- the difference in the statistics used for outlier suppression, which excludes leads differing too much from the mean value, as too difficult to be analyzed.

Consequently, the results are not reproducible from one machine to another, and the serial comparison or follow-up are manufacturer dependent.

The QT dispersion is meant to reveal re-polarization changes in various zones of the heart muscle tissue; so is the measure of the absolute differences of all QT

Figure 8.5. Details on T wave maximum and T-end point measurements

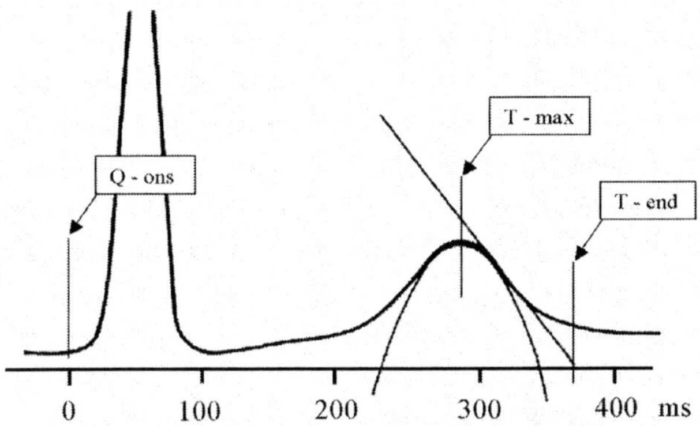

sections in all of the 12-lead recordings. As recommended in the literature (Laguna, Mark, Goldberger, & Moody, 1997; Davey, 1999; Risk, Bruno, Llamedo Soria, Arini, & Taborda, 2005), our algorithm uses a second-order approximation of T wave maximum and a maximum slope approximation of T wave end (Figure 8.5). The approximation techniques allow for sampling frequency-independent processing for a wide range of acquired signals.

The Prototype Service

The prototype of the service was build with use of a Linux-based Web server. Concerning human access, a standard Web site is developed in order to upload the signal, launch the processing thread, and present the diagnostic outcome. For the machine access, an automatic login and identification procedure is provided, and the returning message contains the diagnostic outcome in binary format. The service test was initially made using the human access because machine access required the manufacturer's approval for the modification of an existing ECG machine by adding communication interfaces, proper data upload, and task request format support. Except for two real ECG machines, the remaining clients were emulated during the test with use of independent PC machines. The other advantage of client simulation was the alternative local implementation of the diagnostic subroutines launched on the PCs in parallel, allowing easy measurement for the delay caused by the remote operation. The delay was thus measured as a difference in performance time with the use of local and remote service.

Experimental Device Setup

The wired connection tests were performed on the prototype QT dispersion service with static IP addresses and 100 Mbps direct Internet connections. A maximum of 10 clients simultaneously requested their computation tasks. This number was limited only by the available IP reserves. Remote computation was nearly as fast as its local counterpart; the systematic delay measurement for the remote processing was 130ms ± 53ms and was found not significant for the diagnostic performance.

A similar test was repeated for the node server connected to the Web out of the institution area domain. The packet routing procedure and consecutive mediation of Internet nodes influence the processing delay, in particular for the first connection (1639ms ± 280ms). Subsequent connections from the same machine are performed much faster (170ms ± 67ms) thanks to access route caching.

The test for wireless client-server connections was performed within the institution's address domain for one wireless-connected client, while the others used a regular cable connection. The separated client used an 802.11g LAN PC Card set for the maximum data transfer of 11 Mbps. Once again, the time necessary to establish the connection was very significant (up to 5s), and the subsequent tasks were processed faster (210ms ± 97ms).

Figure 8.6. Block diagram of the experiments diagnostic Web-service operation: (a) LAN connections; (b) WAN connections; (c) wireless LAN to WAN connection

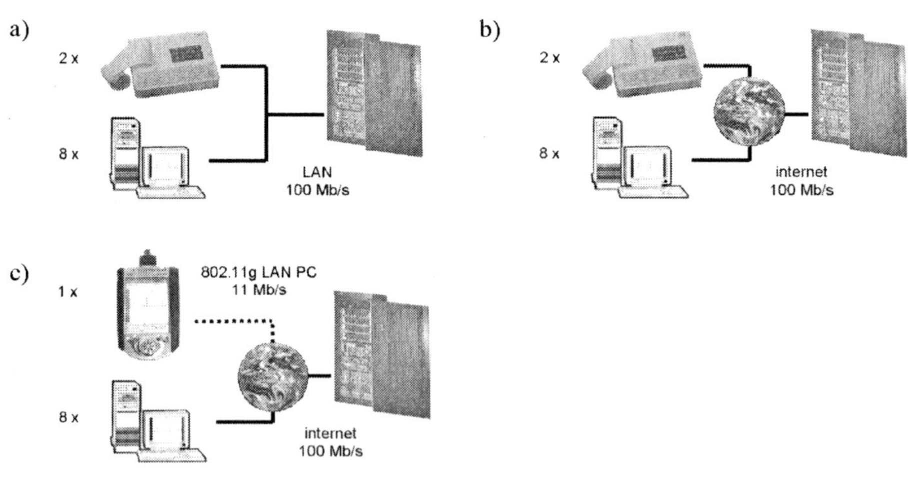

Results and Observations

The delay was measured by the client computer as a difference of completion time between the remote and local task performance on the same signal section. Table 8.1 summarizes all the mean values and standard deviations of the delay caused by the remote operation of QT dispersion interpretation.

Three sources of delay were identified during the analysis of remote tasks:

1. remote service connection and file transfer;
2. client recognition, data verification, and result buffering and
3. interpretive computation in a multitask environment.

The contributions of a particular component depend on the service scale, Internet connection quality, computation power, and so forth. Because of high specialization, the service scale and the server resources may be adjusted according to medical demand.

The experimental part confirmed the hope for the practical usefulness of the service. Except for the first request, tasks performed by the remote service were not noticeably longer than those carried out by the local subroutine. In the case of multiple different interpretation tasks ordered in parallel from specialized services, processing may be completed even faster than in a sequential local analysis performed by an interpretive electrocardiograph with limited computational power.

The subscriber service may replace specialized medical centers or may be supported by them under the supervision of qualified cardiologists. In the future

Table 8.1. Statistics of the QT dispersion interpretation delay (remote processing vs. local processing)

Connection method	average delay [ms]	standard deviation [ms]
100 Mbps Ethernet connection, same address domain	130	53
100 Mbps Ethernet connection, different address domains (first look-up)	1,639	280
100 Mbps Ethernet connection, different address domains (subsequent connection)	170	67
802.11g LAN PC Card 11 Mbps infrastructure mode (first look-up)	4,105	880
802.11g LAN PC Card 11 Mbps infrastructure mode (subsequent connection)	210	97

they may evolve into complex services tailored to individual needs and centers for specialized calculations using rare methods. In further experiments, we plan to use a GPRS client connection that closer approximates communication conditions in a busy, worldwide network. The third generation of global telecommunication should definitely solve the problem of clients in motion (e.g., ambulance services) or people living in remote areas who do not have access to the Internet.

REFERENCES

AHA. (1967). *AHA ECG database.* Available from Emergency Care Research Institute, Plymouth Meeting, PA.

Algra, A., Le Brunand, H., & Zeelenberg, C. (1987). An algorithm for computer measurement of QT intervals in the 24 hour ECG. *Computers in Cardiology, 14,* 117-119.

Augustyniak, P. (2003). From databases to knowledge spaces for cardiology. *International Journal of Bioelectromagnetism, 5.*

Benhorin, J., Merri, M., Alberti, M., Locati, E., Moss, A. J., Hall, W. J., & Cui, L. (1990). Long QT syndrome. New electrocardiographic characteristics. *Circulation, 82,* 521-527.

Berger, R. D. (2003). QT variability. *Journal of Electrocardiology, 36*(5), 83-87.

Berger, R. D., Kasper, E. K., Baughman, K. L., Marban, E., Calkins, H., & Tomaselli, G. F. (1997). Beat-to-beat QT interval variability novel evidence for repolarization liability in ischemic and nonischemic dilated cardiomyopathy. *Circulation, 96*(5), 1557-1565.

CardioSoft. (2005). *Version 6.0 operator's manual.* Milwaukee, WI: GE Medical Systems Information Technologies.

Christov, I., Otsinsky, I., Simova, I., Prokopova, R., Trendafilova, E., & Naydenov, S. (2006). Dataset of manually measured QT intervals in the electrocardiogram. *Biomedical Engineering Online, 31*(5), 5-31.

Coumel, P., Maison-Blanche, P., Catuli, D., Neyroud, N., Fayn, J., & Rubel, P. (1995). Different circadian behavior of the apex and end of the T wave. *Journal of Electrocardiology, 28*(supplement), 138-142.

Daskalov, I. K., & Christov, I. I. (1999). Automatic detection of the electrocardiogram T-wave end. *Medical and Biological Engineering and Computing,* 37, 348-353.

Davey, P. (1999). QT interval measurement: Q to T apex or Q to T end . *Journal of Internal Medicine, 246,* 145-149.

Extramiana, F., Maison-Blanche, P., Badilini, F., Pinoteau, J., Deseo, T., & Coumel, P. (1999). Circadian modulation of the QT rate dependence in healthy volunteers. *Journal of Electrocardiology, 32*(1), 33-43.

HP. (1994). *M1700A interpretive cardiograph physician's guide* (4th ed.).

Jensen, B. T., Abildstrom, S. Z., Larroude, C. E., Agner, E., Torp-Pedersen, C., Nyvad, O., Ottesen, M., Wachtell, K., & Kanters, J. K. (2005). QT dynamics in risk stratification after myocardial infarction. *Heart Rhythm, 2,* 357-364.

Kardys, I., Kors, J. A., van der Meer, I. M., Hofman, A., van der Kuip, D. A. M., & Witteman, J. C. M. (2003). Spatial QRS-T angle predicts cardiac death in a general population. *European Heart Journal, 24,* 1357-1364.

Laguna, P., Mark, R. G., Goldberger, A., & Moody, G. B. (1997). A database for evaluation of algorithms for measurement of QT and other waveform intervals in the ECG. *Computers in Cardiology, 24,* 673-676.

Lang, C. C. E., Neilson, J. M. M., & Flapan, A. D. (2004). Abnormalities of the repolarization characteristics of patients with heart failure progress with symptom severity. *Annals of Noninvasive Electrocardiology , 9*(3), 257-264.

Maison-Blanche, P., Catuli, D., Fayn, J., & Coumel, P. (1996). QT interval, heart rate and ventricular tachyarrhythmias. In A. J. Moss & S. Stern (Eds.), *Noninvasive electrocardiology: Clinical aspects of Holter monitoring* (pp. 383-404). London, W. B. Saunders Co.

Malik, M., & Batchvarov, V. (2000). QT dispersion In J. Camm (Ed.), *Clinical approaches to tachyarrhythmias.* Armonk, NY: Futura.

Marciano, F., Cuomo, S., Migaux, M. L., & Vetrano, A. (1998). Dynamic correlation between QT and RR intervals: How long is QT adaptation to heart rate? *Computers in Cardiology, 25,* 413-416.

Merri, M., Moss, A. J., Benhorin, J., Locati, E., Alberti, M., & Badilini, F. (1992). Relation between ventricular repolarization duration and cardiac cycle length during 24-hour Holter recordings: Findings in normal patients and patients with long QT syndrome. *Circulation, 85,* 1816-1821.

Moody, G., & Mark, R. (1988). *MIT-BIH arrhythmia database directory.* Cambridge, MA: MIT Biomedical Engineering Center.

Murabayashi, T., Fetics, B., Kass, D., Nevo, E., Gramatikov, B., & Berger, R. D. (2002). Beat-to-beat QT interval variability associated with acute myocardial isquemia. *Journal of Electrocardiology, 35*(1), 19-25.

Nihon Kohden. (2001). *ECAPS-12C user guide: Interpretation standard* (revision A).

Pueyo, E., Malik, M., & Laguna, P. (2005). Beat-to-beat adaptation of QT interval to heart rate. *Proceedings of the 27th Annual International Conference of the IEEE Engineering in Medicine and Biology Society* (pp. 2475-2478).

Pueyo, E., Smetana, P., Malik, M., & Laguna, P. (2003). Evaluation of QT interval response to marked RR interval changes selected automatically in ambulatory recordings. *Computers in Cardiology, 30,* 157-160.

Risk, M. R., Bruno, J. S., Llamedo Soria, M., Arini, P. D., & Taborda, R. A. M. (2005). Measurement of QT interval and duration of the QRS complex at different ECG sampling rates. *Computers in Cardiology, 32,* 495-498.

Sosnowski, M., Czyz, Z., Leski, J., Petelenz, T., & Tendera, M. (1996). The coherence spectrum for quantifying beat-to-beat adaptation of RT intervals to heart rate in normal subjects and in postinfarction patients. *Computers in Cardiology, 23,* 669-672.

Strumillo, P. (2002). Nested median filtering for detecting T-wave offset in ECGs. *Electronic Letters, 38*(14), 682-683.

Tadeusiewicz, R. (2004). Automatic understanding of signals. In M. A. Kłopotek, S. T. Wierzchoń, & K. Trojanowski (Eds.), *Intelligent information processing and Web- mining* (pp. 577-590). Berlin: Springer-Verlag.

Willems, J. L. (1990). *Common standards for quantitative electrocardiography: 10th CSE progress report.* Leuven, Belgium: ACCO.

Willems, J. L. (1991). *SCP-ECG project manager. Standard communications protocol for computerized electrocardiography. Final specifications and recommendations.* Final Deliverable AIM Project #A1015. Leuven, Belgium: ACCO.

Wirth, N. (1976). *Algorithms + data structures = programs.* Englewood Cliffs, NJ: Prentice Hall.

Zareba, W. (2001). Digital Holter in drug studies. *Proceedings of the FDA Meeting on Digital ECGs.*

Zareba, W., Nomura, A., & Perkiomaki, J. (2001). Dispersion of repolarization: Concept, methodology and clinical experience. In W. Zareba, P. Maison-Blanche,

& E. H. Locati (Eds.), *Noninvasive electrocardiology in clinical practice.* Armonk, NY: Futura.

Chapter IX
Dynamic Task Distribution in Mobile Client-Server Cooperation

Wearable ECG recorders are conceived as miniature versions of bedside electrocardiographs. Although contemporary micro-electronic technologies have made it possible for wearable recorders to be smaller, the other limitations of wearable recorders are even more manifested.

This chapter discusses the technical limitations of remote wearable recorders. These are caused mainly by high expectations of mobility and manifest themselves through short autonomy time, low computational power, limited resources, and unacceptable physical size.

Interpretation software is usually rigid-designed, a universal variant of clinical application, and meets the average diagnostic requirements of the medium patient. The aim of personalizing interpretation software is to provide accurate information of highest importance, depending on the variable status of the patient. The secondary benefit is the standardization of devices at the design and manufacturing stage, followed by its further customization by the software when in use according to patient-specific features and in the context of a specified disease.

This chapter provides details about the re-programmability of the remote device allowing for replacement of diagnostic procedures via wireless connections. The supervising center manages the remote device resources and applies the most suitable interpretation procedure to determine the expected diagnosis. The interpretation chain architecture is partially modified while the software is running, so this adaptation must consider all the events and delays that may occur in both devices and in the transmission channel.

A decision about software adaptation is expected to yield a diagnostic result that approximates the absolute correct values. Assuming that the server resources are unlimited and the machine may run a very complicated algorithm for a certain strip of signal, the diagnostic result calculated by the server is taken as a reference close enough to the correct values. Then, the assessment of the dynamic task distribution is based on the convergence of remote computed parameters to the reference computed by the server. The software adaptation needs to redefine diagnostic parameter quality and employ the quality description to the software functional modulation.

The remote software performance is controlled automatically by a multi-criteria decision process running on the server. The rules for such a process were defined very strictly, taking interpretation standards as a first reference. Investigations and queries in the medical world yielded further knowledge about the behavior and preferences of cardiologists.

TECHNICAL LIMITATIONS OF REMOTE WEARABLE ELECTROCARDIOGRAPHS

Telemedicine based on the remote acquisition of various vital signs (Chiarugi et al., 2002; Nelwan, van Dam, Klootwijk, & Meil, 2002) opens up a wide application area ranging from equipment for clinical use to the home care devices (Gouaux et al., 2002; Maglaveras et al., 2002). Several commercial tele-diagnostic services in the United States and Europe offer the continuous monitoring of cardiac risk people. Such services typically use restricted-access wireless networks of star topology. The interpretive intelligence aimed at the derivation of diagnostic features from recorded time series is implemented either in the recorder or in the supervising server. Both approaches have serious limitations.

The *central intelligence* model uses the communication channel continuously to report raw signals of high data volume, so it needs the uninterrupted carrier availability, which makes the transmission cost very high. The *spread intelligence* model assumes that the recording device interprets the signal and issues an alert message in case of abnormalities. Although the *spread* interpretation *intelligence* reduces communication costs, the diagnostic quality is affected due to resource limitations typical to a wearable computer. Other alternatives, like a triggered acquisition method typical for the ECG event recorders, suffer from poor reliability since a manually operated device risks missing an event when the patient in pain is unable to start the recording session. Our research aims at combining the advantages of both interpretive intelligence models.

At first glance, the advantages of remote controlled recording devices are two-fold:

- The signal is interpreted online and if necessary transmitted without delay, so that the medical intervention (e.g., rescue action) may start immediately if necessary.
- The acquisition is controlled by experienced staff with the support of an almost unlimited knowledge base and with reference to previous results.

When considering the additional features of remote programmability, two dimensions should be pointed out: the levels and the aspects of adaptation.

Levels of software adaptation quantitatively describe the interference of the management procedure into the ECG interpretation process. According to the adaptation level, various kinds of programming technology are used to achieve the adaptation aim. The main adaptation levels are software update based on the modification of selected computation coefficients and software upgrades based on the dynamical re-linking of function libraries.

Aspects of software adaptation provide a qualitative description of the changes and the choice of procedures selected for modification in order to achieve overall improvement in the diagnostic quality of a given patient's status. The management of the software adaptation aspects is complicated by the dependencies between the diagnostic parameters originating from a common branch of the interpretation tree.

In a typical topology of surveillance network (Figure 9.1), remote wearable recorders are supervised and controlled by a node archiving the captured information. Assuming both device types are equipped with signal interpretation software, the analysis of other constraints leads to the following remarks, which are a background for the proposed adaptive concept:

- Higher interpretation performance of the wearable device results in higher power consumption and shorter autonomy time assuming a specified hardware.
- Lower interpretation performance of the wearable device augments the datastream and increases the costs of digital communication, assuming costs to be proportional to data volume.
- The interpretation requisites and priorities vary with time and patient; they not only depend on many factors known before the examination starts, but also on previous examination results.

- The supervising server does not need to be mobile, but it benefits from world-wide knowledge resources and can be supported by human experts.

Considering these remarks, a new concept of the adaptive wearable vital signs monitor was developed in our laboratory. This concept joins the artificial intelligence approach to both device types in the network and employs the generalized division of tasks practiced by medics. The main assumptions of our concept are:

- The interpretation is done partially in the remote device and partially by a complementary software thread running on the server computer. Results are prioritized following changes in the diagnostic goals and current patient state.
- The actual data contents and format results from negotiations between the central server and the remote monitor. The negotiation process may be driven by distributed optimizations of power consumption, transmission channel use, and diagnosis quality.
- The high flexibility of a vital signs monitor may be achieved remotely in real time.

Size

The essential feature of wearable devices is reduced size and weight. The device should not influence the everyday activity of the patient and preferably it should not

Figure 9.1. Typical topology of surveillance network using wireless digital communication

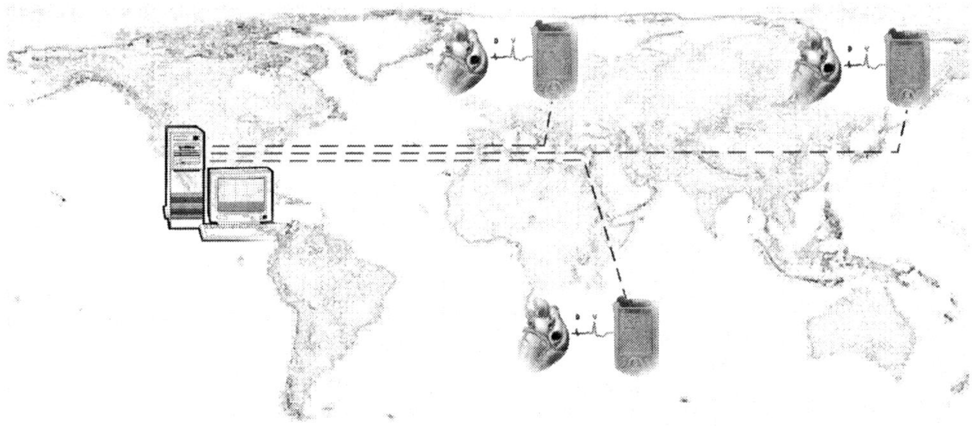

even be noticed. A good example and probably the only wearable device currently commonly known is the watch. Electronic watches, thanks to the flexibility and size-reduction of current electronics, are equipped with sophisticated functions like altimeter or DCS radio synchronization.

The habit of wearing a watch has also inspired the designers of some simple paramedical devices (e.g., pulse recorders for joggers). Some serious medical equipment of controlled quality also is manufactured in this form. In many such applications a reduction in the circuitry size is easier to achieve than a reduction in the required power, and consequently the power source is the heaviest part of the device and occupies the majority of its volume. A good example of such device is the implantable pacemaker.

Autonomy Time

Because power source capacity in relation to physical volume ratio is limited by technology, autonomous operation time is a compromise between the size and the current drain. Therefore, a good design of electronic circuitry should be power-saving oriented and include intelligent methods of power dissipation reduction. Nevertheless, currently used solutions—in particular for biosignal inputs and conditioning—should operate at high signal values in order to achieve required immunity against noise. Similarly, radio transmitting modules must be supplied by a considerable amount of power to achieve the necessary communication range. If intelligent power management is used, the power at the aerial is reduced in the case of good transmission quality or disconnected in periods when no transmission is performed. Cellular phones, certainly the most common mobile communication device, have reached the limits of technology with regard to power source capacity (Li-Ion batteries) and digital radio communication solutions. New concepts, design guidelines, and semiconductor technologies are necessary to put biomedical wearable devices into even smaller cases and to extend their autonomy time.

Computational Power

It is a common observation that every computation or logical operation in digital circuitry needs switching power. The switching power is used to move the electrical charge representing binary information, and due to the electrical capacitance intrinsic to all electronic devices, the power increases with the computation speed. Computational capacity is therefore limited by the size, but an even more important factor is power availability. Although modern technology may reduce the electrical capacitance, the electrical charge used for the reliable representation of digital information may not be reduced below a certain value and the computational power is always reduced in wearable devices. Since signal interpretation may be considered as a data reduction process, an interesting issue partly discussed hereafter is the balance between the energy required for autonomous signal processing in the wearable recorder and the energy required for the radio transmission of the unprocessed data.

Electromagnetic Compatibility

Medical electronic devices should not harm the function of other adjacent devices and must be immune to any environmental interference. Electromagnetic fields of high energy and interferences of this nature freely propagate in the space. Internal information integrity is guaranteed by the amount of electrical charge representing the unit information in the circuit. If the charge is insufficient, the interference-induced charge overwrites the usable data and the information integrity is distorted. On the other hand, all the abrupt current switching in the circuitry is the source of the electromagnetic field because the resistance, capacitance, and inductance are unavoidable for any physical realization of the computer. Limiting the electromagnetic field energy dissipation would require smooth current switching, which would limit the computational power. The alternative solution consisting of shielding of the system kernel implies increase of the weight and size of the device.

The issue of electromagnetic compatibility concerns not only the device itself, because of the existence of an external closed loop including the aerial and patient's body. Many studies report the influence of the electromagnetic field on humans at both the organ and cell levels. These phenomena have an impact upon the electrical properties and the activity of the living tissues being measured by the wearable device. The electromagnetic field emitted by the aerial also induces electrical potentials in leads and interferes with the measured organ's activity. Since the aerial is a common element for all these interference distribution paths, its proper design and use have been found to be essential for every radio-communicating wearable device.

Mutual Dependencies of Recorder Limiting Factors

The wearable recorder is a very complex electronic device facing many compromises towards the best compliance of its role in an integrated mobile health monitoring system. The fundamental aspect of its performance has been declared in the following order:

- *Usability understood as the influence of the device on the patient's comfort*— Low usability, difficult maintenance, complicated operation, or continuous attention requirement will lower the acceptance of the recorder by the patient and leads to the failure of continuous surveillance.

- *Reliability seen as maximum performance in medical data interpretation in given recording conditions*—Poor reliability decreases the confidence level of the medical result and limits the surveillance application to the raw screening of the main vital signs.
- *Economic interest expressed by the average cost of distant monitoring in relation to expenses for an alternative diagnosis* (e.g., personal contact with the doctor)—High costs for maintenance of the device, transmission channel use, medical staff supervision, and so forth, as well as high unit production costs of the recorder, will limit the potential application area and user population.

Except for these considerations, the wearable recorder requires a very thorough design and prototyping with consideration for the mutual dependencies of the limiting factors. Some of them are intrinsic features of the analog and digital data representation or are unavoidable because of their physical nature. Others are limited by current electronic materials and chemical technologies, and hopefully may be improved in the future. Finally, the influence of several limiting factors may be reduced by the optimization of the use of device resources. Similarly, some relations, like the ratio of data quality to resource use or the ratio of autonomy time to transmission channel use, may be optimized.

It is important to note that thanks to the use of software for remote device management via a bi-directional digital communication channel, optimization may be carried out beyond the device production stage. The main novelty of our approach is the continuous optimization of ECG interpretation following patient status changes and the variability of diagnostic goals.

ADJUSTMENT AND PERSONALIZATION OF THE INTERPRETATION SOFTWARE

Telemedical systems are currently considered as very interesting applications because of their direct impact on the life quality. Actually, in the area of vital signs-based diagnoses and monitoring, the difference between the stationary or bedside recorder (Klingeman & Pipberger, 1967; Pordy et al., 1968; Macfarlane, Lorimer, & Lowrie, 1971; IBM, 1974; HP, 1994; DRG, 1995; Nihon Kohden, 2001; CardioSoft, 2005) and the telemedical recorder (Fayn et al., 2003; Chiarugi et al., 2003; Banitsas, Georgiadis, Tachakra, & Cavouras, 2004; Bar-Or, Healey, Kontothanassis, & Van Thong, 2004) consists of just applying a wireless digital data link. In several developed countries, the commercial offer of telemedical surveillance or home care include continuous or semi-continuous distant interpretation of the electrocardiogram, respiration, or blood oxygenation (SpO_2). In the case of the ECG, however, conventional systems must meet a compromise. The centralized signal interpretation involves significant costs to the datastream transmission, while the remote interpretation has low reliability in a wearable battery-operated recorder with limited resources. In that case no personalization or diagnosis-oriented processing is possible. Disregarding the patient status and diagnostic aims, the interpretation always uses rigid procedures based on commonly applicable medical knowledge.

Home-care ECG recorders are found to be extremely useful when a long-term acquisition is necessary from a remote or sparsely populated area. However, common are complaints about the high cost of telecommunication services and poor performance manifested mainly by the huge number of false-positive alerts (Gouaux et al., 2002; Pinna, Maestri, Gobbi, La Rovere, & Scanferlato, 2003). Due to the fact that the remote interpretation runs as an unsupervised process, the diagnostic results cannot be verified and their reliability is influenced by the compromise between computational power and energy consumption.

The use of standardized interpretation criteria for all patients regardless of diagnostic goals and patient status is common today, however it is starting to be considered as an important limitation factor. Certainly the criteria are set as optimal for the most expected patient, although the individuals of statistically mean normal diagnostic value can rarely be found. Sometimes alternative computational constants are considered depending on subject age (neonate, pediatric, adult) or sex. For some parameters, independent diagnostic criteria are used depending on race; however, up until now serious race-dependent investigations are rarely reported.

The current widespread computer-assisted interpretation of electrocardiograms implies standardization of the diagnostic procedure (IEC 60601-2-51, 2003). However, uniform procedure does not take into account human expert behavior, thus it has two considerable drawbacks:

- prefers an average instead of a patient-oriented approach, and
- neglects the rules of information flow established in the course of the history of medicine and also does not consider the latest achievements of medical sciences.

The use of agile software (Augustyniak & Tadeusiewicz, 2006) removes the main technological constraints for patient-oriented interpretation and opens up the opportunity for a better simulation of human expert assistance by the machine.

The principle of the network operation is conceptually based on the following generalized rules of human relations often concluded from the observation and analysis of interpersonal relations in cardiology:

- General practitioners interpret a wide range of easy records on they own; in the case of doubt they ask experts for an interpretation.
- Cardiology experts interpret not only more specialized but also more difficult records; they often report their findings to general practitioners.
- Repeated problems enlarge general practitioner knowledge supported by expert findings and advice; consequently, general practitioners are becoming more specialized.
- Expert knowledge is based on experience in dealing with similar records successfully interpreted in the past; since patients look for the best diagnosis available, an increase in expertise increases the chance of encountering similar records in the future.

The authors believe that during the history of medicine, interpersonal relations and pathways for knowledge exchange were created optimally. Now, in an era of artificial intelligence, significant improvements in diagnostic quality may be achieved by reproducing these relations in a network of cooperating diagnostic-oriented computers.

It is worth noting that the turn towards constantly adaptive interpretation systems was made possible with the introduction of programmable micro-electronics. The interpretation software exists in multiple variants at the origin, and the manufacturer uploads the desired version upon necessity. As far as all software complies with diagnostic safety and accuracy requirements, there is no medical objection to tailor the final software package with regard to client needs. The end user usually estimates his needs from experience and historical factors, and rarely has a justified background for his prediction. With the aim of not suffering from the lack of some options and facing even very rare problems, the needs are usually overestimated. The current market offers devices with a dozen rarely used, obsolete, or even useless diagnostic parameters.

Thanks to the use of flash technology, the device's program memory, formerly called 'read only memory' (ROM), may be rewritten up to a million times. The previous name is now justified only because in opposite to the random access memory (RAM) or data memory, the software itself only reads the code and does not use the program memory as storage space for variables. Flash technology also makes the re-programming easier than ever. A supervisory procedure stored in a safe non-erasable area allows for the update of embedded software in many home computers (e.g., BIOS), entertainment (e.g., DivX or MP3 players), or communication devices (e.g., mobile phones). On the other hand, the coexistence of code and data in a common storage area is typical for a von Neuman system architecture. In systems using RAM as program memory (e.g., personal computers), there are no technical constrains for software to be updated dynamically when it is being utilized. Two *modification levels* are considered in the case of the interpretive systems: heuristic constants update and executable code replacement. The modification of system hardware with the use of FPGAs (field programmable gate arrays), although possible with current technology, was not included in our further considerations.

REAL-TIME SOFTWARE REARRANGEMENTS AND THE DYNAMIC LINKING OF PROCEDURES AND LIBRARIES

Novelty Highlights

The approach presented in this chapter assumes re-programmability of the remote recorder and the adaptation of the signal interpretation process to several prioritized criteria of a medical and technical nature (Augustyniak, 2005). The ECG interpretation is designed as a distributed process performed partially by a separated thread on the supervising center and partially by the adaptive software of the remote recorder (Augustyniak, 2005). The digital wireless link is used in a bi-directional mode, not only for patient and device status reporting, but also for control of the remote software, for requesting for the adaptation of report contents and data priority, and for reloading of software libraries as necessary. This innovation assumes deep modulation of remote recorder functionality by the software, and its main challenge is the simulation of the continuous presence of a cardiology expert without limiting patient mobility.

The auto-adaptive surveillance system for cardiology, unlike its predecessors, uses a closed feedback loop modifying the performance of interpretation subroutines on the basis of recently calculated diagnostic results. The issues of stability, data convergence, and final result inaccuracy, as known from the classical control theory, should be defined and solved in a proposed system. We also used mathematical models of complex dependencies in the system for detection of unwanted behavior and for the estimation of its medical consequences.

Technical Details

Technically speaking, the remote recording adaptability was reached with the use of two layers of dedicated software. The basic layer contains unalterable modules: data acquisition and wireless communication services, as well as fundamental user interface procedures. The flexible overlay includes all interpretation and report formatting procedures programmed as diagnosis-oriented dynamic libraries, which may be charged and released upon request. This approach not only personalizes the remote recorder with patient-specific signal features, but it also allows for an unprecedented flexibility required for pertinent real-time reactions to unexpected events. The most common and frequent signals are fully interpreted by the wearable device software and issue only a tiny and cost-acceptable datastream. The occurrence of any difficult or unresolved event is reported as a short strip of raw signal for the interpretation by the supervising center software automatically, or in very rare cases with the assistance of an expert cardiologist (Figure 9.2).

The basic cell of the auto-adaptive surveillance system uses a star topology network and consists of three kinds of devices: supervising server (SuSe), remote recorder (PED), and wireless link (WL). Since patients supervised in parallel are independent, we can limit the consideration to a single PED, corresponding WL, and a separate software thread run on SuSe. Some functions are destined uniquely for the SuSe, some uniquely for the PED, and some may be assigned to the PED or SuSe by the task-sharing procedure (Figure 9.4). The randomly assignable procedures should have fully compatible versions despite significant platform differences.

The SuSe is not only managing the data archive, but performs many important tasks including the monitoring of result quality, estimating the optimal description of patient status, and managing randomly assignable interpretation procedures. The PED buffers the raw ECG signal and performs basic interpretation procedures necessary for emergency detection. Further processing, report contents, and frequency depend on the configuration request received from the SuSe. It consists of signal and data transmission, loading and unloading specialized libraries of interpretation software, and prioritized data-dependent reporting. The role of WL is limited to a passive transmission medium and described by variable transmission speed

Figure 9.2. Elements of cooperation between the remote recording device and the node server

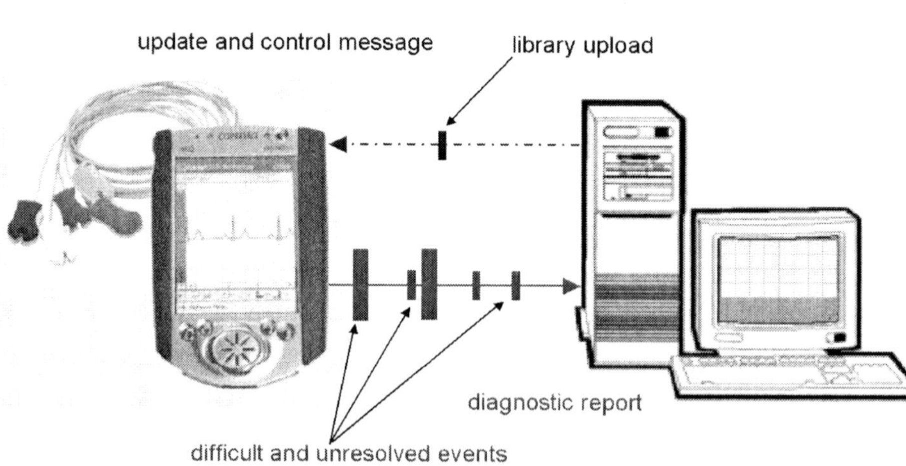

Figure 9.3. Scheme of dependencies between the remote recorder basic knowledge layer and examples of optional dynamically linked libraries

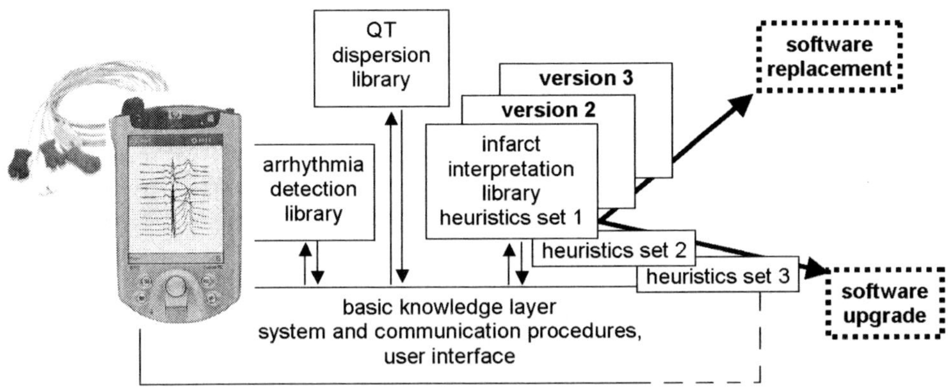

Figure 9.4. Task assignment in a distributed interpretive cardiac surveillance system

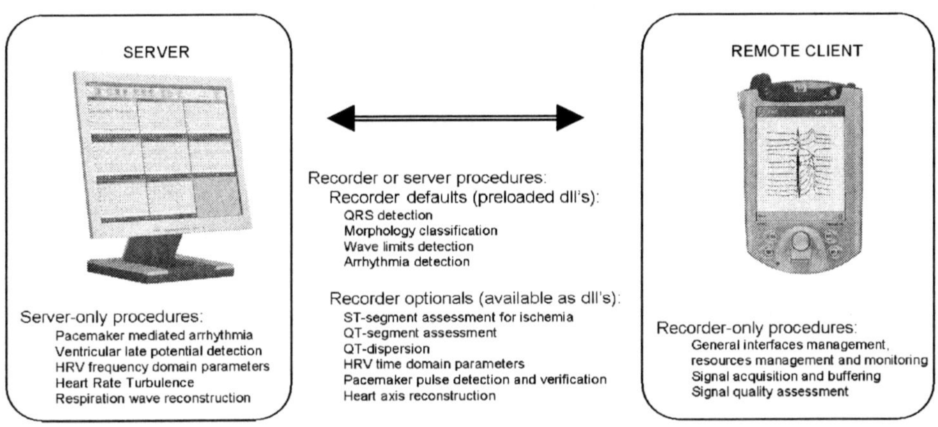

increasing with the reduction of data packet size, and by transmission cost increasing proportionally with the data packet size and the priority of messages.

Interfacing and Cross-Dependencies of Libraries

Interpretive software management is based on the raw assumption that the result reliability is proportional to the computational complexity and to the use of remote resources. It is common practice that a software manufacturer has a repository of several subroutines for the calculation of each specific diagnostic parameter in order to use them alternatively depending on system purpose (handheld recorders, interpretation workstations, real-time exercise monitors, etc.; see Figure 9.5).

The automatic replacement of the procedures while the interpretation is running must observe the following rules:

- The procedure thread is not currently running (i.e., allocate memory or use the stack).
- The other dependent procedures allow for the exchange (upgrade, downgrade, or absence) of the procedure being replaced.
- The interface (gateway) of all procedures of the same purpose is standardized within the system.

The first issue is easily managed with the use of software semaphore masking the exchange request for the time the procedure is called. The complete vector of currently used procedures (usage status) is a system variable stored in the flags area of the memory. The dependency tree is also stored as an aggregate variable (structure) build and updated each time the software is modified. The tree is specific for each procedure and may be generated automatically with the use of scanning the external calls in the source code. In the prototype system the tree was fixed for each subroutine and written in the code description area.

Figure 9.5. Structure of example repository of QT interval analysis procedures; each procedure is described by statistical parameters: result reliability and accuracy, expected memory usage, and computation complexity

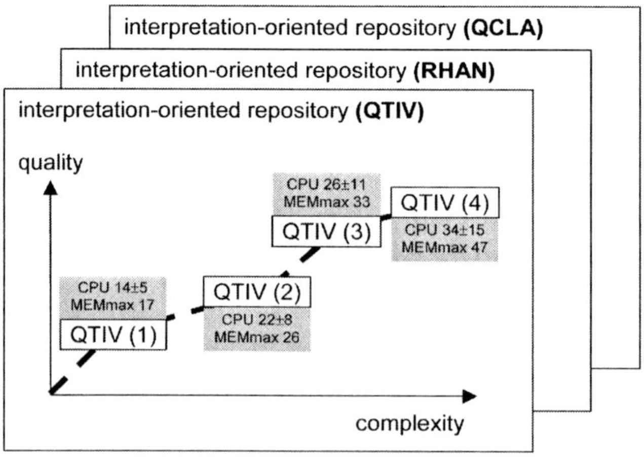

For the reason of compatibility, all procedures of the same type must use a common communication structure (gateway) supporting all external data flow. This structure was designed as optimal for the most advanced procedure used. This choice does not limit the performance of most advanced interpretation procedures; however, for the simplest versions the gateway is oversized.

ADAPTIVE REPORTING

Relations Between Processing and Reporting Adaptiveness

Non-uniform reporting is an intrinsic result of the non-uniform ECG processing performed by the agile software. Nevertheless, non-uniform reporting may be set up independently from the processing even in the case of rigid interpretation software. In the case of agile software, there exists a technically possible, but very impractical option of uniformize the report; however, for adaptive process, non-uniform reporting is a natural consequence. Non-uniform reporting resulting from the re-programmability of the ECG interpretation process is discussed in this section. Details of the non-uniform report format are provided in Chapter X, and other aspects of non-uniform reporting are considered in Chapter XI.

The cooperation of the network elements is conceptually based on a model of human relations often observed in cardiology: numerous general practitioners interpret most of the cases on their own, reporting only the most difficult problems to the expert and getting from him hints as to how to increase their diagnostic skills.

The re-programmable overlay in the remote recorder architecture also contains report formatting procedures (Augustyniak, 2004), therefore the report content, data priority, and reporting interval can be adjusted remotely. Here again, the decision is justified by patient status determined from previous diagnostic results, but the patient with the 'event button' occasionally can also trigger a report regardless of the current configuration-dependent reporting interval. The use of circular memory buffers provides a short strip of signal directly preceding the event button press for the analysis and reporting. The data communication format contains mandatory data description fields and optional data containers of variable size. This approach creates space for future extensions of diagnostic signals, data, patient communication, patient positioning coordinates, JPEG pictures, and so forth.

One of the principal issues is data priority in the report. The term has two different meanings: one concerning the global report urgency attribute, and the second a description of data order within the report packet.

One of the consequences of interpretation programmability is the multitude of output signal formats ranging from raw electrocardiograms to the sparse data (e.g., heart rate). The modifiable transmission protocol is very useful for the optimization of wireless channel use aimed at keeping monitoring costs at an acceptable level. As a general rule, we propose the transmission of basic interpretation results for all the monitoring times and more detailed reports for short time intervals. Occurrence or suspicion of any event results in a more detailed report, even including the corresponding strip of raw signal. This approach was conceived as a result of observation and analysis of cardiologists' behavior. It can be remotely programmed upon request.

The adaptability of the remote monitor goes far beyond the functional or economic aspects. Four issues were considered within the framework of the research project on content-adaptive signal and data format:

1. reporting frequency;
2. report content and data priority in a report;
3. signal sampling variability; and
4. the supervising of adaptability, including negotiation rules for the exchange of processing abilities, for report volume, and for reliability.

Aspects of Non-Uniform Reporting

Reporting frequency is independently controlled by the SuSe for each cooperating PED. In typical cases, all reports are issued with the frequency calculated by the SuSe from the diagnostic data. Since the reporting interval value is included in the report, missing reports are easily detected by the SuSe and the data can be recovered by a supplementary report request. For difficult signals, a similar solution supports the report of unexpected cases. In case the PED cannot interpret the signal, the complementary processing thread running on the SuSe issues both the interpretation and the report interval imposed on the remote device.

Continuous reporting is supervised by the SuSe only, because in real time the PED issues only basic diagnostic parameters (e.g., heart rate) accompanied by the raw signal, so the main interpretation is performed by the server thread. Figure 9.6 summarizes all modes of reporting frequency control.

From a signal-theory viewpoint, frequency of patient status recording should fulfill the Shannon rule. Temporal variability significantly differs for particular diagnostic parameters, and the occurrence of critical values increases the variation expectancy. Thus, the maximum time interval for the next measure point should be determined individually considering the past and present values of each parameter. Irregularly sampled datastreams may be interpolated in case the mid-point samples need to be estimated.

Figure 9.6. Examples of reporting frequency control: (a) and (b) pathological ECG interpreted remotely; (c) unexpected event causing raw signal transmission and server-side interpretation

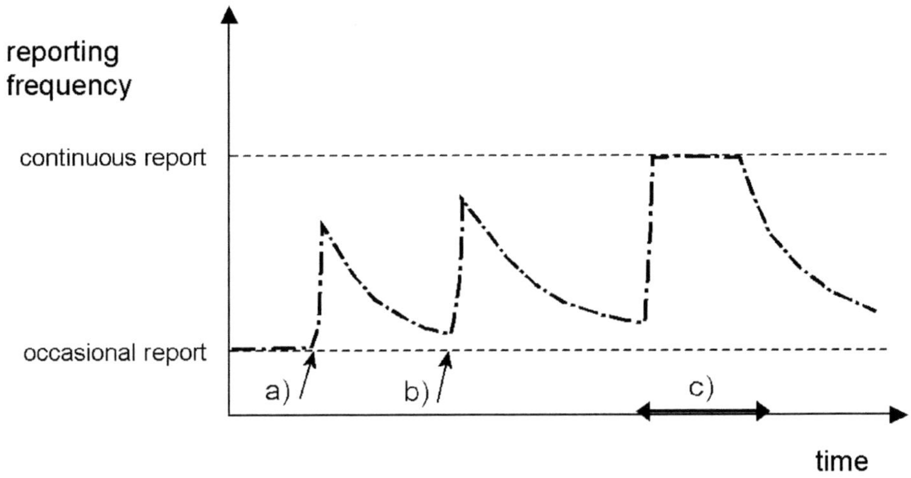

During the ECG interpretation process, medical information is represented in various data forms: signals, diagnostic parameters, and metadata. The distributed architecture of interpretive software with adaptive task sharing involves the transmission of data at various processing stages. Consequently, the data communication format contains data description fields, specifying data containers of variable size (see Chapter XI). The report of a normal finding may include supplementary data, and larger delay is tolerable without affecting the diagnosis consistency.

The adaptive ECG signal sampling is based on the P, QRS, and T waves recognition. Its usage is thus restricted to cases when the remote recorder correctly recognizes the waves, but fails in further signal interpretation. The raw ECG signal is compressed before the transmission with the use of the information on expected local bandwidth in particular sections representing the cardiac cycle. Because the methodology is based on a physiological background, the compression is expected to fully preserve the signal diagnostability, although the reconstructed data sequence is not bit-accurate (Figure 9.7) (Augustyniak, 2002). Technically speaking, the signal is re-sampled to a non-uniform sequence with the use of cubic splines. The time interval between samples and the cut-off frequency of the anti-aliasing filter strictly follow the local bandwidth of each section detected in the ECG (see Chapter VI).

Results

Three aspects of ECG reporting adaptability were implemented in a prototype client-server configuration using a PDA computer (Hewlett-Packard) running the WindowsCE operating system. The ECG conditioning and digitizing module is connected through the Bluetooth interface and performs 12-lead standard acquisition (frequency: 500Hz, accuracy: 10bits). The transmission is based on an embedded mobile phone module with a GPRS connection to the Internet. The SuSe was a PC-standard computer connected to the Internet via a 100 Mbps Ethernet card. At the reported stage of the experiment, multi-threading interpretation was not implemented, consequently sever accessibility was limited to the specified remote recorder.

The interpretation software source code was written in C++ programming language. The interpretive software architecture was redesigned for a complementary run on both platforms. The processing chain contains multiple exit and entry points at which the interpretation process may be transferred to the server (Figure 9.8.A-C).

Except for the soft customization of the general-purpose low-cost device with the specific tasks, in particular patient status and diagnostic goals, the adaptability

Figure 9.7. Comparing a heartbeat in the regular and in the variable sampling rate signals

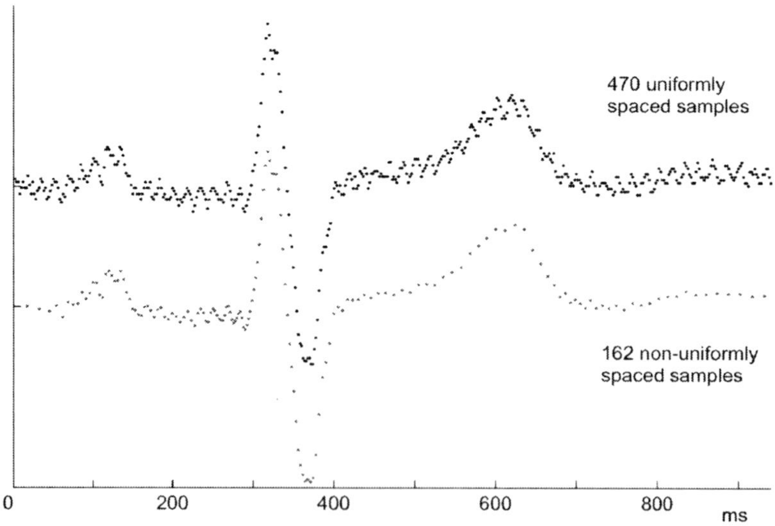

of the remote interpretive software has several measurable advantages over the fixed procedures used today. Two of them are:

- extending the remote recorder autonomy achieved by avoiding unnecessary computation and data transmission to a considerable extent, and
- reducing the costs of digital communication achieved by content-adaptive signal and data representation.

Figure 9.8. (a) Distant ECG processing chain in 'central intelligence' variant

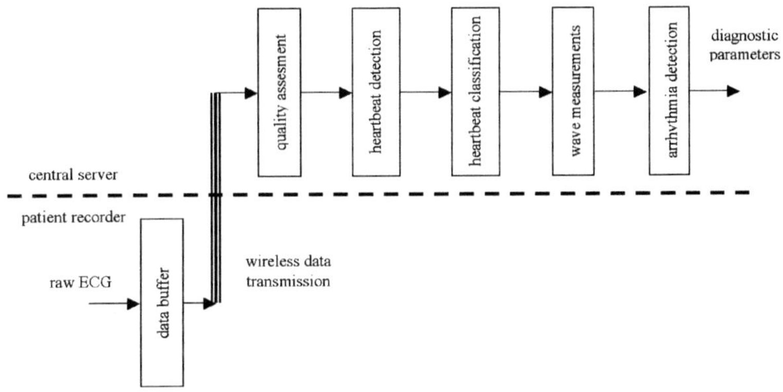

Figure 9.8. (b) Distant ECG processing chain in 'remote intelligence' variant

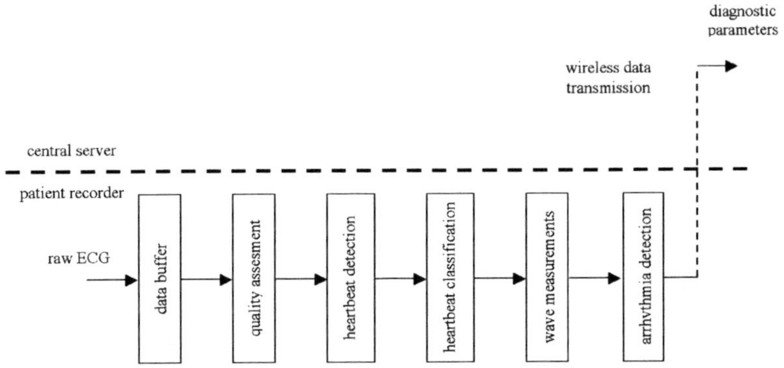

continued on following page

Figure 9.8. (c) Distant ECG processing chain in 'distributed intelligence' variant

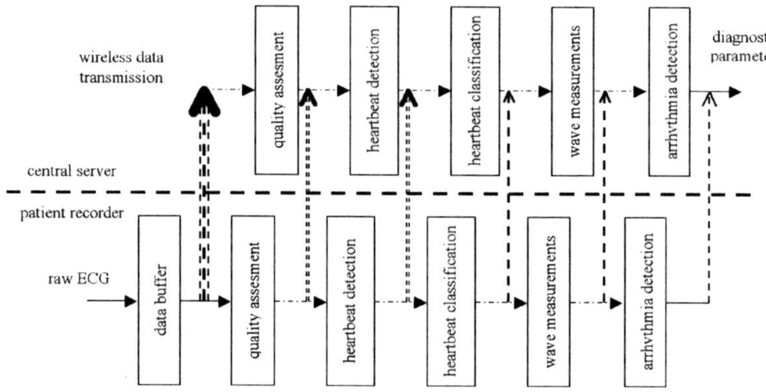

Because of our concern with information reliability and consistency, the data quality parameters and transmission delays were measured according to typical procedures (IEC 60601-2-51, 2003).

All tests were performed on 58 artificial signals originating from looped normal CSE records with inserts of pathological CSE records (Willems, 1990). The inserts were made with regard to the corrected baseline points on each record. With regard to test integrity, signals of duration of 1-1.5 hour were reproduced by a multi-channel programmable generator conceived for the advanced testing of interpretive ECG recorders.

In comparison with the uniform regular reporting, our tests show a data reduction ratio of 5.6 times (average) as a result of report content management. In some cases, employing raw signal transmission, an additional data reduction of 3.1 times was achieved thanks to the non-uniform signal sampling in selected records. Furthermore, data reduction of 2.6 times (average) is a result of irregular reporting with the use of the prediction of diagnostic parameter variability.

By avoiding unnecessary computation and data transmission, report content management also extends the remote recorder battery life on average by 65% compared to the software of a standard architecture running on the same PDA.

All diagnostic data were reconstructed by the recipient using interpolation techniques and stated that they fall within the respective standard deviation accuracy limits. Regular report messages were delayed on the Internet up to 20 seconds, while in the worst case of abnormal finding message, the total delay falls below 1.3 seconds thanks to the priority attribute and a concise form.

Discussion and Conclusions

Considering the human interpretation-derived directions, we rearranged a typical machine interpretation software to simulate human reasoning. Several aspects of the data are adjusted according to the automatic rough estimate of the record contents: the interpretation process flow, the result priority, the report content and frequency, and the local sampling frequency of the reported ECG strip.

The content-adaptive signal and data format have a considerable impact on the diagnostic quality because of the following features:

- The monitoring and auto-alerting parameters are adjustable to patient-specific signals anytime during the recording.
- The reporting can follow any unexpected event, and the interpretation is flexible enough to cover a variety of diagnostic goals, changed or updated remotely.
- The reporting closely follows the medical practice of personal interactions optimized during the centuries of the history of medicine.

Additionally, the adaptive report may include audio-visual communication with the patient or his or her supervisors supporting the transmission of instructions necessary in the case of technical troubles (e.g., electrode replacement), medical risk (e.g., physical overload), medication intake, or remote modification of monitor function.

The adaptive ECG formats may also be considered for other applications typical for the digital age:

- message optimization and prioritizing;
- pre-selection of abnormalities—facilitating a doctor's interpretation; and
- data fingerprinting—faster and more reliable management of databases.

The most problematic issue is now the compatibility of the interpretive software designed for different platforms. The SuSe-side thread could not be designed optimally, due to creating multiple entry points where the interpretation could be taken up from the remote recorder. Consequently, the processing chain of the SuSe thread must follow several design requisites resulting from the restrictions on its counterpart in a PED.

AUTOMATIC VALIDATION OF DYNAMIC TASK DISTRIBUTION

Introduction

Quality control is an aspect of principal importance in all diagnoses supported automatically. The automatic system should allow the end-user to pay more attention to the patient, without the necessity of fully supervising the behavior of the software. Professional organizations like cardiology societies implement strict certification procedures for medical electronic equipment (Willems, 1990). In the domain of automated ECG interpretation software testing, worldwide standard databases with reference signals and data are used to measure whether the diagnostic parameters issued by the software under test fall within the tolerance margin around the corresponding reference value (gold standard; IEC 60601-2-51, 2003).

Research towards adaptive distributed ECG interpretation networks not only revealed unprecedented advantages, but also standardization requirements not previously considered. Such networks show high flexibility of interpretation task sharing, eliminating the unnecessary computation and data flow, and finally they adapt to the variable status of the patient and diagnostic goals (Augustyniak, 2006). Until today, there was no standard to test these new features beyond the parameters common to the rigid software. Our proposal aims to fill this gap and to implement a multidimensional hyperspace of quality. Since the target system under test is adaptive and time plays a crucial role in life-critical cardiac events, quality estimation must support the dynamic behavior of the system and include transient description parameters.

Unfortunately, medical guidelines and testing standards (e.g., AHA, 1967; IEC 60601-2-51, 2003) describe only stable pathologies and provide stationary (in the medical sense) reference records. This is sufficient for off-line interpretation systems attempting each part of the signal with the same assumption and thus guaranteeing high repeatability of results. Human experts, however, behave differently, taking into account not only a limited section of cardiac electrical records, but also a much wider context of history, including extracardiac events. Staying in touch with their patients, human experts often witness medical emergencies and modify their further diagnostic goal. Design of a remote adaptive interpretation system that is expected to simulate the presence of a doctor must consider new criteria of adaptiveness and assessment of diagnostic quality present in everyday clinical life, but not formally covered by current standards. These criteria should refer to the present patient status and cover:

- specific areas of interest for further diagnosis (the optimal hierarchy of diagnostic parameters) in patient description,

- expected data variability and resulting minimum update frequency of each parameter,
- tolerance of each parameter value,
- possible subsequent diagnoses (patient status) ordered by the likelihood of occurrence, and
- reference records containing example transient signals.

Concept of Multi-Dimensional Quality Estimate

While conventional rigid software must be evaluated in the domain of result accuracy, adaptive software may be assessed in multidimensional hyperspace. Initially, let us assume that three dimensions are sufficient:

- asymptotic accuracy,
- adaptation delay, and
- convergence (adaptation correctness).

Asymptotic accuracy is the absolute value of diagnostic error when the transient-evoked software adaptation is completed. Assuming no other transient is present in the subsequent signal, it may be expressed as:

$$Q = \lim_{t\to\infty} \left| v(t) - v_0 \right| \tag{9.1}$$

where $v(t)$ is the subsequent diagnostic outcome and v_0 is the absolute correct value.

Adaptation delay is defined as the time period from the transient occurrence t_0 to the moment t_D when the diagnostic outcome altered by the interpreting software modification starts falling into a given tolerance margin ε around its final value.

$$D = t_D - t_0 : \forall t > t_D \; v(t) \in (v(\infty) - \varepsilon, v(\infty) + \varepsilon) \tag{9.2}$$

The *convergence* represents the correctness of decisions made by the management procedure about the interpretation processing chain. Taking the analogy from the theory of control, the software adaptation plays the role of feedback correcting the diagnoses made automatically. If the software modification decisions are correct, the outcome altered by the interpreting software modification approaches the true value, the modification request signal is removed in consequence of decreasing error, and the system is stable. Incorrect decisions lead to the growth of diagnostic outcome error and imply an even stronger request for modification. The outcome value may stabilize on an incorrect value or swing the measurement range in response to subsequent trials. In the last case, the system is unstable and the diagnostic outcome does not converge to the true value.

The Concept of Weighted Accuracy Estimate

There is no general estimate of diagnostic quality in a system composed of several procedures responsible for each parameter. The quality estimates need to correspond to the procedures selected for modification. Usually in the ECG interpretation chain, there is a complex dependency among the diagnostic parameters and interpreting procedures (Figure 9.9). Each final outcome is influenced by several procedures and each procedure usually affects multiple parameters. The range of influence depends on the interpretation stage at which the procedure is applied. The quality of early processing stages affects all of the diagnostic parameters and the influence range narrows at subsequent stages. Each kind of diagnostic procedure is attributed by a static list of influenced diagnostic parameters.

The system makes its decision about the software modification with regard to all the diagnostic parameters that may be concerned. The list of influenced diagnostic parameters is hierarchically scanned in order to detect any conflict of interest between simultaneously affected data. This hierarchy is, however, variable depending on patient status. Following the dependence of the diagnostic parameters' medical relevance on the patient status, we propose the use of the same list of relevance factors to modulate the contribution of particular parameter errors to the general estimate of diagnostic quality.

Standardization of Data

Non-uniform asynchronous updating of particular diagnostic parameters is an intrinsic advantage of adaptive interpretation systems. However, due to the non-uniformity, a direct comparison of their outcome to the reference values is not possible. Patient status must be estimated from the irregular series of data issued by the adaptive system under test at each data point when the reference results are available.

The diagnostic outcome of the adaptive interpretation being a non-uniformly sampled time series $N_j(\{n, v(n)\})$ was first uniformized with the use of the cubic spline interpolation (Aldroubi & Feichtinger, 1998), given by a continuous function:

$$S_i(x) = a_i + b_i(x - x_i) + c_i(x - x_i)^2 + d_i(x - x_i)^3 \qquad (9.3)$$

$x \in [x_i, x_{i+1}]$, $i \in \{0, 1, \ldots n\text{-}1\}$ best fitted to the series N_j.

The interpolation yielded a uniform representation of each parameter by sampling the $S_i(x)$ at the time points m corresponding to the results of the fixed software:

$$N'_j(m) = \sum_m S_i(x) \cdot \delta(x - mT) \quad (9.4)$$

The values estimated at regularly distributed time points were finally compared to the reference. The assessment of data conformance must consider three quality factors:

1. tested data accuracy at their individual sampling points,
2. interpolation error, and
3. reference data accuracy.

*Figure 9.9. The illustration of reciprocal dependencies of diagnostic parameters and interpretation procedures. According to patient status, parameter priority influences the final decision on remote software management. A bad parameter **A** triggers the replacement of only the procedures '2. beats clustering' and '4. wave axes' affecting parameters of lower priority **K** and **Y**.*

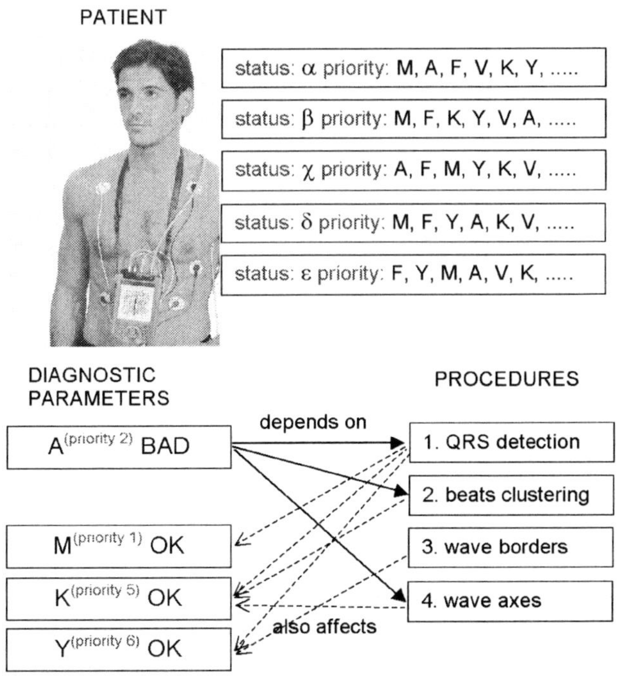

Quality Estimation in a Prototype Limited Scale Network

The behavior of the limited-scale network prototype of an ECG monitoring system with auto-adaptive software was investigated with the use of the proposed tools. The PED (remote recorder) was based on a PDA-class handheld computer with bi-directional GPRS connection. Instead of ADC module, a computer-based ECG simulator (8 channels, 12 bits, 500 sps) was connected via Bluetooth interface. The SuSe (supervising server) was a PC-class desktop computer with a static IP address and 100 Mb Internet access running Linux OS.

The test database contained 857 signals composed of artificially joined physiological ECG and a signal representing one of 14 selected pathologies considered as most frequent. The main goal of the test was the assessment of the software adaptation correctness. The process of remote software update is initiated if PED-issued diagnostic results differ from the SuSe-calculated reference by more than a threshold defined according to the diagnosis priority in four categories: 2% for QRS detection and heart rate, 5% for wave limits detection and ST segment assessment for ischemia, 10% for morphology classification, and 20 % for the remaining parameters.

In cases where the result after a single software modification step is still outside of the given tolerance margin, the decision about the next update is made by the SuSe depending on whether the new value is closer to the reference. The prototype allows for up to four consecutive update steps.

The values of the adaptation delay presented in Table 9.2 were measured with the use of wireless GPRS connection. An estimate of the longest delay is crucial for the design of data buffer length in the remote recorder and for the assessment of non-response time when a cardiac event occurs during system reconfiguration.

Conclusions

The presented method offers estimations of various new properties emerging due to the adaptation of ECG interpretation. Several concepts presented in this chapter (multi-dimensional quality estimate, weighted accuracy estimate) reveal the high complexity of the problem and some areas not covered by the medical procedures and recommendations. These topics were presented for discussion in cardiologists' forums.

The principal elements of the proposed quality estimation method were used in the assessment of a prototype cardiac monitoring network. In this application our method contributed to a final adjustment of the system's properties in particular automatic decision making about further processing and reporting in the PED.

Table 9.1. Results of test for the convergence of remote diagnostic results after the consecutive steps of interpretation software modification

calculation constants update steps	cumulative percentage	
	converging	non-converging
First	63.1	36.9
Second	74.5	25.5
Third	79.1	20.9
Fourth	80.7	19.3

Table 9.2. Delay to the remote recorder adaptation for various adaptation modalities of ECG interpretation software (in seconds)

adaptation modality	longest delay	average delay	standard deviation
calculation constants update	17.1[a]	4.3	1.3
software upgrade	6.0	4.4	1.5
software replacement	5.9	4.5	1.5
relocation the erroneous task to the server [b]	2.4	0.8	0.3

a *four steps of calculation constants update*
b *to the remote device software modification*

CONTROL RULES FOR AUTOMATIC SOFTWARE MANAGEMENT

General Remarks

A specialized supervisory process is necessary for optimal information management and task sharing. Such a procedure, aimed at diagnosis quality assessment, is designed as a part of each interpretive function running on the PED. At this point the software decides what was reliably interpreted by the recorder and what is too difficult and needs further processing by the server. Another supervisory procedure is running on the SuSe within each processing thread in order to manage the interpretive libraries for each cooperating PED. At this point the SuSe software analyzes PEDs errors, and estimates the probability of event repetition and the available remote computational power in order to decide about uploading a complementary interpretive library to the PED.

The concept and prototype of the adaptive PED for seamless ECG monitoring makes the assumption that the interpretation task sharing between the remote device and the central server is asymmetric.

Every ECG interpretation software consists of a processing chain following a given sequence of executed procedures. Procedures initiating the chain transform the raw signal to meta-parameters, while procedures terminating the chain issue diagnostic outcomes based on meta-parameters fed to their inputs. For the sake of supporting a wide range of medical cases, the processing chain conditionally branches into paths following some medically justified assumptions.

The statistics of procedures use and data flow in the ECG interpretation software from different independent manufacturers reveals three common rules:

1. Data volume is reduced at subsequent interpretation stages.
2. The interpretation reliability for common diseases is significantly higher than for very rare ones.
3. Simple procedures are commonly used, whereas sophisticated and computationally complex procedures are rarely used.

Observing these remarks, our concept assumes that the interpretation process is adaptively distributed between the PED and the SuSe (see Figure 9.4). The task distribution is asymmetrical in two aspects:

- The resources of the PED are limited, and technical constrains must be considered while planning task-sharing rules; the SuSe resources are virtually unlimited and may be supervised by the human expert.
- The diagnostic information flow is uni-directional, thus the PED initiates the interpretation process and completes it when possible, while the SuSe supports the interpretation at any stage of advancement and completes it when necessary.

Various implementations imply individual approaches to the interpretation task sharing specifying the processes running on a remote device, on a central server, or on either of these devices. The important point is that the procedures implemented for both platforms have to perform accordingly, regardless of the hardware and operating system differences. Otherwise, the complementary task allocation or redundant signal re-interpretation for assessment of result reliability would produce ambiguous results.

It is worth noting that the asymmetrical task sharing is very advantageous, at least in the following aspects:

- The PED performs easier and most common operations, require less computational power, and the results are less susceptible to errors.
- The captured datastream is fairly reduced at the initial stages of interpretation in the PED, and the required wireless channel bandwidth is fairly low.

The task sharing in the distributed ECG interpretation system is an important problem because it influences monitoring costs and diagnostic reliability. The compromise is pursued perpetually with consideration of results of research on human expert-derived diagnosis priority, statistic-based automatic assessment of result reliability, and machine estimations of available remote resources.

Expert-Derived Diagnosis Priority

It seems obvious that for a human expert, selected diagnostic results are more important than others. However, systematical research on the diagnostic statement hierarchy can hardly be found. For the purpose of building such a priority list, we studied the Cardiology Societies Standards and analyzed doctors' choices about report contents in a series of clinical trials.

Many standards issued by Cardiology Societies formally define the diagnostic path with conditional branches that direct the subsequent steps of ECG analysis depending on the results of precedent stages. Although different approaches were found in the literature, a rough common diagnostic path was estimated and rearranged as a binary tree. Its nodes define medically justified conditions for selecting a particular way recommended as optimal for further ECG interpretation efficiency.

The established interpretation priority is used as fuzzy selection criteria modulating the contribution from errors of a particular diagnostic parameter to the global estimate of patient description quality. This global value is a subject for further optimization depending on patient status. In practice it highlights even a small inaccuracy of important parameter values and suppresses a much larger divergence of diagnostic data not being relevant for the current description. Studies about the parameter priority are reported in Chapter X.

Automatic Assessments of Result Reliability

In a typical case, the ECG is completely interpreted by the PED, and thus only the diagnostic results of minimum data volume are transmitted to the center. Unfortunately, the PED's resources are limited, and occasionally the interpretation of an altered signal may not be as reliable as required for medical diagnosis.

Two processes are proposed for the continuous monitoring of remote interpretation reliability: random redundant signal re-interpretation and knowledge base similarity check.

Redundant signal re-interpretation uses bi-directional transmission and begins with the raw signal request issued by the SuSe. The PED does the interpretation independently, and besides the diagnostic result returns the raw electrocardiogram as well. As the signal is coded into a large data packet of low priority, it may reach the server with a significant delay. The requested signal is next interpreted by the SuSe software thread in a virtually unlimited environment. The results are considered as reference for comparison with the outcome received form the remote interpretation. Any difference is carefully analyzed, statistically processed, and compared to tolerance thresholds. Every outstanding value is a background for modification of the PED interpretation software. This process requires an additional load of the

Figure 9.10. An example of a processing tree in the ECG rhythm classification

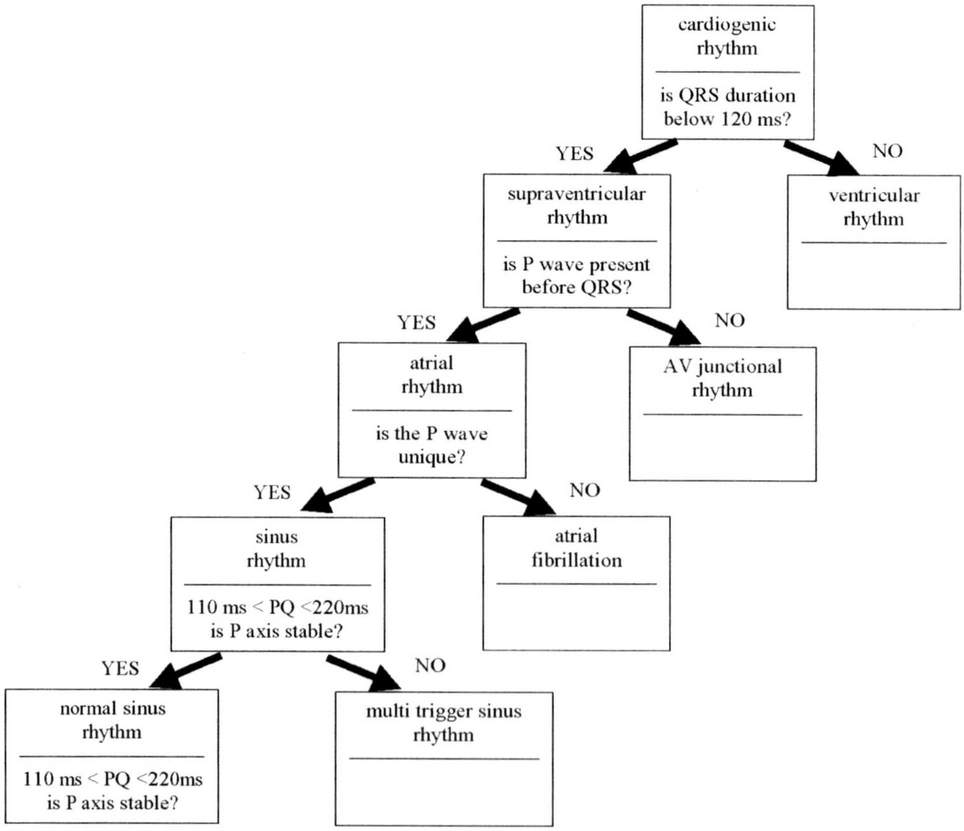

wireless channel and slightly increases the computational complexity assigned to the particular client. Therefore, the redundant re-interpretation rate should not be performed more often than once per 20 regular report packages.

Knowledge base similarity check is much simpler for implementation and does not overload the transmission channel. Therefore, it is performed for every received data packet. Each time a new packet arrives, the SuSe accesses the database for two reasons: verifying the consistency of the received data by comparing it to the most similar database record and estimating the trends of diagnostic parameters from changes observed in similar records. In order to reduce the database search, the compared data are prioritized by disease history, sex, and fundamental ongoing findings (e.g., heart rate or rhythm type). If the packet contains 'expected' data, no action is taken and the remote diagnostic results are considered reliable. In any suspicious case, often triggered by the sudden nature of cardiac events, the SuSe assumes that the remote interpretation failed and issues a raw signal request. Since the raw ECG is buffered in the PED, the signal behind suspicious data is retrieved, transmitted, and then interpreted by the SuSe for reference.

An Estimation of Available Remote Resources

The remote recording device is based on a PDA-class computer running mobile version of an operating system. During the monitoring process, the execution of any third-party software is excluded in order to enable the proper management of all available resources. The biggest part of the system memory is allocated for the raw ECG buffer. Raw signal buffering is used for delayed signal transmission in the case of central re-interpretation and for repeated remote interpretation each time the recorder software is modified. The second largest memory block is allocated for the executable code of interpreting software. Since many interpreting modules are programmed as dynamically linked libraries (dlls), the size of the program memory is variable and thus high functional flexibility is achieved at the price of constant resources monitoring.

The resources report included in the PED's status word is a mandatory part of every data packet. Whether the diagnostic packet rate may be set very low, there is an independent way to pool remote status on the server-issued request. The resources report (Figure 9.12) contains a few variables representing battery drain and status, ambient temperature, connection quality, processor usage, memory allocation, and codes of linked libraries. Receipt of this information is for the SuSe a background for the estimation of available resources and the modification of remote interpreting software according to the current diagnostic goal and to the extent it was fulfilled by the recorder. In the case of poor reliability or inconsistency found in automatic assessment diagnostic outcomes, the PED software adaptiveness provides us with a choice of four procedures according to the problem severity and available resources (Table 9.3).

The decision about the adaptation of remote interpretive software is always taken by the SuSe software. With the use of the bi-directional wireless channel, the modifying data are sent to the PED. Data exchange takes a considerable amount of time (up to several seconds), thus the monitoring system response time may be insufficient for sudden cardiac events. However, thanks to signal buffering, the continuity of monitoring is maintained.

Results

The ECG interpretation task-sharing rules were designed, programmed in C++ language, and tested in a prototype implementation in the PDA-based ECG monitor

Figure 9.11. Flow diagram of knowledge base similarity check and redundant signal re-interpretation for automatic assessment of result reliability

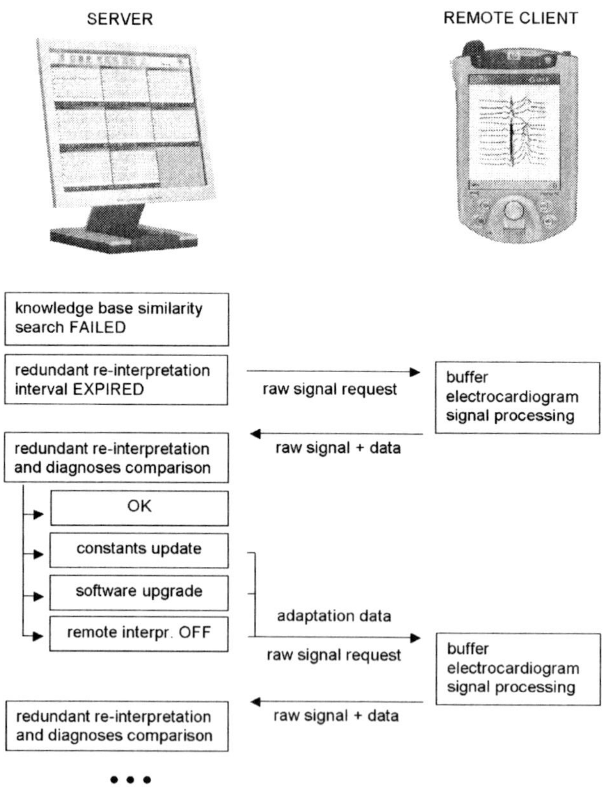

and the PC-class server for the set of standard test signals. The reference medical findings were known from the test signal database. However, the tests were focused on the task-sharing rules and thus the diagnostic correctness was of secondary importance. Several aspects were investigated during the test procedure:

- the convergence of remote-issued diagnostic results with the central-computed results on the same signal after the remote calculation constants update;
- the correctness of software upgrade and replacement in the technical and medical aspects;
- the delay since the first detection of remote interpretation inaccuracy to the completion of a PED's adaptation in the case of calculation constants update, software upgrade, and assignment of erroneous tasks to the SuSe; and
- the correctness of software replacement decisions with regard to expert-derived diagnosis priority.

The quantitative results of software modification tests including outcome convergence, accuracy, and delay were reported above (Tables 9.1 and 9.2). Because

Figure 9.12. Resources report format

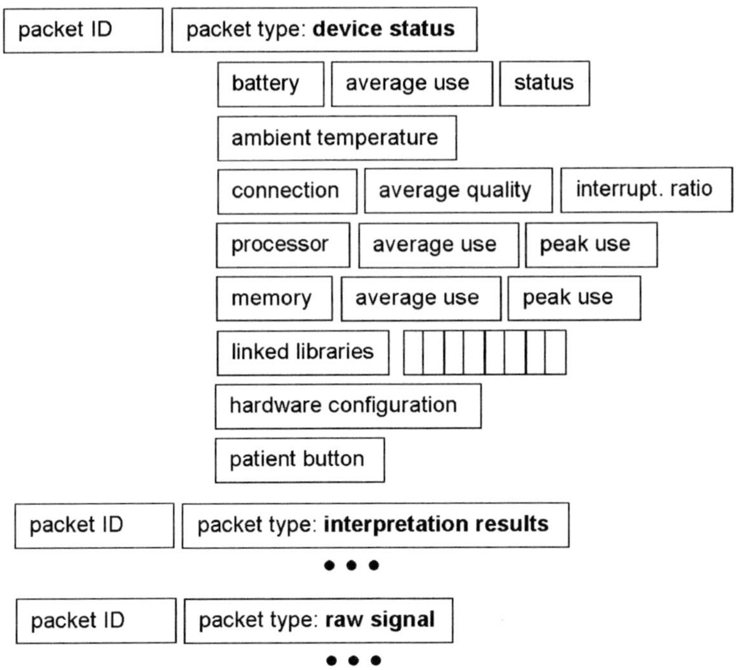

the value of relevance is not equivalent for particular diagnostic outcomes, software replacement favors certain procedures over others; the diagnostic parameter error was also modulated by diagnostic priority values. In more than 80% of the cases, software replacement resulted in diagnostic result improvement.

With regard to the technical aspect, the correctness of software upgrade and replacement is expressed by the percentage of incorrect adaptation attempts. Considered incorrect were *resources overestimation,* leading to memory allocation violation, and *underestimation,* resulting in the suspension of the software upgrade when the upgrade was feasible (Table 9.4). The correct results are displayed in the upper left and lower right corners, and the incorrect results are displayed in the upper right and lower left corners. The medical correctness was investigated only for all the technically correct modification attempts (768 cases, Table 9.5). With regard to the medical aspect, the correctness of the interpretive software upgrade and replacement is expressed by the percentage of adaptation attempts leading to diagnostic parameters converging on the reference values. The overall distance in the diagnostic parameter hyperspace is expressed by the values of the diagnostic parameter errors weighted by diagnosis priority.

Table 9.5 shows that the software upgrade provides for the smooth adjustment of diagnostic procedures and in a large majority of cases is made correctly. Unfor-

Table 9.3. Simplified decision matrix for the adaptation of remote interpretive software

interpretation error severity	resources available memory+processing / transmission yes / yes	yes / no	no / yes	no / no
low	CU	CU	CU	CU
intermediate	SU	SU	CI	SR
high	CI	SU	CI	SR

Abbreviations:

CU – calculation coefficients (heuristics) update

SU – software upgrade; linking supplementary interpretive library

CI – central interpretation; the remote interpretation is overwritten by the results issued by the server

SR – software replacement; unlinking an existent interpretive library of lower results priority and linking supplementary interpretive library

Note that CU, SU, and SR always require remote re-interpretation of buffered ECG and a redundant central re-interpretation for the automatic assessment of result reliability

tunately, its usability is limited by the range of values approved for the calculation coefficients. In cases where slight improvement is necessary, the software upgrade is an optimal choice because of the continuous use of the same computation algorithm. The software replacement is a significant intervention into the software architecture, computation algorithms, and possibly the calculation coefficients. Therefore, it should be reserved for cases when a sudden change of patient status or recording conditions require severe modification of PED functionality.

Discussion

Software adaptation and customization of a remote interpretive ECG recorder during seamless monitoring—which takes place based on automated diagnosis verification and resources assessment—is a complicated and responsible task. Particular procedures were programmed, implemented, and tested separately. The software adjustment and test process not described in this section lasted for 14 months. A total of 2,751 one-hour 12-lead ECG records were processed in the system in real time. With regard to 857 records (31.2%), software adaptation was required; the next 86 records (3.1%) were found to be too complicated for interpretation by the PED. A total of 768 (89.6%) of the software adaptation attempts were correct, while the remaining 89 (10.4%) failed due to the incorrect estimation of available PED resources. The overestimation of resources resulted in an operating system crash and thus monitoring discontinuity occurred in 27 (3.2%) cases. Future versions of

Table 9.4. Technical correctness of software upgrade and replacement

action	upgrade possible	upgrade impossible
upgrade performed	647 (75.5%)	27 (3.1%) resource overestimation
upgrade suspended or library replacement	62 (7.3%) resource underestimation	121 (14.1%)

Table 9.5. Medical correctness of software adaptation

action	diagnosis improvement	diagnosis degradation
software upgrade	643 (99.4%)	4 (0.6%)
software replacement	97 (80.2%)	24 (19.8%)

PEDs are expected to support the data buffer protection that allows for the re-interpretation of the ECG even after system restart.

Thanks to adaptive remote recorders, wireless pervasive cardiovascular monitoring networks provide new opportunities and new challenges. Adaptation alone does not guarantee improvement; it must be justified by medical procedures and must consider technical constraints. Adaptation is realized by remote software modification resulting in the flexible sharing of interpretation tasks between the remote recorder and the central server. Our approach combines the advantages of the two solutions in use today:

- The transmission channel load is nearly as low as when remote interpretation was used.
- The interpretation reliability and difficult case handling resemble a common centralized interpretation architecture, not excluding a human expert assistance.

In the authors' opinion, significant progress was made when formulating the ECG interpretation task-sharing rules, implementing them as software controlling the distributed monitoring system and testing their properties. The test results show considerable improvement of diagnosis quality in comparison to a rigid software. However, for further development the analysis of outliers is advisable. The rules just established must pass extensive clinical tests before use, and at present may not yet be applicable. More important than the rules themselves may be the description of our investigation of them, and in this work we hope to initiate a discussion and inspire other scientists to express their ideas. We believe that with this research a new investigation direction has been pointed. The history of biomedical engineering shows that automatic ECG interpretation software was developed to follow human expert reasoning. Today, multiple intelligent devices collaborate together, and they are expected to follow human expert collaboration rather than to emulate multiple independent doctors.

REFERENCES

AHA. (1967). *AHA ECG database.* Available from Emergency Care Research Institute, Plymouth Meeting, PA.

Aldroubi, H., & Feichtinger, J. (1998). Exact iterative reconstruction algorithm for multivariate irregularly sampled functions in spline-like spaces: The Lp theory. *Proceedings of the American Mathematical Society,* 126(9), 2677-2686.

Augustyniak, P. (2002). Adaptive discrete ECG representation—comparing variable depth decimation and continuous non-uniform sampling. *Computers in Cardiology, 29,* 165-168.

Augustyniak, P. (2004). Optimizing the machine description of electrocardiogram. *Journal of Medical Informatics and Technology, 8,* :MM-41-MM48.

Augustyniak, P. (2005). Content-adaptive signal and data in pervasive cardiac monitoring. *Computers in Cardiology, 32,* 825-828.

Augustyniak, P. (2006). The use of selected diagnostic parameters as a feedback modifying the ECG interpretation. *Computers in Cardiology, 33,* 825-828.

Augustyniak, P., & Tadeusiewicz, R. (2006). Modeling of ECG interpretation methods sharing based on human experts relations. *Proceedings of the 28th IEEE EMBS Annual International Conference* (pp. 4663-4669).

Banitsas, K. A., Georgiadis, P., Tachakra, S., & Cavouras, D. (2004). Using hand-held devices for real-time wireless teleconsultation. *Proceedings of the 26th Annual International Conference of the IEEE EMBS* (pp. 3105-3108).

Bar-Or, A., Healey, J., Kontothanassis, L., & Van Thong, J. M. (2004). BioStream: A system architecture for real-time processing of physiological signals. *Proceedings of the 26th Annual International Conference of the IEEE EMBS* (pp. 3101-3104).

CardioSoft. (2005). *Version 6.0 operator's manual.* Milwaukee, WI: GE Medical Systems Information Technologies.

Chiarugi, F. et al. (2002). Real-time cardiac monitoring over a regional health network: Preliminary results from initial field testing. *Computers in Cardiology, 29,* 347-350.

Chiarugi, F. et al. (2003) Continuous ECG Monitoring in the Management of Pre-Hospital Health Emergencies. *Computers in Cardiology, 30,* 205-208.

DRG. (1995). *MediArc premier IV operator's manual* (v. 2.2.).

Fayn, J. et al. (2003), Towards new integrated information and communication infrastructures in e-health. Examples from cardiology. *Computers in Cardiology, 30,* 113-116.

Gouaux, F. et al. (2002). Ambient intelligence and pervasive systems for the monitoring of citizens at cardiac risk: New solutions from the EPI-MEDICS project. *Computers in Cardiology, 29,* 289-292.

HP. (1994). *M1700A interpretive cardiograph physician's guide* (4th ed.).

IBM. (1974). *Electrocardiogram analysis program physician's guide* (5736-H15) (2nd ed.).

IEC 60601-2-51. (2003). *Medical electrical equipment: Particular requirements for the safety, including essential performance, of ambulatory electrocardiographic systems.* First edition 2003-02, International Electrotechnical Commission, Geneva

Klingeman, J., & Pipberger, H. V. (1967). Computer classification of electrocardiograms. *Computers and Biomedical Research, 1,* 1.

Macfarlane, P. W., Lorimer, A. R., & Lowrie, T. D. V. (1971). 3 and 12 lead electrocardiogram interpretation by computer. A comparison in 1093 patients. *British Heart Journal, 33,* 226.

Maglaveras, N. et al. (2002). Using contact centers in telemanagement and home care of congestive heart failure patients: The CHS experience. *Computers in Cardiology, 29,* 281-284.

Nelwan, S. P., van Dam, T. B., Klootwijk, P., & Meil, S. H. (2002). Ubiquitous mobile access to real-time patient monitoring data. *Computers in Cardiology, 29,* 557-560.

Nihon Kohden. (2001). *ECAPS-12C user guide: Interpretation standard* (revision A).

Pinna, G. D., Maestri, R., Gobbi, E., La Rovere, M. T., & Scanferlato, J. L. (2003). Home telemonitoring of chronic heart failure patients: Novel system architecture of the home or hospital in heart failure study. *Computers in Cardiology, 30,* 105-108.

Pordy, L., Jaffe, H., Chesky, K. et al. (1968). Computer diagnosis of electrocardiograms, IV, a computer program for contour analysis with clinical results of rhythm and contour interpretation. *Computers and Biomedical Research, 1,* 408-433.

Willems, J. L. (1990). *Common standards for quantitative electro-cardiography: 10th CSE progress report.* Leuven, Belgium: ACCO.

Chapter X
Optimization and Prioritization of Cardiac Messages

This chapter presents a signal theory viewpoint concerning diagnostic parameter datastreams. Particular diagnostic parameters are considered as a time sequence representing certain medical variables as time-dependent. Since the parameters represent various aspects of electrical heart activity (e.g., the depolarization rate, the re-polarization speed, etc.), their variability, and therefore the bandwidth of the corresponding signal, is limited by physiological relations. For example, a sinoatrial node stimulation rate may accelerate or decelerate by up to 20% on a beat-to-beat basis, while the ST segment depression representing heart cell re-polarization is dependent on blood oxygenation in the coronary arteries and thus is not expected to significantly change within a five-minute period. The minimum sampling frequency is estimated by analyzing the maximum expected variability. Due to the nature of the parameters, the sampling frequency ranges from 0.0000118 Hz (once a day) to 4 Hz, which is a maximum physiological heart rate.

The observation of the patient-doctor relationship justifies the common belief identifying two main reasons for medical examinations as: (1) expiry of the validity period of the precedent examination, and (2) sudden deterioration of the patient's condition (subjective or objective). Currently, the dependence of the patient examination frequency on his or her status has no analogy in automated diagnostics. This chapter presents a proposal of medically justified modulations of the frequency of cardiac reporting, implemented in a client-server distant cooperation model. The supervising center analyzes incoming messages and other conditions, and issues the desired reporting interval back to the remote device. As a result of the authors' tests and simulations, this method may reduce wireless channel usage and increase remote autonomy up to three times.

Although the raw electrocardiogram is digitized with a constant frequency, the medical importance of particular signal strips varies significantly. Similar to a paper record, the cardiac message may be a confirmation of a patient's state of health as well as being a carrier of an emergency alert. That constitutes a background for another scientific challenge in electrocardiography. We explore the opportunities opened up by the modification of content of the data packet and its priority in the network as depending on diagnostic data. The patient-oriented analysis performed by the PED separates all unexpected patterns, as well as divergences of parameters marked by a newly proposed interest attribute. Such processing favors singularities as an indication of abnormal heart activity of unknown origin and potential danger. On the other hand, the hypothesis-driven analysis is oriented to detect minor changes in selected parameters that may be also considered as severe. Beyond the regular report packages, these alerts are transmitted to the SuSe with a high priority attribute set. This adaptation reduces the cost of long-term monitoring and speeds up messages in urgent cases.

VARIABILITY ANALYSIS OF MOST COMMON DIAGNOSTIC PARAMETERS IN ECGS

The electrocardiographic signal is the carrier of all diagnostic parameters derived from it, and the need for high sampling frequency is justified by expectation of high-fidelity digital representation of analog signals. Within the ventricle contraction period represented by the QRS complex, the signal frequency is occasionally high, but for the rest of the signal there is a considerable redundancy of adjacent samples (Bailey et al., 1990; Augustyniak, 2002). This redundancy was the key point of the family of algorithms for the ECG compression based on a temporal similarity of samples. Although it is theoretically possible, there is no diagnostic parameter showing variability as high as the raw representation of a cardiac electrical field.

Although changes in electrical heart activity are continuous, they are rarely observed and reported within a heartbeat. The only exception is probably a baseline and noise level estimation that should reflect abrupt changes in noise power and thus alter the ECG measurement conditions. These measurements are used in the compensation or improvement of the signal within short strips (a few samples), however their local values are rarely stored in the internal database and included in the report. In most cases the signal quality estimate and the baseline level are stored once per heartbeat. The first value is used to assess the reliability of heartbeat-derived diagnostic parameters or optimal choices of geometrical aspects in the case of multilead recordings. The second is used for baseline compensation in wave borders and electrical axes determination procedures.

As stated previously, the highest variability of diagnostic parameters is limited to the frequency corresponding to a beat-to-beat rate. Nevertheless, multiple parameters are computed at that rate, but due to known physiological limitations, high variability is assumed to be caused by external sources (e.g., noise or measurement uncertainty) and eliminated. The reported value is a result of averaging the adjacent beat-derived components over a specified period of time or over a given number of heartbeats. Arrhythmia sequences also belong to that range of variability, since they cannot be detected more precisely than with the accuracy of a few heartbeats. The other group of parameters shows the variability reflecting slow changes in conduction, re-polarization conditions like those influenced by chemical or hormonal signals.

The general classification of parameter variability includes three groups:

1. *Parameters of High Variability (0.8-3Hz)*—RR-interval, wave axes, PQ-interval, baseline level and noise, T wave alternans, respiration-induced changes, intermittent morphology changes.
2. *Parameters of Medium Variability (0.03-1.5Hz)*—Dominant rhythm, heart rate, arrhythmia.
3. *Parameters of Low Variability (0.00067-0.03Hz)*—ST-level and slope changes, QT-interval, block and infarct changes, drug-induced morphology changes.

The diagnostic parameters variability within the confines specified above shows a significant degree of dependency on patient status. As a general rule, good or stable patient status implies a lower probability of change and therefore the necessary frequency of update for a majority of parameters. Taking the normal sinus rhythm (NSR) as an example, to fulfill the medical definition, four parameters must meet specified criteria: P wave existence and uniqueness, PQ intervals within the range of 60-220ms, PQ interval stability, and P wave axis stability. Considering all physiological conditions, once the NSR is detected and confirmed, the sudden occurrence of similar non-NSR rhythm not satisfying a single of these criteria is very improbable. This presents the opportunity to limit the criteria under consideration to two alternately selected from within the four.

Since the investigation of proper reporting contents and frequency dependent on patient condition is still not concluded, we had to report some preliminary results together with assumptions on the remaining outcomes specifying the reporting frequency separately for each ECG parameter (Table 10.1).

Table 10.1. Excerpt of the cross-reference table describing the data validity period as a function of patient condition

Parameter Validity Period rt [s]	Patient Status Estimate heart rate	rhythm type	extrasystoles	PQ-interval
rhythm type	>110 bpm, rt = 160-HR <60 bpm, rt = 3*(HR-40)	normal: rt = 60 atrial: junct.: rt = 10 ventric.: rt = 3	absent: rt = 60 atrial: junct.: rt = 5 ventric.: rt = 2	> 180 ms rt = 240-PQ < 60 ms rt = PQ
heart rate	>100 bpm, rt = 55-HR/4 <60 bpm, rf = HR-30	normal: rt = 30 atrial: junct.: rt = 10 ventric.: rt = 3	absent: rt = 30 any: rt = 1	-
wave axis	-	normal: rt = 60 atrial: junct.: rt = 5 ventric.: rt = 1	absent: rt = 60 any: rt = 1	ΔPQ > 40ms rt = 1 ΔPQ > 15ms rt = 15

IRREGULAR REPORTING DRIVEN BY PATIENT STATUS

Irregular Reporting as a Consequence of Adaptive Processing

Considering the distributed cardiac monitoring system with the intelligent management of remote processing involves the use of a flexible data report format including raw signal strips, metadata, and diagnostic parameters. As the signal interpretation is modulated by the patient's status, the inclusion of a result for particular diagnostic parameters is selectable. Modulation of report content may follow one of the following scenarios:

- inclusion or exclusion of automatically selected diagnostic parameters;
- attributing the diagnostic parameters with priority and validity period specification, followed by inclusion in the report of only a limited subset of most relevant data; and
- continuous regular reporting (as performed by most of today's wireless monitoring systems).

The distributed computing design (Figure 10.1) assumes that processing is initiated in the PED immediately after the signal capture and continues as far as necessary and possible. The patient-specific adaptation of the remote interpretation procedure is achieved with the use of specialized subroutines uploaded from the supervising software thread running on the SuSe (Augustyniak, 2005; Tadeusiewicz & Augustyniak, 2005). Technical limitations of the PED are compensated by a complementary interpretation thread running on the SuSe that clarifies any ambiguous or unresolved records. The adaptation is locally controlled by the PED procedure and additionally monitored by the SuSe software with the option of human assistance in critical cases.

Adaptability of the distributed interpretation process involves continuous and dynamic control of the task share and the data flow. Consequently, the signal and medical data reported by the PED depend on many medical and technical circumstances including:

- the diagnostic goals,
- the current status of the subject,
- interpretation performance and reliability, and
- environmental dependencies.

The main aspects of the dynamic update of recorder capability are discussed in Chapter IX, and the studies on the structural re-arrangement of interpretive software targeted to a wearable device are presented in Chapter VII. The proposed architecture considers estimated reliability and error propagation factors oriented towards the improvement of remote interpretation quality and datastream optimization (Augustyniak, 2006). The present chapter highlights the concept and selected details of the proposed adaptive report format.

It is worth recalling that the principle of task sharing is conceptually based on the generalized rules of interpersonal relations often observed in cardiology. Reproducing these relationships in a network of cooperating computers has a significant impact on diagnosis quality. Following these relations, the most common and frequent episodes are interpreted by the PED software, and consequently, the wearable device issues a cost-acceptable datastream. The occurrence of any difficult or unresolved event is reported as a short strip of raw signal to be automatically interpreted by the SuSe software or, in very rare cases, with the assistance of a human expert.

Investigations of Irregular Reporting

Following the principal rule, the measurement should not affect the observed phenomena. Because our aim was to gather cardiologists' preferences for the content of the final report, the best way was to observe human behavior during the parameter selection act. Usually, once the automatic interpretation is completed by the computerized system, the final report selection window appears on the screen and

Figure 10.1. The principles of auto-adaptive system design

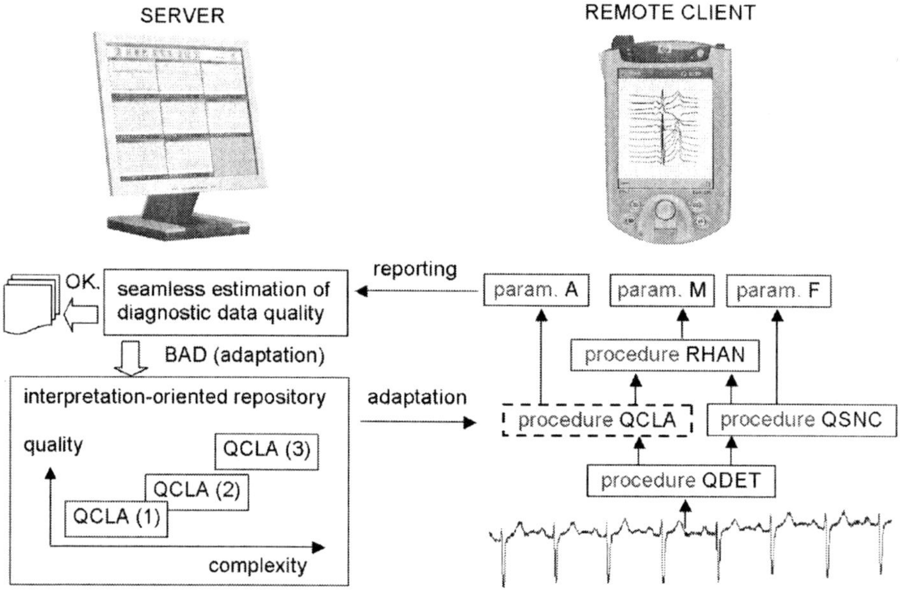

the doctor, according to patient status, selects the necessary items to be included in the paper or electronic report. In commercial software, the items are displayed in a static ordered list, and some of them are selected by default.

For the studies concerning doctors' behavior, we asked the ECG software manufacturer to modify the selection window properties and to add a spy procedure that can record the operator's activity. The modified software was then released for up to seven months of tests to a restricted group of testing cardiologists. The modification lies in replacing the default order and pre-selection attributes of each report item with random values (Figure 10.2). Each time the interpretation is completed, all possible report items appear together on the screen randomly pre-selected and the doctor is prompted to include or exclude items to/from the report contents. His or her interaction with the report proposal was recorded in the context of the diagnosis. Each time an expert selects an unselected item, we increase the relevance factor of corresponding parameters. On the other hand, each de-selection act de-values the relevance factor. The order of selection and the preferred items are memorized along with the diagnostic outcome, and thus after the statistical processing of this data we had knowledge about doctors' preferences with regard to the most common diseases.

Considering the relative frequency F of occurrence of parameter p, the rank C:

$$F = \frac{\sum C : L_C = L}{\sum (C \cdot |L - L_C|) : L_C \neq L} \tag{10.1}$$

The *diagnostic relevance* is represented by the weighting coefficient W_p including the rank L and the frequency F:

$$W_p = \frac{F}{L} \tag{10.2}$$

Finally, the weighting coefficients were normalized so their sum equals the unity:

$$\sum_p W_p = 1 \tag{10.3}$$

During the experiment we investigated 1,730 visual ECG interpretations performed by humans of different expertise. Twelve diseases appeared frequently enough for the statistical processing of the results of expert preferences (16 to 323 cases). Seventeen other pathologies were recorded too rarely, and the statistical generalization could not be expected to yield a reliable conclusion.

Figure 10.2. The selection window for the contents of final diagnostic report; in modified software, each display resulted with a different order of items and preselection mark

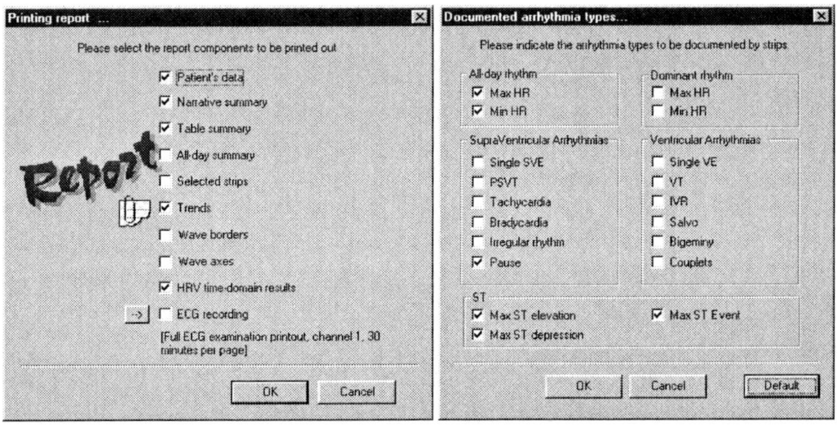

Results

As a result of our investigation of preferences with regard to most important diagnostic parameters in the context of the diagnosis, we distinguished 12 items in the patient status domain and 22 parameters ranked by the relevance coefficient W_p given by Equation 10.2. Table 10.2 displays the upper left corner of the result matrix.

Table 10.2 does not include the complete set of experimental results, but the most important feature of the relevance coefficients may be easily observed. Even for a heart rate (HR), usually considered as a basic ECG parameter, the relevance factor varies depending on the patient health status.

Discussion

The relevance coefficients derived experimentally for the main ECG diagnostic parameters in the context of most frequent diseases is new knowledge reproducing the dynamic aspect of human expert reasoning. Considering the patient and the doctor as two mutually dependent objects in regards to the control theory, we have the following principal relationships:

- The doctor acts according to many factors, mainly to patient status which is represented in ECG diagnostic parameters.
- The patient status depends on many external factors, with a considerable impact of doctor influence (therapy), as far as the environment is controlled.

These remarks lead to the conclusion that in the loop-back presented above, relevance coefficients may have a significant practical application in the:

- control of ECG processing, in particular in automated auto-adaptive systems based on prioritized computation and data storage; and
- assessment of the ECG diagnostic data quality, in particular in systems using data compression.

The second topic, although not considered in this work, was widely discussed in the context of lossless compression of the ECG signal and a proper estimate of the distortion and signal quality. Except for one proposal from Zigel (Zigel, Cohen, & Katz, 1996; Zigel & Cohen, 1999), concerning the weighted diagnostic difference (WDD) as a signal distortion measure, all other investigations and reports assumed equal relevance of the ECG diagnostic parameters.

It is not surprising that the time sequence of ECG diagnostic parameters has quite similar properties to the raw signal (Table 10.3; see also Chapter VI).

Table 10.2. Excerpt of the diagnostic parameter relevance matrix in the context of the current diagnosis

Diagnostic Parameter	Patient Status Space						
	111	normal sinus rhythm	163	persistent supraventricular tachycardia	508	ST suppression heart muscle ishemiae	.....
heart rate (HR) [1/min]		0,15		0,35		0,22	.....
dominant trigger rate (%)		0,25		0,21		0,07	.....
PQ section [ms]		0,12		0,17		0,03	.....
.....		.....		.....		.....	.....
SUM		**1**		**1**		**1**	

Although medically justified, weighting functions (see Table 10.2) may have to be corrected in the future. Here we used the experimental data to test technical aspects of the request-driven interpretation algorithm, and we successfully demonstrated the correctness, feasibility, and expected benefits of such systems.

Quality Aspects of Rigid and Agile Interpretation

The term *quality control* is often raised in the context of automatic interpretation of medical data and specifically for images and signals. Quality is understood as a strength of the relationship between automatically derived parameters and their counterparts issued by human experts. An assessment of the interpretation quality is a statistical process fully independent from the interpretation itself (Willems, 1990; IEC, 2001; Khoór et al., 2003; Pinna et al., 2003). It is performed with the use of general-purpose computers in any convenient time after the interpretation has been validated. This meaning of interpretation quality assessment is only a departing point for our approach of quality assessment aimed at the continuous validation of patient description accuracy and relevance used for automatically modifying the processing and reporting in the distributed network.

The diagnostic report is the final stage of the ECG signal process and reflects the computations made by the PED. As such, the report is expected to provide the necessary information for the correct and reliable assessment of patient status. The aim of this assessment is twofold:

1. *medical,* being stored in the database and considered as a resource for therapy; and

Table 10.3. Comparison of raw signal and diagnostic outcome time series

	Raw Signal Time Series	**Diagnostic Parameter Time Series**
Multichannel Time Series	the sampling frequency and quantization parameters are equal for all channels, but may be irregular according to the heart evolution, common for all simultaneous ECG channels.	Sampling frequency and quantization parameters are equal for all channels in regular systems, but may be independently irregular with reference to global estimates of patient status.
Variable Channel Relevance	Relevance is considered as constant unless a specific event is detected in a particular channel, which makes that channel more important.	Relevance is equal in rigid systems, but may be modulated with regard to global estimates of patient health status.

2. *technical,* being background for the automated human-like or human-supported decisions about further diagnostic needs consequently realized as the functional modulation of a PED's functionality by means of the agile software.

This chapter provides proof that a statistical or signal theory-based approach yields a much oversized bandwidth estimate in the case of ECG diagnostic datastreams. Nevertheless, a great deal of work must be done to convince the medics and their technology-oriented collaborators to abandon rigid processing and data formats, which are perceived as 'safe', and accept adaptive procedures and formats that are economically interesting, promising unprecedented flexibility but requiring more research. Such research has been requested from medical societies; however, cardiologists appear to have little interest in this area. The main reason could be indicated in trends towards the uniformity, often caused by standardization of procedures and data formats in both human and electronic diagnostics.

REFERENCES

Augustyniak, P. (2002), Adaptive discrete ECG representation—comparing variable depth decimation and continuous non-uniform sampling. *Computers in Cardiology, 29,* 165-168.

Augustyniak, P. (2005). Content-adaptive signal and data in pervasive cardiac monitoring. *Computers in Cardiology, 32,* 825-828.

Augustyniak, P. (2006). The use of selected diagnostic parameters as a feedback modifying the ECG interpretation. *Computers in Cardiology, 33,* 825-828.

Bailey, J. J., Berson, A. S., Garson, A. et al. (1990). Recommendations for standardization and specifications in automated electrocardiography: Bandwidth and digital signal processing. *Circulation, 81,* 730-739.

IEC 60601-2-51. (2003). *Medical electrical equipment: Particular requirements for the safety, including essential performance, of ambulatory electrocardiographic systems.* First edition 2003-02, International Electrotechnical Commission, Geneva.

Khoór, S. et al. (2003). Internet-based, GPRS, long-term ECG monitoring and non-linear heart-rate analysis for cardiovascular telemedicine management. *Computers in Cardiology, 30,* 209-212.

Pinna, G. D. et al. (2003). Home telemonitoring of chronic heart failure patients: Novel system architecture of the home or hospital in heart failure study. *Computers in Cardiology, 30,* 105-108.

Tadeusiewicz, R., & Augustyniak, P. (2005). Information flow and data reduction in the ECG interpretation process. *Proceedings of the 27th Annual IEEE EMBS Conference.*

Willems, J. L. (1990). *Common standards for quantitative electrocardiography: 10-th CSE progress report.* Leuven, Belgium: ACCO.

Zigel, Y., & Cohen, A. (1999). On the optimal distortion measure for ECG compression. *Proceedings of the European Medical & Biological Engineering Conference.*

Zigel, Y., Cohen, A., & Katz, A. (1996). A diagnostic meaningful distortion measure for ECG compression. *Proceedings of the 19th Convention of Electrical & Electronic Engineers in Israel* (pp. 117-120).

Chapter XI
Future Perspective:
Data Validity-Driven Report Optimization

This chapter first presents the description of a common approach to ECG interpretation triggering, assuming that the parameters are updated each time the input data is available. The heartbeat detector runs for each acquired sample, and all heartbeat-based diagnostic parameters (e.g., arrhythmias) are calculated immediately after a positive detection of a heartbeat. This approach keeps the diagnostic parameters up to date with the frequency of the physical variability limit of their source at the cost of unnecessary computation. Slowly changing parameters are significantly over-sampled and consecutive values show high redundancy.

As mentioned in Chapter X, each diagnostic parameter has a physiology-originated variability limitation and consequently also a specific validity period in which it should be updated. Non-uniform reporting assumes that the parameters are calculated and reported only by the expiry (i.e., end of the validity) of previous values. In this approach, computational costs are much lower compared to uniform reporting. The lack of uniformity has no significant influence on the diagnostic quality, as long as the parameter-specific update frequency (or validity period) is set correctly. Besides the economic aspect, this approach provides the opportunity for modulation of the update frequency by the patient health status as mentioned in Chapter X. Data validity-driven reporting closely reflects a doctor's activity when requesting parameters and refreshing their values with an optimized workload, taking into consideration the patient status.

At the end of the chapter, we present a concept of a packet-content manager. This procedure collects all requests concerning diagnostic parameter update and computation, supervises the propagation of the validity attribute backwards through the processing chain, and provides an exceptional pathway for all abnormality alerts emerging in the processing chain. As a result, all parameters are reported as rarely as possible without breaking the Shannon rule. The sampling frequency may be individually modulated in a wide range depending on the patient's status, and computation costs are reduced, providing longer battery life for the wearable recorder.

For transmission, the data are organized into packets, each containing some overhead data depending on the protocol. To be independent, each packet should be described at least by its origin, target, time stamp, and references to other packets. Additionally, the data packet has a minimum length and growth quanta that must be filled even with invalid data when not used. Considering the overhead, it is evident that the transmission of a few data bytes in the network is unprofitable, so should be avoided, except for emergency messages. From that point the necessity of the packet-content manager is more evident. This procedure collects data size and validity periods for all parameters and estimates the content of the nearest report as well as the time point it was generated. Because the validity of particular diagnostic parameters is not synchronous, the procedure reserves space in the nearest packet for diagnostic parameters' values in the order of their expiry up to a certain filling ratio. Then, based on nearest parameter update time, the update request is also generated for other parameters, even if their update time point is later. This task becomes even more complicated, when considering the data priority in the report.

UNIFORM REPORTING BASED ON SOURCE DATA AVAILABILITY

Introduction

Early wearable cardio-monitor solutions used modern micro-electronic technology, but their functional aspect followed bedside interpretive electrocardiographs (HP, 1994; Nihon Kohden, 2001; Gouaux et al., 2002; Maglaveras et al., 2002; Bousseljot et al., 2003; Banitsas, Georgiadis, Tachakra, & Cavouras, 2004; Paoletti & Marchesi, 2004; CardioSoft, 2005; González, Jiménez, & Vargas, 2005). Similarly, surveillance networks were conceptually closer to a group of independent cardiologists than to a hierarchy established during the history of medicine. Moreover, the traditional approach assumes unconditional signal acquisition based on uniform time-interval, rigid processing, including all available computation stages. Most of the processing branches end up with a conclusion of no relevant change since the last diagnostic report, because the variability of the diagnostic parameters is much lower than the variability of the signal itself.

Regular Updates of the Input and Program State

Computer programs could be considered as deterministic sequential machines, whose outputs (described as the current state) are dependent on the inputs and the previous state. Following this scheme most software is built including the automatic ECG interpretation program. The scheme assumes that each change of input could potentially influence the "machine" status and the output values. Following this reasoning, calculations are triggered for each new sample of incoming raw ECG signal. Formally, all internal data is updated and in practice, fortunately for the computation complexity, most of the processing is launched conditionally upon the detection of a new heartbeat (QRS complex).

The recording of a new heartbeat in the internal database launches measurements like electrical axes, wave borders detection, arrhythmia detection, heart rate variability assessment, update of ST segment description, and many others. Here again, the appearance of new input results in the launch of every computation in order to update the output.

The analysis of data flow in a typical ECG interpretation chain leads to three main sources of events being prospective triggers for computation:

1. *the acquisition of new signal samples,* implying the update of local signal buffers, filtered signal, heartbeat detectors, and pacemaker detector inputs and other signal-dependent calculations; the sampling rate is high (100-1000sps) and constant;
2. *the appearance of new positive QRS detector outcomes,* causing the subsequent computation of all heartbeat-based parameters, beat measures, beat sequence detections, and sequences of beat-to-beat measures; the beat rate is low (0.8-3bps) variable and subject to physiological limitations like tissue-dependent stimulus conduction velocity and cell refraction time; and
3. *the presence of new pacemaker pulses or patient button inputs,* resulting in the launch of alternative or auxiliary procedures aimed at the correlation of spikes and stimulated contractions; the pulse rate is low and subjected to technical limitations, however a burst of spikes could be expected in the case of pacemaker failure.

The characteristics of the events specified above are used in the estimation of the expected processing workload and reporting frequency.

Regular Reporting as a Consequence of Source Data-Triggered Computation

As the program state is expected to be changed by every sample of the source signal, new reports should be generated frequently. No ECG parameter really follows the variability of the raw signal, so no device is expected to issue a report at the example frequency of 400Hz. Let us consider QRS detection as a source of new data and a detector procedure as a transform of the raw signal to the internal database ECG representation. This transform has a multi-dimensional heartbeat representation in its output, initially consisting of a single detection point reference and then completed in the domains of other parameters in the course of further processing. Considering separately every parameter describing the heartbeat, we can define time series as inputs to corresponding diagnostic data-oriented procedures. Despite two considerable drawbacks—(1) these procedures are launched for each data-point even if, given an assumption of lower variability of represented parameters, their final outcome is usually averaged; and (2) the heartbeat-based time series are irregularly sampled in time domain (0.83-2.67Hz for heart rates 50-160 bpm, respectively)—these time series are commonly accepted as the basis of report triggering. Consequently, high redundancy is present in the diagnostic reports, and many calculations are performed unnecessarily. Both these aspects are crucial for wearable monitoring systems using a wireless communication channel for reporting, so uniform reporting, based on source data availability, will be challenged thereafter.

NON-UNIFORM REPORTING BASED ON RECIPIENT REQUESTS AND DATA VALIDITY

Introduction

Our investigation of non-uniform signal representation (Augustyniak, 2002) and irregular reporting in the wireless cardiac monitoring network (Augustyniak, 2005a, 2005b) concluded with an estimation of specific band limit values for each basic diagnostic parameter. The bandwidth itself is also variable and dependent on patient status. Generally, worse patient health status implies the necessity for more frequent reporting.

The concept of adaptive ECG interpretation and reporting is based on prioritized irregularly timed requests for diagnostic parameters (see Chapters IX and X). That concept was consequently developed for a request-driven ECG interpretation method presented in this chapter. It considers two issues crucial for wearable devices with

Figure 11.1. Main principle of request-driven ECG interpretations: (a) traditional interpretation scheme and (b) request-driven interpretation scheme

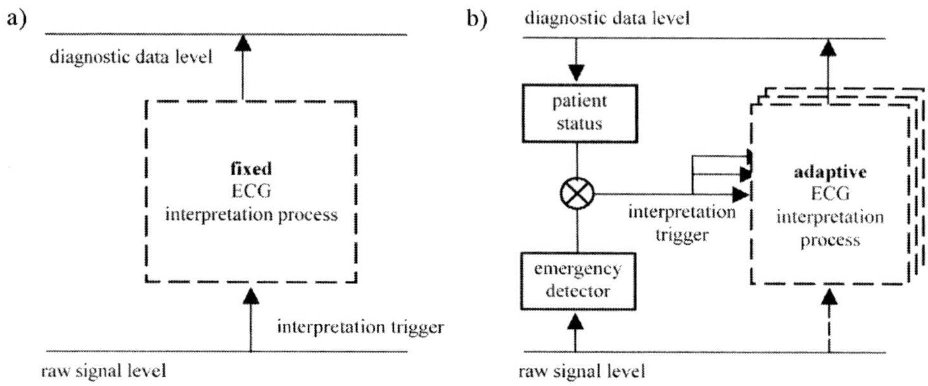

a wireless connection: maximized autonomy and minimized transmission channel costs.

The main novelty of our method consists of irregular ECG processing triggered and defined by two sources: patient status and emergency detectors.

In the remote recorder these sources launch a subset of interpretation subroutines necessary to provide requests for diagnostic parameters (Figure 11.1). Unnecessary processing is limited, thus the interpretation is relatively fast and the outcome contains highly relevant data transmitted in smart packets.

Besides the economic aspect, the additional advantage of this approach is closer simulation of human expert behavior.

Estimating and Using Data Validity Periods

Human experts usually perform hypothesis-driven interpretation task sequences and limit the diagnostic set to the most relevant results. The introduction of data priority attributes adapted to diagnostic goals has a significant impact on the automatic interpretation process, with regard to the aspect of economy and similarity to human reasoning.

The appropriate selection of the update interval or the data validity period is an extension of the data priority concept. Depending on data variability and current patient status, each component of the diagnostic result must be calculated and transmitted not earlier than its expiry time. In cardiology, an example of a high-frequency parameter is the heart rate (HR), whereas an example of a low-frequency parameter is the ST segment depression.

Data validity periods are estimated by a supplementary cross-reference procedure (see Table 10.1) and included in the diagnostic parameter set. Unfortunately, no currently available medical information storage and interchange standard provides data fields of such types.

Patient Status as an Interpretation Trigger

The data type-specific validity periods depend on patient status represented in the parameter under consideration and other parameters as well (Figure 11.2). Detailed investigations of correlations between diagnostic parameters and multidimensional nonlinear regressions describing their contribution to the data validity period exceed the framework of presented research. For example, the QT dispersion must be reported once every five minutes if the measured value falls in the physiological norm, otherwise the reporting frequency should be increased and reaches the beat-to-beat rate.

Because the validity periods specific for patient status-dependent data types are a main source of interpretation triggers, all relevant parameters should be calculated in real time upon the availability of diagnostic parameters.

Figure 11.2. Cross-dependence scheme of the validity period for diagnostic parameter α_2 and current values of diagnostic parameters

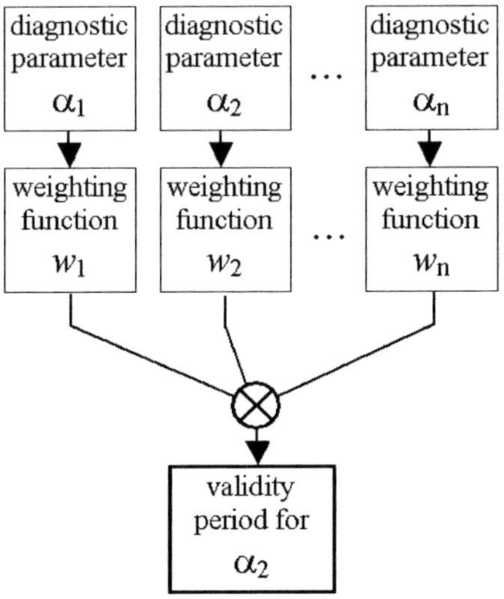

Emergency Detector as Interpretation Trigger

Even if data validity periods are estimated as relatively long, the system must support sudden changes in a patient's conditions. The emergency detector consists of a significantly limited set of interpretation procedures and balances between two contradictory criteria:

1. It issues a meta-parameter, shortening the validity period of any diagnostic parameter.
2. From a computational aspect it is as simple as possible, and preferably it uses only initial stage subroutines of the interpretation chain in order to maximize the reliability.

Having medical standards, examples of open-source software, and a few cardiology experts' opinions as a background, we finally selected the heart rate variation as a parameter most suitable for emergency detection. Figure 11.3 demonstrates two stages of emergency detection.

Request-Driven Interpretation Testing Areas

Fixed interpretation software is usually tested for yielding results within the tolerance margins specified on a physiological background. In adaptive software, more

Figure 11.3. The detection of sudden abnormality occurrences: (a) data validity periods are long corresponding to physiological data, emergency detectors trigger the interpretation which issues the pathology alert signal; (b) pathological diagnostic data shortens data validity periods and triggers the interpretation more frequently

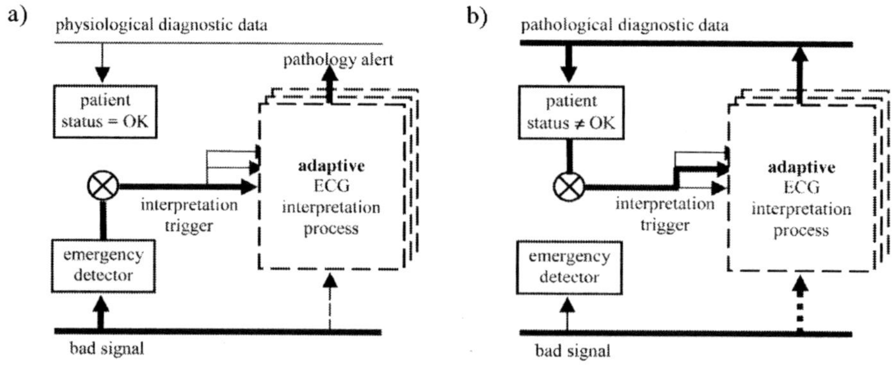

interesting is the dynamic aspect of adaptation, and thus new parameters should be added to the global estimate of method performance:

- convergence delay and coherence of fixed and adaptive interpretation results;
- static divergence of uniformly reported fixed interpretation results and their sparsely reported counterparts from adaptive interpretation;
- disease-domain sensitivity of the emergency detectors;
- technical and economic advantages of request-driven ECG interpretation; and
- the correctness of data validity period estimations.

Because these areas and appropriate test methodology are rarely reported in the literature, we mainly focused here on the delay and coherence test and the estimation of technical advantages. Other areas require additional research, also in the medical sciences, and will be considered in future works. In order to complete the agile software testing described in Chapter IX, two trigger description parameters were added to the testing dimension: sensitivity of emergency detectors and data validity period estimations.

Test Signals and Results Conditioning

Adaptive interpretation methods, having been recently introduced, are not considered by worldwide-recognized standard databases. These databases contain annotated examples of specific pathologies, but transient or unexpected events are rarely represented.

Long-term databases like MIT-BIH (Moody & Mark, 1990) rarely contain more than two channels. Thanks to long recording times, the probability of transient occurrence is fairly high and the wide spectrum of transient rhythm signals (arrhythmia, heart rate variability, pacemaker failures, or even death ECG) is represented. Unfortunately, two leads provide heart representations not precise enough to perform a contour analysis. This type of interpretation usually requires a 12-channel lead set, however, 4-channel EASI recordings (Dower, Yakush, Nazzal, Jutzy, & Ruiz, 1988) or 3-channel VCGs have also been reported as sufficient. For the contour analysis, multilead databases were issued like CSE (Willems, 1990). Conversely, multilead recordings lasts for a short time (usually 10s), which limits the probability of transient occurrence. In fact, the CSE database represents rather stationary (in a medical sense) signals, however the exact meaning of stationarity is fulfilled only by the artificial CSE recordings (group Ma).

Because the available transient signals were not reliably annotated, we decided to artificially combine several strips of original database recordings into transient ECG test signals representing various pathologies.

Because of the lack of guidelines on testing the adaptive ECG interpretation software, we applied our custom test procedure, taking the diagnostic outcome of fixed software as the reference. A direct comparison of values was not possible, because the diagnostic outcome of the adaptive system is non-uniform. Each parameter is updated at different time points, with the frequency varying relatively to the values of previous estimates of patient status. The diagnostic outcome of the adaptive interpretation, which was a non-uniformly sampled time series, was first uniformized with the use of the cubic spline interpolation (Aldroubi & Feichtinger, 1998), described in detail in Chapter IX.

Convergence Tests of Fixed and Adaptive Interpretation Results

The adaptive interpretation is expected to issue diagnostic results whose quality corresponds to results of fixed methods. Comparing diagnostic data quality is a complex issue, which needs the consideration of:

- dependence of convergence delay and final coherence with reference to the stimulus represented in the ECG signal alteration and the precedent configuration of the interpretation process,
- different convergence properties for particular diagnostic parameters, and
- a different medical relevance of the adaptation delay and final divergence between particular parameters and corresponding references.

As a general estimate of convergence quality, we propose the value Q, a weighted sum of relative error of the 12 most frequently used ECG diagnostic parameters (HR, rhythm estimates, wave lengths and axes, etc.). Weighting coefficients are calculated based on the use of statistics, and their sum is normalized to 1.

$$Q = \sum_{i=1}^{12} \Delta p_i \cdot w_i, \text{ where } \sum_{i=1}^{12} w_i = 1 \qquad (11.1)$$

Results for the general quality of diagnostic data issued by the request-driven ECG interpretation for a sample of sudden cardiac events simulated in test signals are summarized in Table 11.1.

Other performed tests aimed at estimating the technical and economic advantages of request-driven interpretations. We assumed that the adaptive interpretation and emergency detector are implemented in a wearable battery-operated device connected

Table 11.1. Results for the general quality of diagnostic data issued by a request-driven ECG interpretation

Transient Simulated in the ECG Signal	Q Initial Value (%)	Q Final Value (%)	Delay to 120% of Final Q Value(s)
normal → atrial fibrillation	19.1	2.4	6.7
normal → ventricular tachycardia	56.3	4.7	3.5
normal → ST depression (150μV)	14.7	1.1	12.2*
normal → bigeminy	27.4	0.7	3.8
normal → persistent supra-ventricular tachycardia	22.1	1.3	5.8
normal → acute myocardial infarction	12.8	2.2	5.5

* *not detected as an emergency*

Table 11.2. Estimates of the technical and economic advantages of request-driven ECG interpretation with respect to the static software of the same interpretation range and with use of identical test signals

Medical Contents Represented in the ECG Signal	Processing Complexity (%)*	Transmitted Data Volume (%)	Processing Time (%)
normal	22	12	27
atrial fibrillation	25	25	37
ventricular tachycardia	33	17	40
ST depression (150μV)	25	28	39
bigeminy	27	25	37
persistent supra-ventricular tachycardia	37	33	42
acute myocardial infarction	57	40	85

* *including the emergency detector thread*

via a digital wireless communication channel with the server collecting diagnostic results and issuing requests. The anticipated advantages consisted of a reduction of resources (i.e., processor time) and transmission channel usage in comparison to the fixed interpretation method. The results are highly dependent on the signal contents, thus in Table 11.2 they are summarized for sample test signals.

Discussion

The request-driven ECG interpretation concept based on individual data validity periods was prototyped and partially tested with the use of standard database-originated signals representing various medical contents and events. In the course of the reported research, we faced many challenges and unprecedented issues implied mainly by the adaptability of the ECG interpretation process. Some of the questions were directed at cardiologists and need intense research in the future, for example, the proper reporting of contents and frequency with regard to patient condition. The lack of medical knowledge and detailed procedures that could be considered as a reference caused us to postpone tests and estimates of some important features available in the adaptive algorithm. In spite of some limitations, our research contributes to the very hot topic of automatic distributed vital signs-based surveillance with several interesting remarks:

- demonstrates the feasibility of an adaptive interpretation system triggered by the data request based on variable validity periods depending on data type and value;
- considers the scenario of emergency and describes the system behavior necessary for the prompt dealing of life-critical events; and
- defines the area for testing of diagnostic parameter quality in the case of adaptive systems.

In our opinion, adaptive systems using request-driven interpretation, except for the technical advantages, more closely approximate human reasoning. They provide prioritized and accurate patient reporting when it is expected.

SETTING THE INDIVIDUAL CONTENT FOR EACH DATA PACKET

Packet Content Description

Common trends in the standardization of medical data format have resulted in several cardiology-oriented protocols for electronic data exchange like SCP-ECG (Willems, 1991; Fisher & Zywietz, 2001), MFER (Hirai & Kawamoto, 2004), and the use of general-purpose patient health records like HL7 (Dolin, Alschuler, Boyer, & Beebe, 2004) or DICOM (DICOM, 2007) in cardiology. Unfortunately, these protocols are all designed for the purpose of regular and uniform reporting, and thus do not support report content variability and irregular reporting. Aiming at greater flexibility of the report content, we proposed a custom reporting protocol simple enough for the implementation in a wearable device of limited computational power (Figure 11.4).

The packet content is composed of three layers of data fields:

1. mandatory header describing the packet and device status,
2. mandatory data description fields with references, and
3. optional data.

The mandatory fields of the header include recorder identifier and status, used for the correct assignment of the incoming data to the central server thread. The next fields represent the report number and reporting interval value, which are key parameters for testing the data integrity. In the network the packets are propagated with undetermined speed and may not reach the target in the same order as they were sent. Moreover, the packet may get lost in the network due to poor connection stability, and then the retrieval of a lost packet from the remote recorder's buffer is performed by referencing its number. The report interval is necessary to verify the temporal continuity of reporting. Since the reporting may be irregular, this field contains the value of delay from the precedent report. The sum of report interval values of the collected reports is expected to be equal to the continuous monitoring time. Other mandatory fields of the header provide the data type description of the first data field content and the pointer to this field in the record. Optionally,

Figure 11.4. Data communication format; mandatory fields are bordered by the solid line, optional fields are bordered by the dashed line

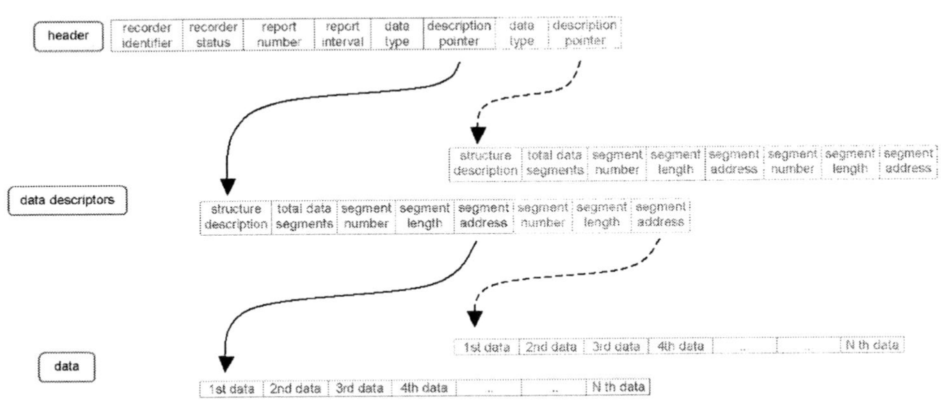

these fields may be repeated in the header if necessary when the report contains multiple data types.

The data description fields are proper for each data type. Because data may be included in the report in various processing stages (raw signal to final diagnostic outcomes) and in various forms (singular values, vectors, matrices), structure description is the first field of this layer. Structure definition supports nested data types, and thus the structure may include other structures defined beforehand. The dynamic definition of data structure occupies a considerable space in the record; thus considering a limited number of possible definitions used in the course of monitoring, the field contains one byte of structure number referencing corresponding data types in the remote recorder and central server. With the use of the remote recorder reprogrammability feature, data types used for reporting may be re-defined before the monitoring session starts, satisfying the need for almost unlimited data flexibility. However, during the monitoring session the variety of data types used is limited to 256. In practical sessions, data structure variability rarely exceeds the use of 16 different data types.

The next mandatory fields in the data description layer correspond to a segment structure of data of the same type. Therefore, the common structure description and the total segment count are followed by triplets of segments' description data containing number, length, and reference. Of these triplets the first one is mandatory with the assumption that the report contains no valid data; the remaining ones are optional.

The serialized data are the only content in the data layer. The first data field is pointed to by the first segment reference of the first defined data type and is thus obligatory, even if it contains only an end-of-file flag. The minimum length of the report is 18 bytes, while the maximum length is unlimited and depends only on the input datastream. For practical reasons, reports below 256 bytes are sent only in the case of emergency alerts, and records exceeding 32kB are split.

Optimizing the Packet Content

Up to this point we assumed every diagnostic parameter was sampled or re-calculated at the end of its validity period, satisfying the lowest sampling frequency acceptable to the Shannon theorem. This raises the necessity of individual reporting for each diagnostic parameter since their expiry intervals are not correlated and vary in time depending on patient health status. The individual reporting of singular values is impractical considering the header data overhead and minimum data packet length, because filling up the record to a minimum length with invalid values would increase transmission channel costs. This mode is used only for emergency messages.

For irregular reporting the packet content manager is used to optimize the data volume and the sampling frequency. This procedure collects data size and validity periods for all parameters and estimates the content of the forthcoming report as well as the time point it is generated. Because the validity of particular diagnostic parameters is not synchronous, the procedure reserves space in the nearest packet for the diagnostic parameters' values in the order of their expiry time up to a given filling ratio. Then, based on the nearest parameter update time, the update request is also generated to the interpretation chain for other parameters even if their update time point occurs later.

The report content optimization task becomes even more complicated when considering the data priority in the report. According to the size and priority of the diagnostic data issued by the interpretation chain, they are going to be included as content in the forthcoming report. Parameters of large size precede the singular values, and parameters having a high value of the importance attribute precede those of low value. Each time a new parameter is included, the cost function is calculated reflecting the remaining report fields not effectively used due to the rigid grid of acceptable data packet length values.

In order to maintain reporting continuity, the report must be sent no later than the expiry time of the earliest parameter validity. All other parameters that may be included in the report are calculated and reported prematurely. According to Shannon's theory it is the same as oversampling, but what is more important, it involves more frequent computations than is implied by the parameter variability. For this reason, the additional cost function is calculated and its value depends on the percentage shrinking of the update interval.

These two cost functions are fed into the packet content manager in order to decide which parameters should be included in the report and when the report should be sent. Because the unused data transmission is balanced against unnecessary power consumption, the weighting of the two cost functions is individually set depending on the recording device and data carrier. It is worth noting that in the practical implementation, the ECG processing is not the only reason for the power requirement and for the limitation of the remote recorder autonomy time. The important contribution to the total power consumption comes also from the wireless transmission module, and because considerable time is necessary to switch from idle to operational states or vice versa, transmitting unnecessary data in irregular, relatively short intervals significantly increases power consumptions.

Practical Considerations

Because a prototype of the intelligent remote monitoring system for cardiology already existed, we first tested the proposed data manager procedure on the simulated data and then in a real system with the implementation of the packet content manager procedure.

The first practical consideration is the minimum packet size as required in TCP/IP protocol. For many cases, including the idle status of the recorder (when only the recorder status is reported at a low rate), the pulse rate report (when the frequent report consists of only few data), and others, the data to be sent expires earlier than the amount of the data for the full data packet (i.e., 256 bytes) is collected. In such cases two options are still available:

1. sending the packets filled with recent data, and
2. switching the transmitter to the off-line mode and filling the packet with subsequent data points of the same type at the price of significant delay.

The second practical consideration is that the remaining data fields, which are not used for current reports, may be filled by any data, in particular with past data from the remote recorder buffer. This approach seems to be very interesting because:

- It combines the advantages of the two options above (i.e., recent data is sent together with historical data to fill up the spare space in the packet).
- Since the report is prioritized, each long report is completed with the most relevant historical data. This helps limit the requests of historical data if the data packet is considered lost (e.g., due to the excess of the delay limits).
- The spare fields in the data packet may be filled with additional data if only their nature allows for irregular reporting. First-hand examples of such data may be recording device status or global positioning (GPS) coordinates of the patient.

Although not implemented yet, we are considering buffering the auxiliary information about the device, the patient, and the environment, and conditionally include it into the report as far as the spare data fields will be available in the data packet being sent.

Discussion

Non-uniform reporting requires complex multi-criteria optimization of data transmission with several constraints. The only 'hard' condition is that the data must be updated before their validity expires. The list of 'soft' conditions includes that:

- the computation should be performed as rarely as it is justified by the parameters' variability,

- the data packets should be filled with valid data only, and
- the calculation of diagnostic parameters should respect the mutual dependency of procedures in the software interpretation chain.

Defining the rules above and testing the model of the report content manager procedure reveals a close similarity between automatic non-uniform reporting and real-life observations. At the optimum, the patient is subjected to an additional examination if necessary and only as rare as possible. This limits both the probable side effects and the costs. On the other hand, the analysis of a particular patient result is not possible without the recall of the whole context, and collecting the examination results is also time consuming for the patient. Therefore, an experienced specialist proposes in advance to perform a set of supplementary examinations including those that are not yet expired. Consequently he has a representation of patient health status valid for a considerable period of time without the necessity of a partial update.

REFERENCES

Aldroubi, A., & Feichtinger, H. (1998). Exact iterative reconstruction algorithm for multivariate irregularly sampled functions in spline-like spaces: The Lp theory. *Proceedings of the American Mathematical Society, 126*(9), 2677-2686.

Augustyniak, P. (2002). Adaptive discrete ECG representation—comparing variable depth decimation and continuous non-uniform sampling. *Computers in Cardiology, 29,* 165-168.

Augustyniak, P. (2005a). Implementing the ECG interpretation procedure in a distributed wearable computer systems. *Folia Cardiologica, 12* (suppl. D, paper 0-199).

Augustyniak, P. (2005b). Content-adaptive signal and data in pervasive cardiac monitoring. *Computers in Cardiology, 32,* 825-828.

Banitsas, K. A., Georgiadis, P., Tachakra, S., & Cavouras, D. (2004). Using handheld devices for real-time wireless teleconsultation. *Proceedings of the 26th IEEE EMBS Conference* (pp. 3105-3108).

Bousseljot, R. et al. (2003). Telemetric ECG diagnosis follow-up. *Computers in Cardiology, 30,* 121-124.

CardioSoft. (2005). *Version 6.0 operator's manual.* Milwaukee, WI: GE Medical Systems Information Technologies.

DICOM. (2007). *Digital imaging and communications in medicine.* Rosslyn, VA: National Electrical Manufacturers Association.

Dolin, R. H., Alschuler, L., Boyer, S., & Beebe, C. (2004). *HL7 clinical document architecture. Release 2.0.* HL7 Health Level Seven, Inc., Ann Arbor, MI. Available online at: www.hl7.org (accessed in November 2008).

Dower, G. E., Yakush, A., Nazzal, S. B., Jutzy, R. V., & Ruiz, C. E. (1988). Deriving the 12-lead electrocardiogram from four (EASI) electrodes. *Journal of Electrocardiology, 21*(Suppl.), S182-S187.

Fischer, R., & Zywietz, C. (2001). *How to implement SCP.* Retrieved from http://www.openecg.net

González, R., Jiménez, D., & Vargas, O. (2005). WalkECG: A mobile cardiac care device. *Computers in Cardiology, 32,* 371-374.

Gouaux, F. et al. (2002). Ambient intelligence and pervasive systems for the monitoring of citizens at cardiac risk: New solutions from the EPI-MEDICS project. *Computers in Cardiology, 29,* 289-292.

HP. (1994). *M1700A interpretive cardiograph physician's guide* (4th ed.).

Hirai, M., & Kawamoto, K. (2004). MFER—a Japanese approach for medical wave form encoding rules for viewer design. *Proceedings of the 2nd OpenECG Workshop* (pp. 35-37), Berlin, Germany.

Maglaveras, N. et al. (2002). Using contact centers in telemanagement and home care of congestive heart failure patients: The CHS experience. *Computers in Cardiology, 29,* 281-284.

Moody, G., & Mark, R. (1988). *MIT-BIH arrhythmia database directory.* Cambridge, MA: MIT Biomedical Engineering Center.

Nihon Kohden. (2001). *ECAPS-12C user guide: Interpretation standard* (revision A).

Paoletti, M., & Marchesi, C. (2004). Low computational cost algorithms for portable ECG monitoring units. *Proceedings of IFMBE Medicon* (paper 231).

Willems, J. L. (SCP-ECG project manager) (1991). *Standard communications protocol for computerized electrocardiography. Final specifications and recommendations.* Final Deliverable AIM Project #A1015. Leuven, Belgium: ACCO.

Willems, J. L. (1990). *Common standards for quantitative electrocardiography: 10th CSE Progress Report.* Leuven, Belgium: ACCO.

Chapter XII
Social Impact of Network-Based Ubiquitous Cardiac Surveillance

This chapter is a summary of the book and attempts to evaluate the social impact of the general idea of ubiquitous cardiology. The project discussed in the book is in fact oriented toward designing wireless bidirectional cooperation of two programmable ECG interpreting devices used for permanent heart monitoring and semi-automatic medical diagnosis. As shown above, the main idea of the project under consideration is to replace the traditional patient-doctor interaction model with a semi-automatic system, which was invented, designed, and developed by the staff of the Biocybernetic Laboratory at AGH University of Science and Technology, Krakow, Poland. The system under consideration offers ubiquitous surveillance without time and distance constraints. In this book we presented and discussed the technological aspects of the ubiquitous cardiology system. Conversely, this chapter is about its social aspects. This is also an important issue because every human-dedicated system must take into account human preferences and human limitations. The ubiquitous cardiology system will be used by patients and accepted by doctors when and only when its properties and parameters will be properly related to patient expectations and doctors demands. These aspects of the project are discussed in this chapter.

INTRODUCTION

The ubiquitous cardiology system must serve the people, so it must be accepted by the people. Talking about the people we must in fact take into account three groups of persons. First and the most important group are doctors (cardiologists working in hospitals and in private offices), who must rely on the system. When the doctors trust the system, the patients will also be ready to use it. Without doctor acceptance the system must be counted as worthless even if its technical parameters are perfect. It will be very difficult to achieve such a level of doctor confidence and acceptance, because disbelief is doctors' prime obligation.

The second group of people who must rely on the system are, of course, patients. Even if doctors recommend the system, the patient must agree to use it. The patient must be confident that under electronic monitoring his or her heart will be really safe. It is also not easy because the typical heart patient is frightened after some kind of cardiological incident and requires close monitoring by qualified medical personnel. Replacing direct doctor contact by using a technical device requires a lot of confidence. Not every person is ready to do that!

The third group of people who are indispensable for the success of ubiquitous cardiology includes the staff employed to operate the system. Technical service of the system will be typical, therefore the work of the technical staff will be the easiest part of the job. However, for the doctors who work in the Central Station being "the brain" of the proposed system, the duty will be very hard and demanding. The role of the doctor in the Central Station is much more difficult than the typical work of a hospital cardiologist or private doctor. The first decisions (e.g., diagnosis, therapy recommendation, emergency service alert, etc.) must be formulated without contact with the patient and only on the basis of the data remotely recorded by the computer. For most doctors such a task is viewed as unfeasible. The second circumstance making doctors' work in the Central Station difficult is that the pre-selection of patients is performed by the supervising server (SuSe). All of the typical problems and easily solvable situations are handled by a computer. This means that for doctors' hands remain only very difficult problems—one by one, without breaks. For somebody it can be the most challenging job, interesting and providing a lot of good practice, but for most doctors such a model is too troublesome.

Let us discuss all the above-mentioned problems more precisely.

UBIQUITOUS CARDIOLOGY FROM THE DOCTOR'S POINT OF VIEW

For many old-fashion doctors, it is strange thinking that some electronic device can really replace the direct monitoring of a patient's heart. Fortunately, in hospitals, electronic and computer devices are becoming a part of intensive care systems, therefore the increase of confidence in electronics and informatics also concerns the exclusive society of cardiologists. Nevertheless, there is a big difference between trusting in a hospital monitoring system, which can be supported at any time by the alarm nurse or the doctor on duty, and the confidence in fully automatic elements of the ubiquitous cardiology system. In many cases the patient electronic device (PED) is expected to help the patient autonomously or by means of tele-informatic consultation with another electronic device (SuSe—the main computer in the Central Station). Such revolutionary changes in the role of electronic devices can be hard to understand and even harder to accept for many cardiologists. Therefore, the development and practical implementation of the ubiquitous cardiology system must be preceded by a great deal of scientific research with full clinical monitoring of the results and with precise statistical analysis of all the conclusions. This kind of research and testing was performed by the authors before writing this book, and the selected results can be found in all the previous chapters. Nevertheless, the general properties and the usability of the ubiquitous cardiology system still require more research.

Doctors are conservative, but step by step move towards the acceptance of the ubiquitous cardiology system because it has many advantages. Most of these advantages are related to the patient's situation, which will be described in the next section. However, some advantages can be found from the doctor's point of view—and such advantages we are discussing here. The first advantage is that the ubiquitous cardiology system provides the doctor with a "third option," making his or her decisions easier and more comfortable. Without the ubiquitous cardiology system, the cardiologist has only two possible solutions: hospitalize the patient or return him or her home. Hospitalization is expensive and not comfortable, but returning home has the concern of a lack of monitoring, which can lead to a dangerous situation when the patient's heart is malfunctioning. Thus the ubiquitous cardiology system provides a third option between home and hospital. Using the ubiquitous cardiology system, the patient can stay where he or she wishes, can work, travel, play, and so forth, without cardiac hazard. Let us recollect the phrasing from the Introduction to this book:

Your heart is with you always and everywhere.

Take the monitoring device always and everywhere with your heart expecting a failure!

According to this phrasing, a doctor (cardiologist) can leave a patient at home, but equipped with the device proposed in this book (individual patient heart signal acquisition kits named PEDs). Using this system the patient can be both mobile and safe. Wide implementation of such technology reduces the number of hospitalized patients, decreases the level of risk of unexpected heart attacks, and increases the quality of life for people with a heart disease.

There are many additional advantages for doctors which are connected with the wide application of the ubiquitous cardiology system. Independent of automatic data interchanges between the PED and the SuSe localized in the Central Station, copies of all (or selected) data registered for a particular patient can also be sent directly to the doctor who recommends the ubiquitous cardiology system to the patient. Then the doctor can collect a large amount of data, both about every particular patient and about a large population of patients. Collected data can next be used for a better diagnosis of the patient's real illnesses, can be used for more precise therapy planning, can provide the basis for credible prognosis of the patient's future condition, and—last but not least—can be used for many official and/or scientific reports.

Forecasting is always a very risky pursuit, but taking into account the many advantages for doctors, connected with heart patient referrals to the ubiquitous cardiology system, we hope that after the initial disbelief and related problems, the system will receive a large number and steady stream of patients from many cooperating doctors.

UBIQUITOUS CARDIOLOGY FROM THE PATIENT'S POINT OF VIEW

The most important (and most complicated) part of the system is the Central Station, equipped with a main computer (SuSe), intelligent software, advanced communication devices, as well as a team of best cardiologists who can deal with any problem. However, from the patient's point of view, the system under consideration can be identified with the personal device described in the book—individual patient heart signal acquisition kits called PEDs. The expectations of a particular patient are concentrated on the apparatus taken into their hands—the PED. Acceptance and good assessment for the whole system depends on the PED's features, which will be pointed out and discussed below.

If the contact device PED should be accepted by the patient first, it must be reliable. That is evident. The most important feature for every patient is his or her safety. The presumption for the ubiquitous cardiology system is—as mentioned in this book many times—the replacement of direct permanent observation of the patient's health by qualified personnel with computer monitoring. Thanks to the use of the ubiquitous cardiology system, the patient does not have to stay in a hospital bed, can walk where he would like, work, play, travel, and so forth; nevertheless his or her heart is under permanent monitoring. This is the greatest benefit for the patient: instead of being trapped in the hospital (which is not comfortable and very expensive), a patient equipped with the discussed system can feel independent and be free. But the price for this freedom cannot be at the expense of security. Therefore, the part of the system seen by the patient ought to be comfortable, easy to use, state of the art from a technological point of view, and have many nice and useful properties, which are described in detail in previous chapters of this book—but must be safe of course. Choosing between freedom and safety, most people chose safety, because in the case of a cardiac hazard, the objective danger and the patient's subjective fear are very high.

Next, we outline the main factors responsible for patient safety when a patient's heart is under permanent observation by the ubiquitous cardiology system.

The initial process in the system and the initial source of danger is connected with ECG signal recording and interpretation methods. This initial step is very important because it is the basis for the functioning of the system. In other words, if the individual patient heart signal acquisition kits cannot record an ECG signal properly or if the quality of the signal cannot be evaluated as "good enough," then all of the most advanced information technologies and even all of the very sophisticated algorithms used in the SuSe cannot repair this situation. The system under consideration can perform signal processing using many methods and many technologies, but if there are no signals, it can do nothing.

As everybody knows, ECG signal quality depends very much on lead localization and on the quality of contact between leads and the patient's skin. During clinical examinations, the correct localization of leads and its good contact is guaranteed by qualified medical staff, which perform all the technical operations connected with ECG signal acquisition. In contrast, the patient using the ubiquitous cardiology system is fully self-serviced. Of course, PED construction addresses this, as wearable ECG sensor modules are used instead of traditional leads. Still, even though wearable sensors are easy to use, they often can fail. Therefore, the alarm signal—activated automatically when the quality of the recorded signal falls under an acceptable level—is very important. Such a signal may be a bit irritating and can lead to some frustration in the case of new users who are not skilled enough during system installation, but anything is better than ignorance when the system is in fact totally blind. PED users must know that only a silent device is a safe device. This is important, because safety (of course related to the patient, not to the technical system) is the most important feature of the ubiquitous cardiology system.

Another source of problems is connected with the wireless communication system used for the exchange of information between the PED and the SuSe. This communication can be solved in both economic and effective ways only by using mobile phone systems, which are now absolutely ubiquitous. However, every mobile phone user knows the "low field" phenomena as well as places where cellular communication does not work at all (e.g., on airplanes). Generally speaking, it should not cause major problems because the PED can control patient hearts by also functioning as an autonomic system. In such cases, the patient must be alerted that the scale of maintenance offered by the system is temporarily limited, as it is without direct bi-directional communication with the Central Station. A key issue in all of these situations is patient awareness, and in case of difficulty, he or she must seek help from the nearest doctor. For similar reasons the patient ought to be informed when the communication between the PED and SuSe is reestablished. The SuSe can then verify all of the patient data recorded within the PED in the period of autonomic (off-line) activity, and the information about this result should be given to the patient.

Simplicity is next important prerequisite connected with patient acceptance of the ubiquitous cardiology system. The inside of the system may be very complicated (in fact, it is very complicated), but from the point of view of every patient, the use of the system must be as easy as possible—in particular, the operating simplicity must be similar to that of a cell phone. In the previous section we discussed a very easy method used for connecting a patient to the system (wearable sensors). Now we take into account patient control of some system functions and communication between the PED processor and patient when advice, recommendations, and other messages given by the system must be read (or heard) by the patient, and more importantly, must be understood.

The whole communication process between patient and system must be as simple as possible. Moreover, the system ought to check if the patient really knows the meaning of the information provided to him or her by the system. All of the words used in the messages generated by the system must be known to the patient well enough to reach his or her mind when the patient is under stress and in pain. The same reasons dictate using a friendly and intelligent user interface when messages originate from patients to the system. For typical situations there should be short, fast, and easy-to-use codes (e.g., answer "all right") that require only one key to be pressed. Moreover, when a patient starts to communicate (indicating that he or she might have a problem) and tries to type something on the PED keyboard or puts a voice message through the system audio input, the system must try hard to understand the sense of the message even though it might be deformed (e.g., words might not be spelled correctly).

During this type of alert communication between patient and system, a multilingual approach must also be taken into account. Of course it is impossible to use every available language. In typical circumstances only one *a priori* selected language (possibly English, Spanish, French, German, Japan, Chinese, etc.) will be used for normal communication between the patient and the system regardless of patient nationality. But in the case of an emergency, we must take into account that under stress, pain, and terror, a patient can use his or her native tongue. Therefore, the system must be able to understand at least some words in many languages. A record of patient data specifying information about his or her nationality would be very helpful in such situations.

An additional aspect connected with patient comfort is automatic geographic localization provided by the PED. This is an important factor when the data recorded about the patient's heart suggests emergency medical attention, so the system can help locate the patient even if he or she is unconscious. Two types of automatic localization can be used. The first is connected with cellular communication systems. The PED has a built-in mobile communication device, therefore the cellular communication provider is aware of its location. This kind of localization is not very precise, but its major advantage results from the fact that it operates almost everywhere, whereas the satellite-based system of global positioning does not. Also popular is a GPS device installed inside the PED which can locate a patient with high accuracy. The same system can determine the directions and velocity of a moving object, which is sometimes very useful. Unfortunately, the GPS needs a clear sky over the patient's head, operates poorly when tall buildings surround the patient, and stops working under any roof or underground. Both localization methods, working together, can be very helpful when the user of the ubiquitous cardiology system needs fast rescue; this is an additional virtue of this system.

THE UBIQUITOUS CARDIOLOGY SYSTEM AND ITS OPERATORS

The ubiquitous cardiology system can work if and only if we can find doctors (very good cardiologists) who decide to serve as experts in the Central Station. It is a sociological problem, but compared with the large number of patients, the number of experts is relatively small. Nevertheless, the group of experts employed in the Central Station "is the last line of defense." If these doctors cannot help the patient, he or she may die. As mentioned above, the work in the Central Station is hard work, requiring immense responsibility, and we are afraid that it will not be possible to find enough highly qualified doctors to take this job. Moreover, not every highly qualified doctor can be a candidate for an expert of the ubiquitous cardiology system. Besides the appropriate medical qualifications, the person must have a good imagination to enable him or her to help a patient without involving physical contact. Therefore, suitable candidates for the ubiquitous cardiology system expert post are very rare, and when such a person is found, we must do everything possible to retain him or her. This means (among other things) a high salary and pleasant work environment. A good aspect of the ubiquitous cardiology system from an expert's perspective is its novelty. Working in the Central Station of the system can be a most challenging step in a medical doctor's career. Moreover, such a job provides the doctor with a rather new and exciting role as a human expert inside a high-technology system. He or she is no longer bored by the multitude of regular cases that affect his or her acuity to the emergency. All of the physiological records and the most common pathologies are serviced automatically, leaving to a human expert only the unusual cases. Doctors get a filtered group of difficult patients, however they are required to consider them more carefully using a significantly higher level of expertise.

The global range of cardiac surveillance, which must be assured for the patient, implies existence of a whole network of Central Stations, located in different cities and different countries around the world. It also can be viewed by doctors as an adventure, because the job can be connected with exotic journeys in contrast to working at the same hospital for one's whole career. Taking into account global communication range possible for every particular patient, we must assure the same (and of course very high!) level of accuracy and efficiency of the maintenance, making no difference to the patient and interpretation center localization.

THE RELATIONSHIP BETWEEN THE UBIQUITOUS CARDIOLOGY SYSTEM AND TRADITIONAL HOSPITALS

It is evident that once the ubiquitous cardiology system is born, it will become target of attacks by traditional hospitals. For every cardiological clinic ubiquitous cardiology system first will be seen as competitor. Also for every 'old-fashion thinking' cardiologist, the system will be treated as an enemy. This is normal, because methods and procedures offered by the system will be seen initially as not compatible with the art of medicine or it may even be considered iconoclastic. We repeat: these kinds of reactions are predictable and must be considered as normal, because every medical innovative technology was initially neglected and discarded by the majority of traditional medical doctors. It is sad but unavoidable.

However, this sad period of disapproval for the system can be relatively short. After some period a new kind of relation between hospitals, private doctors, patients, and also other players within healthcare (e.g., life insurance companies) must be established. In fact, in the case of the ubiquitous cardiology system, all the above-mentioned partners should be allies and not competitors, because all parties have the same goal: to assure a long and happy life for as many patients as possible. This goal is honest, noble, and worth every effort; thus we wrote this book.

SYSTEM COST AND THE LIKELIHOOD OF ITS REALIZATION

Last but not least we must talk about money. It is natural that for every patient the PED's cost is important along with the cost of subscribing to the system's services. The ubiquitous cardiology system as a whole is a very expensive investment, mainly because of the high value of the Central Station equipment and because of high salaries that must be paid to the Central Station staff (see below). Also early PEDs will not be inexpensive, because of the high expectations of this device, along with its various functionalities and its sophisticated character. Therefore, we are sure that at least initially, this technology will be too expensive for almost every patient, leading us to question the likelihood of the ubiquitous cardiology system being put into use. Even the best idea cannot be realized by itself, and for practical implementation of the system a lot of money is necessary.

Nevertheless, we are optimistic. The idea described in this book—and proven during many years of scientific, technological, and medical research—is accurate. The system is well designed, can work properly, and most importantly is necessary for saving the lives of many people and for improving the quality of life of many heart patients. Therefore, the system should be implemented.

The beginning will not be easy. During the first year or two, the ubiquitous cardiology system must be financially supported by government or private investors, otherwise it cannot be implemented. But in its mature form, the ubiquitous cardiology system will not only be socially useful, but also very profitable. This is guaranteed, as funding can be taken from patients' standing charges or service fees and will rise quickly when the number of patients increases.

Very helpful in the promotion and development of the ubiquitous cardiology system can be life insurance companies. It is evident that a good, functioning ubiquitous cardiology system can dramatically increase the profits of such enterprises because of the prolongation of the lives of many cardiovascular patients who would have died a short time after their first heart attack, if it weren't for the system. It might be wise for these companies to combine a life insurance policy with a subscription to the ubiquitous cardiology system.

Summarizing this issue: We hope that global availability of cardiac surveillance provided by mass-produced remote PED devices may be inexpensive and widely available. While the interpretation centers are unique and may be very expensive to operate, their services can also be inexpensive because of the large number of users.

Compilation of References

Abenstein, J. P. (1978). Algorithms for real-time ambulatory ECG monitoring. *Biomedical Sciences Instrumentation.* Vol. 14 . pp.73-77.

Abenstein, J. P., & Thakor, N. V. (1981). A detailed design example—ambulatory ECG monitoring. In W. J. Tompkins & J. G. Webster (Eds.), *Design of microcomputer-based medical instrumentation.* Englewood Cliffs, NJ: Prentice Hall.

AHA. (1967). *AHA ECG database.* Available from Emergency Care Research Institute, Plymouth Meeting, PA.

Ahlstrom, M. L., and Tompkins, W. J. (1981) An inexpensive microprocessor system for high speed QRS width detection. *Proceedings of the 1st Annual IEEE Compmedicine Conference* (pp. 81-83).

Akay, M. (1995). Wavelets in biomedical engineering. *Annals of Biomedical Engineering, 23,* 531-542.

Akselrod, S., Norymberg, M., Peled, I. et al. (1987). Computerized analysis of ST segment changes in ambulatory electrocardiograms. *Medical and Biological Engineering and Computing, 25,* 513-519.

Aldroubi, A., & Feichtinger, H. (1998). Exact iterative reconstruction algorithm for multivariate irregularly sampled functions in spline-like spaces: The Lp theory. *Proceedings of the American Mathematical Society, 126*(9), 2677-2686.

Algra, A., Le Brunand, H., & Zeelenberg, C. (1987). An algorithm for computer measurement of QT intervals in the 24 hour ECG. *Computers in Cardiology, 14,* 117-119.

Aloimonos, Y., Weiss, I., & Bandyodaphyay, A. (1987). Active vision. *Proceedings of the 1st ICCV* (pp. 35-54), London.

American Heart Association. (2005). *Heart disease and stroke statistics—2005 update.* Dallas.

Armstrong, W. F., & Morris, S. N. (1983). The ST segment during ambulatory electrocardiographic monitoring. *Annals of Internal Medicine, 98,* 249-250.

Augustyniak, P. (2002), Adaptive discrete ECG representation—comparing variable depth decimation and continuous non-uniform sampling. *Computers in Cardiology, 29,* 165-168.

Augustyniak, P. (2003). From databases to knowledge spaces for cardiology. *International Journal of Bioelectromagnetism, 5.*

Augustyniak, P. (2003). Time-frequency modelling and discrimination of noise in the electrocardiogram. *Physiological Measurement, 24*(3), 753-767.

Augustyniak, P. (2004). Optimizing the machine description of electrocardiogram. *Journal of Medical Informatics and Technology, 8,* :MM-41-MM48.

Augustyniak, P. (2005). Content-adaptive signal and data in pervasive cardiac monitoring. *Computers in Cardiology, 32,* 825-828.

Augustyniak, P. (2005). Implementing the ECG interpretation procedure in a distributed wearable computer systems. *Folia Cardiologica, 12* (suppl. D, paper 0-199).

Augustyniak, P. (2005). Content-adaptive signal and data in pervasive cardiac monitoring. *Computers in Cardiology, 32,* 825-828.

Augustyniak, P. (2006). Scanpath analysis in objective evaluation of reading skills. *Proceedings of the Symposium on Medical Informatics and Technologies* (pp. 261-266).

Augustyniak, P. (2006). The use of selected diagnostic parameters as a feedback modifying the ECG interpretation. *Computers in Cardiology, 33,* 825-828.

Augustyniak, P., & Tadeusiewicz, R. (2006). Modeling of ECG interpretation methods sharing based on human experts relations. *Proceedings of the 28th IEEE EMBS Annual International Conference* (pp. 4663-4669).

Baddeley, A. (1986). *Working memory.* Oxford: Clarendon Press.

Badilini, F., Zareba, W., Titlebaum, E. L., & Moss, A. J. (1986). Analysis of ST segment variability in Holter recordings. In A. Moss & A. Stern (Eds.), *Noninvasive electrocardiology—clinical aspects of Holter monitoring.* London: Saunders Co.

Bailey, J. J., Berson, A. S., Garson, A. et al. (1990). Recommendations for standardization and specifications in automated electrocardiography: Bandwidth and digital signal processing. *Circulation, 81,* 730-739.

Bailón, R., Sörnmo, L., & Laguna, P. (2006). ECG-derived respiratory frequency estimation. In G. D. Clifford, F. Azuaje, & P. E. McSharry (Eds.), *Advanced methods and tools for ECG data analysis* (pp. 215-244). Boston, Artech House.

Bailón, R., Sörnmo, L., & Laguna, P. (2006). A robust method for ECG-based estimation of the respiratory frequency during stress testing. *IEEE Transactions on Biomedical Engineering, 53,* 1273-1285.

Bajcsy, R. (1988). Active perception. *Proceedings of IEEE 76* (pp. 996-1005).

Balda, R. A., Diller, G., Deardorff, E., Doue, J., & Hsieh, P. (1977). The HP ECG analysis program. In J. H. van Bemmel & J. L. Willems (Eds.), *Trends in computer-processed electrocardiograms* (pp. 197-205). Amsterdam: North Holland.

Ballard, D. H., Hayhoe, M. M., & Pelz, J. B. (1995). Memory representations in natural tasks. *Journal of Cognitive Neuroscience, 7*(1), 68-82.

Banitsas, K. A., Georgiadis, P., Tachakra, S., & Cavouras, D. (2004). Using handheld devices for real-time wireless tele-consultation. *Proceedings of the 26th Annual International Conference of the IEEE EMBS* (pp. 3105-3108).

Bar-Or, A., Healey, J., Kontothanassis, L., & Van Thong, J. M. (2004). BioStream: A system architecture for real-time processing of physiological signals. *Proceedings of the 26th Annual International Conference of the IEEE EMBS* (pp. 3101-3104).

Batsford. W. (1999). Pacemakers and antitachycardia devices. In: B.L. Zaret, M. Moser & L.S. Cohen (Eds.) *Yale University School of Medicine Heart Book,* pp. 331-338. Hearst Books. New York. Available online at http://www.med.yale.edu/library/heartbk/ (accessed in November 2008)

Bayes de Luna, A., & Stern, S. (2001). The future of noninvasive electrocardiology In W. Zareba, P. Maison-Blanche, & E. H. Locati (Eds.), *Noninvasive electrocardiology in clinical practice.* Armonk, NY: Futura.

Becker, W. (1989). Metrics. In M. E. Goldburg & R. H. Wurtz (Eds.), *The neurobiology of saccadic eye movements.* Englewood Cliffs, NJ: Elsevier Science.

Becker, W. (1991). Saccades. In R.H.S. Carpenter (Ed.), *Vision and visual dysfunction* vol. 8: *Eye movements.* Boca Raton, FL: CRC Press.

Benhorin, J., Merri, M., Alberti, M., Locati, E., Moss, A. J., Hall, W. J., & Cui, L. (1990). Long QT syndrome. New electrocardiographic characteristics. *Circulation, 82,* 521-527.

Berger, R. D. (2003). QT variability. *Journal of Electrocardiology, 36*(5), 83-87.

Berger, R. D., Kasper, E. K., Baughman, K. L., Marban, E., Calkins, H., & Tomaselli, G. F. (1997). Beat-to-beat QT interval variability novel evidence for repolarization liability in ischemic and nonischemic dilated cardiomyopathy. *Circulation, 96*(5), 1557-1565.

Biagini, A., Mazzei, M. Z., Carpeggiani, C. et al. (1982). Vasospastic ischemic mechanism of frequent asymptomatic transient ST-T changes during continuous electrocardiographic monitoring in selected unstable patients. *American Heart Journal, 103,* 4-12.

Biblo, I. A., & Waldo, A. L. (1986). Supraventricular arrhythmias. In A. Moss & A. Stern (Eds.), *Noninvasive electrocardiology—clinical aspects of Holter monitoring.* London: Saunders Co.

Bilgin, A., Marcellin, M. W., & Altbach, M. I. (2003). Compression of electrocardiogram signals using JPEG2000. *IEEE Transactions on Biomedical Engineering, 50*(4), 833-840.

Boccignone, G. (2001). An information-theory approach to active vision. *Proceedings of the 11th International Conference on Image Analysis and Processing.*

Bonner, R. E., & Schwetman, H. D. (1968). Computer diagnosis of the electrocardiogram II. *Computers and Biomedical Research, 1,* 366.

Bousseljot, R. et al. (2003). Telemetric ECG diagnosis follow-up. *Computers in Cardiology, 30,* 121-124.

Bowman, B. R., & Schuck, E. (2000). Medical instruments and devices used in the home. In J. D. Bronzino (Ed.), *The biomedical engineering handbook.* Boca Raton, FL: CRC Press.

Bradie, B. (1996). Wavelet packet-based compression of single lead ECG. *IEEE Transactions on Biomedical Engineering, 43,* 493-501.

Bronzino, J. D. (2000). Regulation of medical, device innovation. In J. D. Bronzino (Ed.), *The biomedical engineering handbook.* Boca Raton, FL: CRC Press.

Bronzino, J. D., Flannery, E. J., and Wade, M. L. (1990) "Legal and Ethical Issues in the Regulation and Development of Engineering Achievements in Medical Technology," Part I *Engineering in Medicine and Biology Magazine, IEEE* vol. 9, no. 1, pp. 79-81

Bronzino, J. D., Flannery, E. J., and Wade, M. L. (1990) "Legal and Ethical Issues in the Regulation and Development of Engineering Achievements in Medical Technology," Part II *Engineering in Medicine and Biology Magazine, IEEE,* vol. 9 no. 2, pp. 53-57

Calderbank, A. R., Daubechies, I., Sweldens, W., & Yeo, B. L. (1997). Lossless image compression using integer to integer wavelet transforms *Proceedings of the IEEE International Conference of Image Processing* (vol. 1, pp. 596599).

CardioSoft. (2005). *Version 6.0 operator's manual.* Milwaukee, WI: GE Medical Systems Information Technologies.

Caro, C. G., Pedley, T. J., Schroter, R. C., & Seed, W. A. (1978). *The mechanics of the circulation.* New York: Oxford University Press.

Carpenter, R. H. S. (1988). *Movements of the eye.* London: Pion Press.

Chen, J., & Itoh, S. (1998). A wavelet transform-based ECG compression method guaranteeing desired signal quality *IEEE Transactions on BME, 45,* 1414-1419.

Chiarugi, F. et al. (2002). Real-time cardiac monitoring over a regional health network: Preliminary results from initial field testing. *Computers in Cardiology, 29,* 347-350.

Chiarugi, F. et al. (2003) Continuous ECG Monitoring in the Management of Pre-Hospital Health Emergencies. *Computers in Cardiology, 30,* 205-208.

Christov, I., Otsinsky, I., Simova, I., Prokopova, R., Trendafilova, E., & Naydenov, S. (2006). Dataset of manually measured QT intervals in the electrocardiogram. *Biomedical Engineering Online, 31*(5), 5-31.

Chronaki, C. E. (2004). Open ECG: Goals and achievements. *Proceedings of the 2nd Open ECG Workshop* (pp. 3-4), Berlin.

Cimino, J. J., Clayton, P. D., Hripcsak, G. et al. (1994). Knowledge-based approaches to the maintenance of a large controlled medical terminology. *Journal of the American Medical Informatics Association, 1,* 35.

Clifford, G. D. (2006). ECG statistics, noise, artifacts and missing data. In G. D. Clifford, F. Azuaje, & P. E. McSharry (Eds.), *Advanced methods and tools for ECG data analysis* (pp. 55-99). Boston, Artech House.

Cohen, A., & Zigel, Y. (1998). Compression of multichannel ECG through multichannel long-term prediction. *IEEE Engineering in Medicine and Biology, 17*(1), 109-115.

Cohen, D., Edelsack, E. A., & Zimmerman, J. E. (1970). Magnetocardiograms taken inside a shielded room with a superconducting point-contact magnetometer. *Applied Physics Letters, 16,* 278-280.

Conforti, F., Micalizzi, M., & Macerata, A. (2004). Collection and development of open tools for ECG interoperability. *Proceedings of the 2nd OpenECG Workshop* (pp. 13-14), Berlin.

Cosby, R. S., & Herman, L. M. (1962). Sequential changes in the development of the electrocardiographic pattern of left ventricular hypertrophy in hypertensive heart disease. *American Heart Journal, 63,* 180.

Coumel, P., Maison-Blanche, P., Catuli, D., Neyroud, N., Fayn, J., & Rubel, P. (1995). Different circadian behavior of the apex and end of the T wave. *Journal of Electrocardiology, 28*(supplement), 138-142.

Cox, J. R., Nolle, F. M., Fozzard, H. A., & Oliver, G. G. (1968). AZTEC, a preprocessing program for real-time ECG rhythm analysis. *IEEE Transactions on Biomedical Engineering, 15,* 128-129.

CSE Working Party. (1985). Recommendations for measurement standards in quantitative electrocardiography. *European Heart Journal, 6,* 815-825.

Cuomo, S., Marciano, F., Migaux, M. L., Finizio, F., Pezzella, E., Losi, M. A., & Betocchi, S. (2004). Abnormal QT interval variability in patients with hypertrophic cardiomyopathy. Can syncope be predicted? *Journal of Electrocardiology, 37*(2), 113-119.

Daskalov, I. K., & Christov, I. I. (1999). Automatic detection of the electrocardiogram T-wave end. *Medical and Biological Engineering and Computing,* 37, 348-353.

Daskalov, I. K., & Christov, I. I. (1999). Electrocardiogram signal preprocessing for automatic detection of QRS boundaries. *Medical Engineering and Physics, 21,* 37-44.

Daskalov, I. K., Dotsinsky, I. A., & Christov, I. I. (1998). Developments in ECG acquisition, preprocessing, parameter measurement and recording. *IEEE Engineering in Medicine and Biology Magazine, 17,* 50-58.

Daubechies, I. (1992). *Ten lectures on wavelets.* CBMS-NSF Conference Series in Applied Mathematics.

Davey, P. (1999). QT interval measurement: Q to T apex or Q to T end . *Journal of Internal Medicine, 246,* 145-149.

Dawson, T. H. (1991). *Engineering design of the cardiovascular system of mammals.* Englewood Cliffs, NJ: Prentice Hall.

de Chazal, P., & Celler, B. G. (1996). Automatic measurement of the QRS onset and offset in individual ECG leads. *Proceedings of the 18th Annual IEEE International Conference on Engineering in Medicine and Biology Society,* Amsterdam.

Dick, A. O. (1980). *Instrument scanning and controlling: Using eye-movement data to understand pilot behavior and strategies.* NASA CR 3306.

DICOM. (2007). *Digital imaging and communications in medicine.* Rosslyn, VA: National Electrical Manufacturers Association.

DiMarco, J. P., & Philbrick, J. T. (1990). Use of ambulatory electrocardiographic (Holter) monitoring. *Annals of Internal Medicine, 113,* 53-68.

Dobbs, S. E., Schmitt, N. M., & Ozemek, H. S. (1984). QRS detection by template matching using real-time correlation on a microcomputer. *Journal of Clinical Engineering, 9,* 197-212.

Dolin, R. H., Alschuler, L., Boyer, S., & Beebe, C. (2004). *HL7 clinical document architecture. Release 2.0.* HL7 Health Level Seven, Inc., Ann Arbor, MI. Available online at: www.hl7.org (accessed in November 2008)

Dower, G. E. (1984). The ECGD: A derivation of the ECG from VCG leads. *Journal of Electrocardiology, 17*(2), 189-191.

Dower, G. E., Yakush, A., Nazzal, S. B., Jutzy, R. V., & Ruiz, C. E. (1988). Deriving the 12-lead electrocardiogram from four (EASI) electrodes. *Journal of Electrocardiology, 21*(Suppl.), S182-S187.

DRG. (1995). *MediArc premier IV operator's manual* (v. 2.2.).

Duda, K., Turcza, P., & Zieliński, T. P. (2001). Lossless ECG compression with lifting wavelet transform. *Proceedings of the IEEE Instrumentation and Measurement Technology Conference* (pp. 640-644).

Duisterhout, J. S., Hasman, A., & Salamon, R. (Eds.). (1991). *Telematics in medicine.* Amsterdam: Elsevier Science.

Extramiana, F., Maison-Blanche, P., Badilini, F., Pinoteau, J., Deseo, T., & Coumel, P. (1999). Circadian modulation of the QT rate dependence in healthy volunteers. *Journal of Electrocardiology, 32*(1), 33-43.

Extramiana, F., Neyroud, N., Huikuri, H. V., Koistinen, M. J., Coumel, P., & Maison-Blanche, P. (1999a). QT interval and arrhythmic risk assessment after myocardial infarction. *American Journal of Cardiology, 83,* 266-269.

Fayn, J. et al. (2003), Towards new integrated information and communication infrastructures in e-health. Examples from cardiology. *Computers in Cardiology, 30,* 113-116.

Fenici, R., Brisinda, D., & Meloni, A. M. (2005). Clinical applications of magneticardiography. *Expert Review of Molecular Diagnostics, 5,* 291-313.

Fisch, C. (2000). Centennial of the sting galvanometer and the electrocardiogram. *Journal of the College of Cardiology, 36*(6), 1737-1745.

Fischer, R., & Zywietz, C. (2001). *How to implement SCP.* Retrieved from http://www.openecg.net

Fischer, R., & Zywietz, C. (2004). Integrated content and format checking for processing of SCP ECG records. *Proceedings of the 2nd OpenECG Workshop* (pp. 11-12), Berlin.

Fogel, R. I., Evans, J. J., & Prystowsky, E. N. (1997). Utility and cost of event recorders in the diagnosis of palpitations, presyncope, and syncope. *American Journal of Cardiology, 79,* 207-208.

Franchini, K. G., & Cowley, A. E., Jr. (2004). Autonomic control of cardiac function. In D. Robertson, I. Biaggioni, G. Burnstock, & P. A. Low (Eds.), *Primer on the autonomic nervous system* (2nd ed., pp. 134-138). Englewood Cliffs, NJ: Elsevier Academic Press.

Friesen, G. M., Jannett T. C. et al. (1990). A comparison of the noise sensitivity of nine QRS detection algorithms. *IEEE Transactions on Biomedical Engineering, 37*(1), 85-98.

Fumo, G. S., & Tompkins, W. J. (1982). QRS detection using automata theory in a battery-powered microprocessor system. *IEEE Frontiers of Engineering in Health Care, 4,* 155-158.

Furth, B., & Perez, A. (1988). An adaptive real-time ECG compression algorithm with variable threshold. *IEEE Transactions on Biomedical Engineering, 35*(6), 489-494.

Gaita, F., Giustetto, C., Bianchi, F., Wolpert, C., Schimpf, R., Riccardi, R., Grossi, S., Richiardi, E., & Borggrefe, M. (2003). Short QT syndrome a familial cause of sudden death. *Circulation, 108,* 965-970.

Garibyan, L. and L. S. Lilly (2006). The electrocardiogram. In L.S. Lilly (Ed.) Pathophysiology of Heart Disease,: *A Collaborative, Project of Medical Students and Faculty,* fourth ed.. pp. 80-117. Lippincott Williams & Wilkins, Philadelphia.

González, R., Jiménez, D., & Vargas, O. (2005). WalkECG: A mobile cardiac care device. *Computers in Cardiology, 32,* 371-374.

Gouaux, F. et al. (2002). Ambient intelligence and pervasive systems for the monitoring of citizens at cardiac risk: New solutions from the EPI-MEDICS project. *Computers in Cardiology, 29,* 289-292.

GPRS. (2007). *General Packet Radio Service.* Retrieved from http://en.wikipedia.org/wiki/General_Packet_Radio_Service

GSM. (2007). *Global System for Mobile Communications.* Retrieved from http://en.wikipedia.org/wiki/Global_System_for_Mobile_Communications

Gulrajani, R. M. (1998). The forward and inverse problems of electrocardiography. Gaining a better qualitative and quantitative understanding of the heart's electrical activity. *IEEE MBE Magazine, 17*(5), 84-101.

Halpern, E. J., Newhouse, J. H., Amis, E. S. J. et al. (1992). Evaluation of teleradiology for interpretation of intra-venous urograms. *Journal of Digital Imaging, 5*(2), 101.

Hamilton, D. J., Thomson, D. C., & Sandham, W. A. (1995). ANN compression of morphologically similar ECG complexes. *Medical and Biological Engineering and Computing, 33,* 841-843.

Hamilton, P. S. (1993). Adaptive compression of the ambulatory electrocardiogram. *Biomedical Instrumentation & Technology,* vol. 27 No. 1 (January), 56-63

Hamilton, P. S., & Tompkins, W. J. (1986) Quantitative investigation of QRS detection rules using the MIT/BIH arrhythmia database. *IEEE Transactions on Biomedical Engineering, 33,* 1157-1165.

Hamilton, P. S., & Tompkins, W. J. (1991). Compression of the ambulatory ECG by average beat subtraction and residual differencing. *IEEE Transactions on Biomedical Engineering, 38,* 253-259.

Hart, G. (1991). Biomagnetometry: Imaging the heart's magnetic field. *British Heart Journal, 65,* 61-62.

Healthsquare. (2007). *Heart disease.* Retrieved from http://www.healthsquare.com/heartdisease.htm

Heron, M. P., & Smith, B. L. (2003). *Deaths: Leading causes for 2003.* Hyattsville, MD: National Center for Health Statistics.

Hilgard, J., Ezri, M. D., & Denes P. (1985) Significance of ventricular pauses of three seconds or more detected on twenty-four-hour Holter recordings. *American Journal of Cardiology, 55,* 1005-1008.

Hilton, M. (1997). Wavelet and wavelet packet compression of electrocardiograms. *IEEE Transactions on Biomedical Engineering, 44,* 394-402.

Hirai, M., & Kawamoto, K. (2004). MFER—a Japanese approach for medical wave form encoding rules for viewer design. *Proceedings of the 2nd OpenECG Workshop* (pp. 35-37), Berlin, Germany.

Hitch, G. J., & Baddeley, A. (1976). Verbal reasoning and working memory. *Quarterly Journal of Experimental Psychology, 28,* 603-621.

Holter, N. (1961). New method for heart studies: Continuous electrocardiography of active subjects over long periods is now practical. *Science, 134,* 1214-1220.

HP. (1994). *M1700A interpretive cardiograph physician's guide* (4th ed.). Hewlett-Packard.

Hsia, P. W. (1989). Electrocardiographic data compression using precoding consecutive QRS information. *IEEE Transactions on Biomedical Engineering, 36,* 465-468.

http://medical.nema.org

http://www.aerotel.com/en/

http://www.burdick.com/products/

http://www.cardguard.com/newsite/index.asp

http://www.cardiocom.net/

http://www.cardiocomm.com/

http://www.cardiolertsystems.com/

http://www.cardiomedix.com/cardiomedix.htm

http://www.cardionet.com/

http://www.centc251.org

http://www.gehealthcare.com/euen/products.html

http://www.healthfrontier.com/

http://www.hl7.org

http://www.ieee1073.org

http://www.iso.ch/tc215

http://www.medtronic.com/

http://www.monitoring.welchallyn.com/

http://www.pdsheart.com/about.html

http://www.qrscard.com/

http://www.qrsdiagnostic.com/

http://www.spacelabshealthcare.com/company/index.html

Hull, E. (1961). The electrocardiogram in pericarditis. *American Journal of Cardiology, 7,* 21.

Hurst, W. (2002). *The heart, arteries, and veins* (10th ed.). New York: McGraw-Hill.

IBM. (1974). *Electrocardiogram analysis program physician's guide* (5736-H15; 2nd ed.).

IEC 60601-2-51. (2003). *Medical electrical equipment: Particular requirements for the safety, including essential performance, of ambulatory electrocardiographic systems.* First edition 2003-02, International Electrotechnical Commission, Geneva,

Irwin, D. E. (1991). Information integration across saccadic eye movements. *Cognitive Psychology, 23,* 420-456.

Irwin, D. E. (1992). Visual memory within and across fixations. In K. Raynor (Ed.), *Eye movements and visual cognition; scene perception and reading.* New York: Springer-Verlag.

Ishijiama, M. (1993). Fundamentals of the decision of optimum factors in the ECG data compression. *IEICE Transactions Information and Systems, E76-D*(12), 1398-1403.

Ishijiama, M., Shin, S., Hostetter, G., & Sklansky, J. (1983). Scan-along polygonal approximation for data compression of electrocardiograms. *IEEE Transactions on Biomedical Engineering, 30*(11), 723-729.

Iwata, A., Nagasaka, Y., & Suzumura, N. (1990). Data compression of ECG using neural network for digital Holter monitor. *IEEE Engineering in Medicine and Biology Magazine*, (September), 53-57.

Iyer V., Edelman E. R. & Lilly L. S. (2006). Basic cardiac structure and function. In L.S. Lilly (Ed.) *Pathophysiology of Heart Disease: A Collaborative Project of Medical Students and Faculty*, fourth ed.. pp. 1-28. Lippincott Williams & Wilkins, Philadelphia.

Jalaleddine, S. M., & Hutchens, C. G. (1990). SAIES—a new ECG data compression algorithm. *Journal of Clinical Engineering, 15*(1), 45-51.

Jalaleddine, S. M., Hutchens, C. G., Strattan, R. D., & Coberly, W. A. (1990). ECG data compression techniques—a unified approach. *IEEE Transactions on Biomedical Engineering, 37*(4), 329-343.

Jayant, N. S., & Noll, P. (1984). *Digital coding of waveforms.* Englewood Cliffs, NJ: Prentice Hall.

Jensen, B. T., Abildstrom, S. Z., Larroude, C. E., Agner, E., Torp-Pedersen, C., Nyvad, O., Ottesen, M., Wachtell, K., & Kanters, J. K. (2005). QT dynamics in risk stratification after myocardial infarction. *Heart Rhythm, 2,* 357-364.

Kandori, A., Hosono, T., Kanagawa, T., Miyashita, S., Chiba, Y., Murakami, M. et al. (2002). Detection of atrial-flutter and atrial-fibrillation waveforms by fetal magnetocardiogram. *Medical and Biological Engineering and Computing, 40,* 213-217.

Kardys, I., Kors, J. A., van der Meer, I. M., Hofman, A., van der Kuip, D. A. M., & Witteman, J. C. M. (2003). Spatial QRS-T angle predicts cardiac death in a general population. *European Heart Journal, 24,* 1357-1364.

Karlsson, S. (1967). Representation of ECG records by Karhunen-Loève expansions. *Proceedings of the 7th International Conference on Medical and Biological Engineering* (p. 105).

Khoór, S. et al. (2003). Internet-based, GPRS, long-term ECG monitoring and non-linear heart-rate analysis for cardiovascular telemedicine management. *Computers in Cardiology, 30,* 209-212.

Kinlay, S., Leitch, J. W., Neil, A., Chapman, B. L., Hardy, D. B. et al. (1996). Cardiac event recorders yield more diagnoses and are more cost-effective than 48-hour Holter monitoring in patients with palpitations: a controlled clinical trial. *Annals of Internal Medicine, 124,* 16-20.

Klingeman, J., & Pipberger, H. V. (1967). Computer classification of electrocardiograms. *Computers and Biomedical Research, 1,* 1.

Kohler, B., Hennig, C., & Orglmeister, R. (2002). The principles of software QRS detection. *IEEE Engineering in Medicine and Biology Magazine, 21*(1), 42-57.

Kowacki, L., & Augustyniak, P. (2007). Implementation of wavelet compression of the electrocariogram in signal processor. *Journal of Medical Informatics and Technologies.*vol. 11 pp. 147–153

Kowler, E. (1990). The role of visual and cognitive processes in the control of eye movement. In K. Kowler (Ed.), *Eye movements and their role in visual and cognitive processes.* Englewood Cliffs, NJ: Elsevier Science.

Kuklinski, W. S. (1983). Fast Walsh transform data-compression algorithm: ECG application. *Medical and Biological Engineering and Computing, 21,* 465-472.

Kuzume, K., & Niijima, K. (2000). Design of optimal lifting wavelet filters for data compression. *Proceedings of the IEEE, 88*(11).

Laguna, P., Jané, R., & Caminal, P. (1994). Automatic detection of wave boundaries in multilead ECG signals: Validation with the CSE database. *Computers and Biomedical Research, 27*(1), 45-60.

Laguna, P., Mark, R. G., Goldberger, A., & Moody, G. B. (1997). A database for evaluation of algorithms for measurement of QT and other waveform intervals in the ECG. *Computers in Cardiology, 24,* 673-676.

Lamberti, C., & Coccia, P. (1988). ECG data compression for ambulatory device. *Computers in Cardiology, 15,* 171-178.

Lang, C. C. E., Neilson, J. M. M., & Flapan, A. D. (2004). Abnormalities of the repolarization characteristics of patients with heart failure progress with symptom severity. *Annals of Noninvasive Electrocardiology , 9*(3), 257-264.

Lass, J., Kaik, J., Karai, D., & Vainu, M. (2001). Ventricular repolarization evaluation from surface ECG for identification of the patients with increased myocardial electrical instability. *Proceedings of the 23rd Annual International Conference of the IEEE Engineering in Medicine and Biology Society* (pp. 390-393).

Lee, H., Cheng, Q., & Thakor, N. (1987). ECG waveform analysis by significant point extraction. *Computers and Biomedical Research, 20,* 410-427.

Levine, M. D. (1985). *Vision in man and machine.* New York: McGraw-Hill.

Levkov, C. L. (1987). Orthogonal electrocardiogram derived from limb and chest electrodes of the conventional 12-lead system. *Medical and Biological Engineering and Computing, 25,* 155-164.

Lombardi, F. (2001). Frequency domain analysis of heart rate variability In W. Zareba, P. Maison-Blanche, & E. F. Locati (Eds.), *Noninvasive electrocardiology in clinical practice.* Armonk, NY: Futura.

Lu, Z., Kim, D. Y., & Pearlman, W. A. (2000). Wavelet compression of ECG signals by the set partitioning in hierarchical trees algorithm. *IEEE Transactions on Biomedical Engineering, 47*(7), 849-856.

Macfarlane, P. W., & Lawrie, T. D. V. (Eds.). (1989). *Comprehensive electrocardiology. Theory and practice in health and disease* (vols. 1-3). Oxford: Pergamon Press.

Macfarlane, P. W., Lorimer, A. R., & Lowrie, T. D. V. (1971). 3 and 12 lead electrocardiogram interpretation by computer. A comparison in 1093 patients. *British Heart Journal, 33,* 226.

Maglaveras, N. et al. (2002). Using contact centers in telemanagement and home care of congestive heart failure patients: The CHS experience. *Computers in Cardiology, 29,* 281-284.

Maison-Blanche, P., Catuli, D., Fayn, J., & Coumel, P. (1996). QT interval, heart rate and ventricular tachyarrhythmias. In A. J. Moss & S. Stern (Eds.), *Noninvasive electrocardiology: Clinical aspects of Holter monitoring* (pp. 383-404). London, W. B. Saunders Co.

Malik, M. (1995). Effect of ECG recognition artefact on time-domain measurement of heart rate variability. In M. Malik & A. J. Camm (Eds.), *Heart rate variability.* Armonk, NY: Futura.

Malik, M., & Batchvarov, V. (2000). QT dispersion In J. Camm (Ed.), *Clinical approaches to tachyarrhythmias.* Armonk, NY: Futura.

Malik, M., & Camm, A. J. (2004). *Dynamic electrocardiography.* Armonk, NY: Blackwell Futura.

Malik, M., Farbom, P., Batchvarov, V., Hnatkova, K., & Camm, J. (2002). Relation between QT and RR intervals is highly individual among healthy subjects: Implications for heart rate correction of the QT interval. *Heart, 87,* 220-228.

Malik, M., Farrell, T., Cripps, T., & Camm, A. J. (1989). Heart rate variability in relation to prognosis after myocardial infarction: Selection of optimal processing techniques. *European Heart Journal, 10,* 1060-1074.

Mallat, S. G. (1989). A theory for multiresolution signal decomposition: The wavelet representation. *IEEE Transactions on Pattern Analysis and Machine Intelligence, 11*(7).

Mallat, S. G. (1996). *A wavelet tour of signal processing.* New York: Academic Press.

Marciano, F., Cuomo, S., Migaux, M. L., & Vetrano, A. (1998). Dynamic correlation between QT and RR intervals: How long is QT adaptation to heart rate? *Computers in Cardiology, 25,* 413-416.

Marcus, F. I. (1986). Ventricular arrhythmias In A. Moss & S. Stern (Eds.), *Noninvasive electrocardiology—clinical aspects of Holter monitoring.* London: Saunders Co.

McDonald, C. T., & Hammond, W. E. (1989). Standard formats for electronic transfer of clinical data. *Annals of Internal Medicine, 110,* 333.

McPherson, C. A. & Rosenfeld L. E. (1999). Heart rhythm disorders. In B.L. Zaret, M. Moser and Cohen L. S., (Eds.) *Yale University School of Medicine Heart Book*, pp. 195-204. Hearst Books. New York. Available online at http://www.med.yale.edu/library/heartbk/ (accessed in November 2008).

Merri, M., Moss, A. J., Benhorin, J., Locati, E., Alberti, M., & Badilini, F. (1992). Relation between ventricular repolarization duration and cardiac cycle length during 24-hour Holter recordings: Findings in normal patients and patients with long QT syndrome. *Circulation, 85,* 1816-1821.

Miaou, S.-G., & Lin, C.-L. (2002). A quality-on-demand algorithm for wavelet-based compression of electrocardiogram signals. *IEEE Transactions on Biomedical Engineering, 49*(3), 233-239.

Miaou, S.-G., Chen, S.-T., & Chao, S.-N. (2005). Wavelet-based lossy-to-lossless ECG compression in a unified vector quantization framework. *IEEE Transactions on Biomedical Engineering, 52*(3), 539-545.

Milliez, P., Leenhardt, A., Maison-Blanche, P., Vicaut, E., Badilini, F., Siliste, C., Benchetrit C., & Coumel, P. (2005). Usefulness of ventricular repolarization dynamicity in predicting arrhythmic deaths in patients with isquemic cardiomyopathy (from the European Myocardial Infarct Amiodarone Trial). *American Journal of Cardiology, 95,* 821-826.

MIT-BIH Database Distribution. (n.d.). *MIT/BIH ECG database.* Cambridge, MA: Massachusetts Institute of Technology.

Moody, G. (1993). *MIT/BIH arrhythmia database distribution.* Cambridge, MA: MIT Division of Health Science and Technology.

Moody, G. B., & Mark R. G. (1990). The MIT-BIH arrhythmia database on CD-ROM and software for use with it. *Computers in Cardiology, 17,* 185-188.

Moody, G. B., Mark, R. G., Zoccola, A., & Mantero, S. (1986). Derivation of respiratory signals from multilead ECGs. *Computers in Cardiology, 13,* 113-116.

Moody, G., & Mark, R. (1988). *MIT-BIH arrhythmia database directory.* Cambridge, MA: MIT Biomedical Engineering Center.

Mori, H., & Nakaya, Y. (1988). Present status of clinical magnetocardiography. *Cardiovascular World Report* 1, 78-86

Morlet, D. (1986). *Contribution a l'analyse automatique des electrocardiogrammes—algorithmes de localisation, classification et delimitation precise des ondes dans le systeme de Lyon* (in French). PhD Thesis, INSA-Lyon, France.

Moss, A. J. (1986). Clinical utility of ST segment monitoring In A. Moss & S. Stern (Eds.), *Noninvasive electrocardiology clinical aspects of Holter monitoring.* London: Saunders Co.

Moss, A. J., Bigger, J. T., & Odoroff, C. L. (1987). Postinfarction risk stratification. *Progress in Cardiovascular Disease, 29,* 389-412.

Moss, A. J., Schnitzler, R., Green, R., & DeCamilla, J. (1971). Ventricular arrhythmias 3 weeks after acute myocardial infarction. *Annals of Internal Medicine, 75,* 837-841.

Mueller, W. C. (1978). Arrhythmia detection program for an ambulatory ECG monitor. *Biomedical Sciences Instrumentation, 14,* 81-85.

Murabayashi, T., Fetics, B., Kass, D., Nevo, E., Gramatikov, B., & Berger, R. D. (2002). Beat-to-beat QT interval variability associated with acute myocardial isquemia. *Journal of Electrocardiology, 35*(1), 19-25.

National Center for Health Statistics. (2005) *Health, United States, 2005 with chartbook on the health of Americans.* Hyattsville, MD.

Nave, G., & Cohen, A. (1993). ECG compression using long term prediction. *IEEE Transactions on Biomedical Engineering, 40,* 877-885.

Nelson, S. D., Kou, W. H., & Annesley, T. (1989). Significance of ST segment depression during paroxysmal superventricular tachycardia. *Journal of the American College of Cardiology, 13,* 804.

Nelwan, S. P., van Dam, T. B., Klootwijk, P., & Meil, S. H. (2002). Ubiquitous mobile access to real-time patient monitoring data. *Computers in Cardiology, 29,* 557-560.

NEMA (National Electrical Manufacturers Association). (2007). *DICOM strategic document* (version 7.2). Retrieved from http://dicom.nema.org

NEMA. (2007). *Digital imaging and communications in medicine (DICOM).* Rosslyn, VA: Author.

Nihon Kohden. (2001). *ECAPS-12C user guide: Interpretation standard* (revision A).

Nikolaev, N., & Gotchev, A. (1998). De-noising of ECG signals using wavelet shrinkage with time-frequency dependant threshold. *Proceedings of the European Signal Processing Conference* (pp. 2449-2453), Island of Rhodes, Greece.

Nikolaev, N., & Gotchev, A. (2000). ECG signal denoising using wavelet domain Wiener filtering. *Proceedings of the European Signal Processing Conference* (pp. 51-54), Tampere, Finland.

Nikolaev, N., Gotchev, A., Egiazarian, K., & Nikolov, Z. (2001). Suppression of electromyogram interference on the electrocardiogram by transform domain denoising. *Medical and Biological Engineering and Computing, 39,* 649-655.

Nikolaev, N., Nikolov, Z., Gotchev, A., & Egiazarian, K. (2000). Wavelet domain Wiener filtering for ECG denoising using an improved signal estimate. *Proceedings of the International Conference on Acoustics, Speech, and Signal Processing* (pp. 2210-2213), Istanbul, Turkey.

Nomura, M., Nakaya, Y., Saito, K., Kishi, F., Watatsuki, T., Miyoshi, H. et al. (1994). Noninvasive localisation of accessory pathways by magnetocardiographic imaging. *Clinical Cardiology, 17,* 239-244.

Norgall, T. (2004). ECG data interchange formats and protocols status and outlook. *Proceedings of the 2nd OpenECG Workshop* (pp. 25-26), Berlin.

Noton, D., & Stark, L. (1971). Eye movements and visual perception. *Scientific American, 224,* 34-43.

Nygaard, R., Melnikov, G., & Katsaggelos, A. K. (2001). A rate distortion optimal ECG coding algorithm *IEEE Transactions on Biomedical Engineering, 48*(1), 28-40.

Ober, J. K., Ober, J. J., Malawski, M., Skibniewski, W., Przedpelska-Ober, E., & Hryniewiecki, J. (2002). Monitoring pilot eye movements during the combat flights the white box. *Biocybernetics and Biomedical Engineering, 22*(2-3), 241-264.

Onaral, B. (2001). Future directions: Biomedical signal processing and networked multimedia communications. In J. D. Bronzino (Ed.), *The biomedical engineering handbook.* Boca Raton, FL: CRC Press.

Pahlm, O., Börjesson, P., & Werner, O. (1979). Compact digital storage of ECGs. *Computer Programs in Biomedicine, 9,* 293-300.

Pan, J., & Tompkins, W. J. (1985). A real-time QRS detection algorithm. *IEEE Transactions on Biomedical Engineering, 32*(3), 230-236.

Paoletti, M., & Marchesi, C. (2004). Low computational cost algorithms for portable ECG monitoring units *IFMBE Proceedings of Medicon 2004* (paper 231).

Parker J.O., di Giorgi S., & West R.O (1966) A hemodynamic study of acute coronary insufficiency precipitated by exercise. *American Journal of Cardiology* 17: pp. 470-483,

Pashler, H., Carrier, M., & Hoffman, J. (1993). Saccadic eye movements and dual-task interference. *Quarterly Journal of Experimental Psychology, 46A*(1), 51-82.

Paul, J., Reddy, M., & Kumar, V. (2000). A transform domain SVD filter for suppression of muscle noise artifacts in exercise ECGs. *IEEE Transactions on Biomedical Engineering, 47,* 654-662.

Peden, J. (1982). ECG data compression: Some practical considerations. In J. Paul, M. Jordan, M. Ferguson-Pell, & B. Andrews (Eds.), *Computing in Medicine.* Macmillan, London.

Pellerin, D., Maison-Blanche, P., Extramiana, F., Hermida, J. S., Leclercq, J. F., Leenhardt, A., & Coumel, P. (2001). Autonomic influences on ventricular repolarization in congestive heart failure. *Journal of Electrocardiology, 34*(1), 35-40.

Pelz, J. B., & Canosa, R. (2001). Oculomotor behavior and perceptual strategies in complex tasks. *Vision Research, 41,* 3587-3596.

Pinna, G. D. et al. (2003). Home telemonitoring of chronic heart failure patients: Novel system architecture of the home or hospital in heart failure study. *Computers in Cardiology, 30,* 105-108.

Pinna, G. D., Maestri, R., Gobbi, E., La Rovere, M. T., & Scanferlato, J. L. (2003). Home tele-monitoring of chronic heart failure patients: Novel system architecture of the home or hospital in heart failure study. *Computers in Cardiology, 30,* 105-108.

Pordy, L., Jaffe, H., Chesky, K. et al. (1968). Computer diagnosis of electrocardiograms IV, a computer program for contour analysis with clinical results of rhythm and contour interpretation. *Computers and Biomedical Research, 1,* 408-433.

Pottala, E. W., Bailey, J. J., Horton, M. R., & Gradwohl, J. R. (1989). Suppression of baseline wander in the ECG using a bilinearly transformed, null-phase filter. *Journal of Electrocardiology, 22*(suppl), 243-247.

Prineas, R., Crow, R., & Blackburn, H. (1982). *The Minnesota code manual of electrocardiographic findings.* Littleton, MA: John Wright-PSG.

Pryor, T. A. (2000). Hospital information systems: Their function and state. In J. D. Bronzino (Ed.), *The biomedical engineering handbook.* Boca Raton, FL: CRC Press.

Pueyo, E., Malik, M., & Laguna, P. (2005). Beat-to-beat adaptation of QT interval to heart rate. *Proceedings of the 27th Annual International Conference of the IEEE Engineering in Medicine and Biology Society* (pp. 2475-2478).

Pueyo, E., Smetana, P., Malik, M., & Laguna, P. (2003). Evaluation of QT interval response to marked RR interval changes selected automatically in ambulatory recordings. *Computers in Cardiology, 30,* 157-160.

Quartero, H. W. P., Stinstra, J. G., Golbach, E. G. M., Meijboom, E. J., & Peters, M. J. (2002). Clinical implications of fetal magnetocardiography. *Ultrasound in Obstetrics and Gynecology, 20,* 142-153.

Ramakrishnan, A.G., & Supratim, S. (1997). ECG coding by wavelet-based linear prediction. *IEEE Transactions on BME, 44*(12).

Reddy, B. R. S., & Murthy, I. S. N. (1986). ECG data compression using Fourier descriptors. *IEEE Transactions on Biomedical Engineering, 33,* 428-434.

Rennels, G. D., & Shortliffe, E. H. (1987). Advanced computing for medicine. *Scientific American, 257*(4), 154.

Reza, A., Moghaddam, A., & Nayebi, K. (2001). A two dimensional wavelet packet approach for ECG compression. *Proceedings of the International Symposium on Signal Processing Application* (pp. 226-229).

Risk, M. R., Bruno, J. S., Llamedo Soria, M., Arini, P. D., & Taborda, R. A. M. (2005). Measurement of QT interval and duration of the QRS complex at different ECG sampling rates. *Computers in Cardiology, 32,* 495-498.

Rolls H. K., Stevenson W. G., Strichartz G. R.& Lilly L. S. (2006) Mechanisms of cardiac arrhythmias. In L.S. Lilly, (Ed.) *Pathophysiology of Heart Disease: A Collaborative Project of Medical Students and Faculty* , fourth ed.. pp. 269-289. Lippincott Williams & Wilkins, Philadelphia.

Ruttiman, U. E., & Pipberger, H. V. (1979). Compression of the ECG by prediction or interpolation and entropy encoding. *IEEE Transactions on Biomedical Engineering, 26,* 613-623.

Salvucci, D. D., & Anderson, J. R. (2001). Automated eye-movement protocol analysis. *Human-Computer Interaction, 16,* 39-86.

Schneck, D. J. (2000). An outline of cardiovascular structure and function. In J. D. Bronzino (Ed.), *The biomedical engineering handbook.* Boca Raton, FL: CRC Press.

Sengupta, S. (2001). Computer networks in health care. In J. D. Bronzino (Ed.), *The biomedical engineering handbook.* Boca Raton, FL: CRC Press.

Skavenski, A. A. (1990). Eye movement and visual localization of objects in space. In E. Kowler (Ed.), *Eye movements and their role in visual and cognitive processes.* Englewood Cliffs, NJ: Elsevier.

Smith, F. E., Langley, P., van Leeuwen, P. et al. (2006). Comparison of magnetocardiography and electrocardiography: A study of automatic measurement of dispersion of ventricular repolarization. *Europace, 8,* 887-893.

Sörnmo, L., & Laguna, P. (2005). *Bioelectrical signal processing in cardiac and neurological applications.* Englewood Cliffs, NJ: Elsevier Academic Press.

Sosnowski, M., Czyz, Z., Leski, J., Petelenz, T., & Tendera, M. (1996). The coherence spectrum for quantifying beat-to-beat adaptation of RT intervals to heart rate in normal subjects and in postinfarction patients. *Computers in Cardiology, 23,* 669-672.

Stern, S., & Tzivoni, D. (1974). Early detection of silent ischemic heart disease by 24-hour electrocardiographic monitoring of active subjects. *British Heart Journal, 36,* 481-486.

Stramba-Badiale, M., Locati, E. H., Martinelli, A., Courvillet, J., & Schwartz, P. J. (1997). Gender and the relationship between ventricular repolarization and cardiac cycle length during 24-h Holter recordings. *European Heart Journal, 18,* 1000-1006.

Straszecka, E., & Straszecka, J. (2004). Uncertainty and imprecision representation in medical diagnostic rules. *IFMBE Proceedings of Medicon 2004* (paper 172).

Strumillo, P. (2002). Nested median filtering for detecting T-wave offset in ECGs. *Electronic Letters, 38*(14), 682-683.

Swain, M. J., Kahn, R. E., & Ballard, D. H. (1992). Low resolution cues for guiding saccadic eye movements. *Proceedings of the Computer Vision and Pattern Recognition Conference,* Urbana, IL.

Swiryn, S., McDonough, T., & Hueter, D. C. (1984). Sinus node function and dysfunction. *Medical Clinics of North America, 68,* 935-954.

Tadeusiewicz, R. (2004). Automatic understanding of signals. In M. A. Kłopotek, S. T. Wierzchoń, & K. Trojanowski (Eds.), *Intelligent information processing and Web- mining* (pp. 577-590). Berlin: Springer-Verlag.

Tadeusiewicz, R., & Augustyniak, P. (2005). Information flow and data reduction in the ECG interpretation process. *Proceedings of the 27th Annual IEEE EMBS Conference.*

Tadeusiewicz, R., & Ogiela, M. R. (2004). Medical image understanding technology. *Studies in Fuzziness and Soft Computing,* 156. Berlin: Springer-Verlag.

Tadeusiewicz, R., Izworski, A., & Majewski, J. (1993). *Biometry.* Kraków: AGH.

Tai, S. C. (1991). SLOPE—a real time ECG data compression. *Medical and Biological Engineering and Computing, 29,* 175-179.

Tai, S. C. (1992). ECG data compression by corner detection. *Medical and Biological Engineering and Computing, 30,* 584-590.

Tai, S.-C., Sun, C.-C., & Yan, W.-C. (2005). A 2-D ECG compression method based on wavelet transform and modified SPIHT. *IEEE Transactions on Biomedical Engineering, 52*(6), 999-1008.

Takahashi, K., Takeuchi, S., & Ohsawa, N. (1993). Performance evaluation of ECG compression algorithms by reconstruction error and diagnostic response. *IEICE Transactions on Information and Systems, E76-D*(12), 1404-1410.

Tanenbaum, A. S. (1988). *Computer networks* (2nd ed.). Englewood Cliffs, NJ: Prentice Hall.

Task Force of the ESC/ASPE. (1996). Heart rate variability: Standards of measurement, physiological interpretation, and clinical use. *European Heart Journal, 17,* 354-381.

Tayler, D. I., & Vincent, R. (1985). Artefactual ST segment abnormalities due to electrocardiograph design. *British Heart Journal, 54,* 11-28.

Thakor, N. V. (1978). Reliable R-wave detection from ambulatory subjects. *Biomedical Sciences Instrumentation, 14,* 67-72.

Thakor, N. V., Webster, J. G., & Tompkins, W. J. (1980). Optimal QRS filter. *Proceedings of the IEEE Conference on Frontiers of Engineering in Health Care* (vol. 2, pp. 190-195).

Thakor, N. V., Webster, J. G., & Tompkins, W. J. (1982). A battery-powered digital modem for telephone transmission of ECG data. *IEEE Transactions on Biomedical Engineering, 29,* 355-359.

Thakor, N. V., Webster, J. G., & Tompkins, W. J. (1983). Optimal QRS detector. *Medical & Biological Engineering & Computing, 21,* 343-350.

Thakor, N. V., Webster, J. G., & Tompkins, W. J. (1984). Design, implementation, and evaluation of a microcomputer-based portable arrhythmia monitor. *Medical & Biological Engineering & Computing, 22,* 151-159.

Thakor, N. V., Webster, J. G., & Tompkins, W. J. (1984). Estimation of QRS complex power spectra for design of a QRS filter. *IEEE Transactions on Biomedical Engineering, 31,* 702-706.

Tompkins, W. J. (1980). Modular design of microcomputer-based medical instruments. *Medical Instrumentation , 14,* 315-318.

Tompkins, W. J. (1982). Trends in ambulatory electrocardiography. *IEEE Frontiers of Engineering in Health Care, 4,* 201-204.

Tompkins, W. J., Tompkins, B. M., & Weisner, S. J. (1983). Microprocessor-based device for real-time ECG processing in the operating room. *Proceedings of AAMI.*

U.S. Congress. (1993). *Protecting privacy in computerized medical information* (Office of Technology Assessment, OTA-TCT-576). Washington, DC: U.S. Government Printing Office.

Uchiyama, T., Akazawa, K., & Sasamori, A. (1993). Data compression of ambulatory ECG by using multi-template matching and residual coding. *IEICE Transactions on Information and Systems, E76-D*(12), 1419-1424.

Unser, M., & Zerubia, J. A. (1998). Generalized sampling theory without band-limiting constraints. *Transactions on Circuits and Systems–II: Analog and Digital Signal Processing, 45*(8), 959-969.

Valensi, P. E., Extramiana, F., Johnson, N. B., Motte, G., Maison-Blanche, P., & Coumel, P. (2002). Influence of cardiac autonomic neuropathy on heart rate dependence of ventricular repolarization in diabetic patients. *Diabetes Care, 25*(5), 918-923.

Van Bemmel, J. H., & Willems, J. L. (1990). Standardization and validation of medical support-systems: The CSE project. *Methods of Information in Medicine , 29* (special issue), 261-262.

Van Leeuwen, P., Hailer, B., Bader, W., Geissler, J., Trowitzsch, E., & Groenemeyer, D. H. (1999). Magnetocardiography in the diagnosis of foetal arrhythmia. *British Journal of Obstetrics and Gynaecology, 106,* 1200-1208.

Van Leeuwen, P., Lange, S., Klein, A., Geue, D., & Gronemeyer, D. H. (2004). Dependency of magnetocardiographically determined fetal cardiac time intervals on gestational age, gender and postnatal biometrics in healthy pregnancies. *BMC Pregnancy Childbirth, 4,* 6.

Van Mieghem, C., Sabbe, M., & Knockaert, D. (2004). The clinical value of the ECG in noncardiac conditions. *Chest, 124,* 1561-1576.

Vera, Z., & Mason, D. T. (1981). Detection of sinus node dysfunction: Consideration of clinical application of testing methods. *American Heart Journal, 102,* 308-312.

Viviani, P. (1990). Eye movements in visual search: Cognitive, perceptual, and motor control aspects. In E. Kowler (Ed.), *Eye movements and their role in visual and cognitive processes. Reviews of oculomotor research V4* (pp. 353-383). Englewood Cliffs, NJ: Elsevier.

Wagner, G. S., & Marriott, H. J. (1994). *Marriott's practical electrocardiography* (9th ed.). Lippincott Williams & Wilkins, Philadelphia

Wakai, R. T., Strasburger, J. F., Li, Z., Deal, B. J., & Gotteiner, N. L. (2003). Magnetocardiographic rhythm patterns at initiation and termination of fetal supraventricular tachycardia. *Circulation, 107,* 307-312.

Weisner, S. J., Tompkins, W. J., & Tompkins, B. M. (1982). A compact, microprocessor-based ECG ST-segment monitor for the operating room. *IEEE Transactions on Biomedical Engineering, 29,* 642-649.

Weisner, S. J., Tompkins, W. J., & Tompkins, B. M. (1982). Microprocessor-based, portable anesthesiology ST-segment analyzer. *Proceedings of the Northeast Bioengineering Conference* (pp. 222-226).

Wi-Fi. (2007). *Wi-Fi.* Retrieved from http://en.wikipedia.org/wiki/Wi-Fi

Willems, J. L. (1990). *Common standards for quantitative electro-cardiography: 10th CSE progress report.* Leuven, Belgium: ACCO.

Willems, J. L. (1991). *SCP-ECG project manager. Standard communications protocol for computerized electrocardiography. Final specifications and recommendations.* Final Deliverable AIM Project #A1015. Leuven, Belgium: ACCO.

Willems, J. L., Arnaud, P., van Bemmel, J. H. et al. (1985). Assessment of the performance of electrocardiographic computer programs with the use of a reference database. *Circulation, 71,* 523-534.

Willems, J. L., Arnaud, P., van Bemmel, J. H. et al. (1985). Establishment of a reference library for evaluating computer ECG measurement programs. *Computers and Biomedical Research, 18,* 439-457.

Willems, J. L., Arnaud, P., van Bemmel, J. H. et al. (1987). A reference database for multilead electrocardiographic computer measurement programs. *Journal of the American College of Cardiology, 6,* 1313-1321.

Willems, J. L., Arnaud, P., van Bemmel, J. H., Bourdillon, P. J., Degani, R., Denis, B., Graham, I., Harms, F. M., Macfarlane, P. W., Mazzocca, G. et al. (1987). A reference data base for multilead electrocardiographic computer measurement programs. *Journal of the American College of Cardiology, 10*(6), 1313-1321.

Willems, J. L., Zywietz, C., Arnaud, P. et al. (1987). Influence of noise on wave boundary recognition by ECG measurement programs. Recommendations for preprocessing. *Computers and Biomedical Research, 20,* 543-562.

WiMAX. (2007). *WiMAX.* Retrieved from http://en.wikipedia.org/wiki/WiMAX

Wireless. (2007). *Wireless network.* Retrieved from http://en.wikipedia.org/wiki/Wireless_network

Wirth, N. (1976). *Algorithms + data structures = programs.* Englewood Cliffs, NJ: Prentice Hall.

Yan, G. X., & Antzelevitch, C. (1998). Cellular basis for the normal T wave and the electrocardio-graphic manifestations of the long-QT syndrome. *Circulation, 98,* 1928-1936.

Yap, Y. G., & Camm, A. J. (2003). Drug induced QT prolongation and torsades de pointes. *Heart, 89,* 1363-1372.

Yarbus, A. F. (1967). *Eye movements and vision.* New York: Plenum Press.

Yasuma, F., & Hayano, J. (2004). Respiratory sinus arrhythmia. Why does the heartbeat synchronize with respiratory rhythm? *Chest, 125,* 683-690.

Zareba, W. (2001). Digital Holter in drug studies. *Proceedings of the FDA Meeting on Digital ECGs.*

Zareba, W., Nomura, A., & Perkiomaki, J. (2001). Dispersion of repolarization: Concept, methodology and clinical experience. In W. Zareba, P. Maison-Blanche, & E. H. Locati (Eds.), *Noninvasive electrocardiology in clinical practice.* Armonk, NY: Futura.

Zaret B.L., Moser M. & Cohen L. S. (medical editors) (1999). Yale, University School of Medicine Heart Book. Hearst Books. New York. Available online at http://www.med.yale.edu/library/heartbk/ (accessed in November 2008)

Zigel, Y. (1998, August). *ECG signal compression.* MSc thesis, Ben-Gurion University, Beer-Sheva, Israel. Retrieved from http://www.ee.bgu.ac.il/~spl/publication

Zigel, Y., & Cohen, A. (1998). ECG signal compression using analysis by synthesis coding and diagnostic distortion. *IEEE Transactions on Biomedical Engineering, 47*(10), 1308-1316.

Zigel, Y., & Cohen, A. (1999). On the optimal distortion measure for ECG compression. *Proceedings of the European Medical and Biological Engineering Conference.*

Zigel, Y., & Cohen, A. (2000). ECG signal compression using analysis by synthesis coding and diagnostic distortion. *IEEE Transactions on Biomedical Engineering, 47*(10), 1308-1316.

Zigel, Y., Cohen, A., & Katz, A. (1996). A diagnostic meaningful distortion measure for ECG compression. *Proceedings of the 19th Convention of Electrical & Electronic Engineering in Israel* (pp. 117-120).

Zigel, Y., Cohen, A., Abu-Ful, A., Wagshal, A., & Katz, A. (1997). Analysis by synthesis ECG signal compression. *Computers in Cardiology, 24,* 279-282.

Zimetbaum, P. J., Kim, K. Y., Josephson, M. E., Goldberger, A. L., & Cohen, D. J. (1998). Diagnostic yield and optimal duration of continuous-loop event monitoring for the diagnosis of palpitations: A cost-effectiveness analysis. *Annals of Internal Medicine, 128,* 890-895.

Zimetbaum, P., Kim, K. Y., Ho, K. K., Zebede, J., Josephson, M. E. et al. (1997). Utility of patient-activated cardiac event recorders in general clinical practice. *American Journal of Cardiology, 79,* 371-372.

Zimmerman, J. E., Theine, P., & Harding, J. T. (1970). Design and operation of stable rf-biased superconducting point-contact quantum devices, etc. *Journal of Applied Physics, 41,* 1572-1580.

Zywietz, C. (2003). *OpenECG certification and conformance testing process.* Retrieved from http://www.openecg.net

Zywietz, C., Joseph, G., & Degani, R. (1990). Data compression for computerized electrocardiography. In J. L. Willems (Ed.), *Digital ECG data communication, encoding and storage.* Proceedings of the 1st Working Conference of the SCP-ECG Project (pp. 95-136). Leuven, Belgium: ACCO.

Further Readings

Abenstein, J. P., & Tompkins, W. J. (1982). A new data reduction algorithm for real-time ECG analysis. *IEEE Transactions on Biomedical Engineering, 29,* 43-48.

Addison, P. S. (2005). Wavelet transforms and the ECG: A review. *Physiological Measurement, 26,* R155-R199.

Ahlstrom, M. L., & Tompkins, W. J. (1983). Automated high-speed analysis of Holter tapes with microcomputers. *IEEE Transactions on Biomedical Engineering, 30,* 651-657.

Ahlstrom, M. L., & Tompkins, W. J. (1985). Digital filters for real-time ECG signal processing using microprocessors. *IEEE Transactions on Biomedical Engineering, 32,* 708-713.

Ahmed, N., Natarajan, T., & Rao, K. R. (1974). Discrete cosine transform. *IEEE Transactions on Computers, 23,* 90-93.

Akay, M. (1996). *Detection and estimation methods for biomedical signals.* San Diego: Academic Press.

Almeida, R., Rocha, A. P., Pueyo, E., Martínez, J. P., & Laguna, P. (2004). Modelling short term variability interactions in ECG: QT versus RR. *Computational statistics* Vol. 19 Nr 4, pp. 597-604. Berlin: Physica-Verlag.

Andersen, J. L., Hallstrom, A. P., Griffith, L. S. et al. (1989). Relation of baseline characteristics to suppression of ventricular arrhythmias during placebo and active antiarrhythmic therapy in patients after myocardial infarction. *Circulation, 79,* 610-619.

Bahoura, M., Hassani, M., & Hubin, M. (1997). DSP implementation of wavelet transform for real time ECG wave forms detection and heart rate analysis. *Computer Methods and Programs in Biomedicine, 52,* 35-44.

Barbieri, R., & Saul, J. P. (1999). Autoregressive modeling for assessing closed-loop feedback and fedforward in the arterial baroreflex. In M. Di Rienzo, G. Mancia, G. Parati, A. Pedotti, & A. Zanchetti (Eds.), *Methodology and clinical applications of blood pressure and heart rate analysis.* IOS Press, Amsterdam, pp. 21-34.

Barbieri, R., Bianchi, A. M., Triedman, J. K., Mainardi, L. T., Cerutti, S., & Saul, J. P. (1997). Model dependency of multivariate autogressive spectral analysis. *Proceedings of the IEEE Engineering in Medicine and Biology Society* (pp. 74-85).

Barbosa, P. R. B., Barbosa-Filho, J., Cordovil, I., Medeiros, A. B., & Nadal, J. (2000). Phase response of the spectral coherence function between heart rate variability and ventricular repolarization duration in normal subjects. *Computers in Cardiology, 27,* 159-162.

Baselli, G., Porta, A., & Ferrari, G. (1995). Models for the analysis of cardiovascular variability signals. In M. Malik & A. J. Camm (Eds.), *Heart rate variability* (pp. 135-145). New York: Futura.

Baselli, G., Porta, A., Rimoldi, O., Pagani, M., & Cerutti, S. (1997). Spectral decomposition in multichannel recordings based on multivariate parametric identification. *IEEE Transactions on Biomedical Engineering, 44*(11), 1092-1101.

Batchvarov, V., & Malik, M. (2002). Individual patterns of QT/RR relationship. *Cardiac Electrophysiology Review, 6,* 282-288.

Batchvarov, V., Ghuran, A., Smetana, P., Hnatkova, K., Harries, M., Dilaveris, P., Camm, J., & Malik, M. (2002). QT-RR relationship in healthy subjects exhibits substantial intersubject variability and high intrasubject stability. *American Journal of Physiology-Heart and Circulator Physiology, 282,* 2356-2363.

Bhaskaran, V., & Konstantinides, K. (1995). *Image and video compression standards: Algorithms and architectures.* Boston: Kluwer.

Bigger, J. T., Kleiger, R. E., Fleiss, J. L., Rolnitzky, L. M., Steinman, R. C., Miller, J. P., & the Multicenter Post-Infarction Research Group. (1988) Components of heart rate variability measured during healing of acute myocardial infarction. *American Journal of Cardiology, 61,* 208-215.

Bigger, J. T. (1990). Clinical aspects of trial design: What can we expect from the cardiac arrhythmia suppression trial? *Cardiovascular Drug Therapy, 4,* 657-664.

Bjerregaard, P. (1984). Continuous ambulatory electrocardiography in healthy adult subjects over a 24-hour period. *Danish Medical Bulletin, 31,* 282-297.

Bjokander, I., Held, C., Forslund, L., Erikson, S., Billing, E., Hjemdahl, P., & Rehnqvist, N. (1992). Heart rate variability in patients with stable angina pectoris. *European Heart Journal, 13*(abstr suppl), 379.

Bronzino, J. D., (1992) Chapter 10 "Medical and Ethical Issues in Clinical Engineering Practice" In J.D. Bronzino, (Ed.) *Management of Medical Technology.* Butterworth-Heinemann, Boston.

Bronzino, J. D., (1999) Chapter 20 "Moral and Ethical Issues Associated with Medical Technology" In J.D. Enderle, S.M. Blanchard, & J.D. Bronzino, (Eds.) *Introduction to Biomedical Engineering.* Academic Press, San Diego, 1062 pages

Capron, A. (1978) Human Experimentation: Basic Issues." In: The Encyclopedia of Bioethics vol. II. The Free Press, Glencoe, IL.

Chronaki C.E. and Chiarugi F. (2005) Interoperability as a Quality Label for portable & wearable Health Monitoring Systems [in:] Personalised Health: The Integration of Innovative Sensing, Textile, Information & Communication Technologies Studies in Health Technology and Informatics Book Series, IOS Press, 2005

Chronaki C.E. and Chiarugi F. (2006) OpenECG: Testing Conformance To CEN/EN 1064 Standard» 5th European Symposium on BioMedical Engineering (ESBME 2006) 7th to 9th July 2006, Patras, Greece

Chronaki C.E., Chiarugi F., Macerata A., Conforti F., Voss H., Johansen I., Ruiz Fernandez R., Zywietz Chr. (2004) Interoperability in Digital Electrocardiography after the OpenECG Project In Computers in Cardiology, 31:49-52.

Chronaki C.E., Chiarugi F., Reynolds M. (2006) Grid-enabled medical devices, innovation in eHealth, and the OpenECG network paradigm. In ITAB 2006, Ioannina 26-28 Oct 2006

Chronaki C.E., Chiarugi F., Sfakianakis S., Zywietz Chr. (2005) A web service for conformance testing of ECG records to the SCP-ECG standard. Proceedings Computers in Cardiology, Lyon, France, September 2005.

Cohen, A. and J. Kovacevic (1996). Wavelets: The mathematical background. Proceedings of the IEEE 84(4), 514-522.

Coumel, P. (1990). Role of the autonomic nervous system in paroxysmal atrial fibrillation. In P. Touboul & A. L. Waldo (Eds.), *Atrial arrhythmias: Current concepts and management* (pp. 248-261). St Louis: C. V. Mosby.

Cripps, T. R., Malik, M., Farrell, T. G., & Camm, A. J. (1991). Prognostic value of reduced heart rate variability after myocardial infarction: Clinical evaluation of a new analysis method. *British Heart Journal, 65,* 14-19.

Daniels, N. (1987). *Just health care.* Cambridge: Cambridge University Press.

Davey, P. (1999a). A new physiological method for heart rate correction of the QT interval. *Heart, 82,* 183-186.

de Chazal, P., & Celler, B. G. (1994). A critical review of the synthesis of the orthogonal Frank lead ECGs from the 12 lead recordings. *Proceedings of the 16th Annual International Conference of the IEEE Engineering in Medicine and Biology Society, Engineering Advances: New Opportunities for Biomedical Engineers, Vol. 2, November, 1994,* 958-959.

Deedwania, P. C. (1994). Ventricular arrhythmias in heart failure: To treat or not to treat? *Cardiology Clinics, 12,* 137-154.

Dobbs, S. E., Schmitt, N. M., & Ozemek, H. S. (1984). QRS detection by template matching using real-time correlation on a microcomputer. *Journal of Clinical Engineering, 9,* 197-212.

Doval, N. C., Nul, D. R., Grancelli, H. O. et al. (1994). Randomised trial of low-dose amiodarone in severe congestive heart failure. *Lancet, 344,* 493-498.

Dubler, N. N., & Nimmons, D. (1992). *Ethics on call.* New York: Harmony Books.

Edenbrandt, L., & Pahlm, O. (1988). Vectorcardiogram synthesized from a 12-lead ECG—superiority of the inverse dower matrix. *Journal of Electrocardiology, 21*(4), 361-367.

Ertl, A. C., Pfeifer, M., & Davis, S. N. (2004). Diabetic autonomic dysfunction. In D. Robertson, I. Biaggioni, G. Burnstock, & P. A. Low (Eds.), *Primer on the autonomic nervous system.* (pp. 328-331). Englewood Cliffs, NJ: Elsevier Academic.

ESVEM Investigations. (1989). The ESVEM trial: Electrophysiologic study versus electrocardiographic monitoring for selection of antiarrhythmic therapy of ventricular tachyarrhythmias. *Circulation, 79,* 1354-1360.

Ewing, D. J., Neilson, J. M. M., & Traus, P. (1984). New method for assessing cardiac parasympathetic activity using 24-hour electrocardiograms. *British Heart Journal, 52,* 396-402.

Fananapazir, L., German, L. D., Callagher, J. J., Lowe, J. E., & Prystowsky, E. N. (1990). Importance of pre-excited QRS morphology during induced atrial fibrillation to the diagnosis and localization of multiple accessory pathways. *Circulation, 81,* 578-585.

Farrell, T. G., Bashir, Y., Cripps, T., Malik, M., Poloniecki, J., Bennett, E. D., Ward, D. E., & Camm, A. J. (1991). A simple method of risk stratification for arrhythmic events in post-infarction patients based on heart rate variability and signal averaged ECG. *Journal of the American College of Cardiology, 18,* 687-697.

Fleg, J. L., & Kennedy, H. L. (1992). Long-term prognostic significance of ambulatory electrocardiographic findings in apparently healthy subjects >=60 years of age. *American Journal of Cardiology, 70,* 748-751.

Fletcher, R. D., Cintron, G. B., Johnson, G. et al. (1993). Enalapril decreases prevalence of ventricular tachycardia in patients with chronic congestive heart failure. *Circulation, 87*(suppl VI), 49-55.

Garcia, J. M., Wagner, G., Sörnmo, L., Olmos, S. G., Lander, P., & Laguna, P. L. (2000). Temporal evolution of traditional versus transformed ECG-based indexes in patients with induced myocardial ischemia. *Journal of Electrocardiology, 33*(1), 37-47.

Goldstein, B., Deking, D., Delong, D. J., Kempski, M. H., Cox, C., Kelly, M. M., Nichols, D. D., & Woolf, P. D. (1993). Autonomic cardiovascular state after severe brain injury and brain-death in children. *Critical Care Medicine, 21,* 228-233.

Graboys, T. B., Lown, B., Podrid, P. et al. (1982). Long-term survival of patients with malignant ventricular arrhythmias treated with antiarrhythmic drugs. *American Journal of Cardiology, 50,* 437-463.

Gritzali, F. (1988). Towards a generalized scheme for QRS detection in ECG waveforms. *Signal Processing, 15,* 183-192.

Guillem, M. S., Sahakian, A. V., & Swiryn, S. (2006). Derivation of orthogonal leads from the 12- lead ECG. Accuracy of a single transform for the derivation of atrial and ventricular wave. *Computers in Cardiology, 33,* 249-252.

Hamill, R. W., & Shapiro, R. E. (2004). Peripheral autonomic nervous system. In D. Robertson, I. Biaggioni, G. Burnstock, & P. A. Low (Eds.), *Primer on the autonomic nervous system* (2nd ed., pp. 20-28). Englewood Cliffs, NJ: Elsevier Academic.

Hnatkova, K., Staunton, A., Camm, A. J., & Malik, M. (1994). Numerical processing of Lorenz plots of RR intervals is superior to conventional time-domain measures of heart rate variability for risk stratification after acute myocardial infarction (abstract). *Pacing and Clinical Electrophysiology, 17,* 767.

Holter, N. (1961). New method for heart studies: Continuous electrocardiography of active subjects over long periods is now practical. *Science, 134,* 1214-1220.

Huffman, D. A. (1952). A method for the construction of minimum redundancy codes. *Proceedings of the Institute of Radio Engineering* (vol. 40, pp. 1098-1101).

IEC 13818. (1994). *Information technology—coding of moving pictures and associated audio* (part 2). Video.

Johnsen, S., & Andersen, N. (1978). On power estimation in maximum entropy spectral analysis. *Geophysics, 43*(4), 681-690.

Jonsen, A. R. (1990). *The new medicine and the old ethics.* Cambridge, MA: Harvard University Press.

Kaufmann, H. (2004). Evaluation of the patient with syncope. In D. Robertson, I. Biaggioni, G. Burnstock, & P. A. Low (Eds.), *Primer on the autonomic nervous system* (2nd ed., pp. 217-220). Englewood Cliffs, NJ: Elsevier Academic.

Kay, G. N., Epstein, A. E., Dailey, S. M., & Plumb, V. J. (1993). Role of radiofrequency ablation in the management of Supraventricular arrhythmias: Experience in 760 consecutive patients. *Cardiovascular Electrophysiology, 4,* 371-389.

Kerr, C. R., Callagher, J. J., & German, L. D. (1982). Changes in ventriculoatrial intervals with bundle branch block aberration during reciprocating tachycardia in patients with accessory atrioventricular pathways. *Circulation, 66,* 196-201.

Khan, M. H., & Sinoway, L. I. (2004). Congestive heart failure. In D. Robertson, I. Biaggioni, G. Burnstock, & P. A. Low (Eds.), *Primer on the autonomic nervous system* (2nd ed., pp. 247-248). Englewood Cliffs, NJ: Elsevier Academic.

Kim, K. (2004). Mechanism of differentiation of autonomic neurons. In D. Robertson, I. Biaggioni, G. Burnstock, & P. A. Low (Eds.), *Primer on the autonomic nervous system* (2nd ed., pp. 6-11). Englewood Cliffs, NJ: Elsevier Academic.

Kinder, C., Tamburro, P., Kopp, D. et al. (1994). The clinical significance of nonsustained ventricular tachycardia: current perspectives. *PACE, 17,* 637-664.

Kleiger, R. E., Miller, J. P., Bigger, J. T., Moss, A. J., & the Multicenter Post-Infarction Research Group. (1987). Decreased heart rate variability and its association with increased mortality after acute myocardial infarction. *American Journal of Cardiology, 59,* 256-262.

Laguna, P., & Sommo, L. (2000). Sampling rate and the estimation of ensemble variability for repetitive signals *Medical and Biological Engineering and Computing, 38,* 540-546.

Lamport, S., Lown, B., Graboys, T. B. et al. (1988). Determinants of survival in patients with malignant ventricular arrhythmias associated with coronary artery disease. *American Journal of Cardiology, 61,* 791-797.

Lees P.J., Chronaki C.E., Chiarugi F. (2004) Standards and Interoperability in Digital Electrocardiography. The OpenECG Project, *Hellenic Journal of Cardiology 45*(6), pp. 364-369

Ljung, L. (1999). *System identification theory for the user* (2nd ed.). Upper Saddle River, NJ: Prentice Hall.

Lombardi, F., Colombo, A., Porta, A., Baselli, G., Cerutti, S., & Fiorentini, C. (1998). Assessment of the coupling between RT apex and RR interval as an index of temporal dispersion of ventricular repolarization. *PACE, 21,* 2396-2400.

Maggioni, A. P., Zuanetti, G., Franzosi, M. G. et al. (1993). Prevalence and prognostic significance of ventricular arrhythmias after acute myocardial infarction in the fibrinolytic era: GISSI-2 results. *Circulation, 87,* 312-322.

Magnano, A. R., Holleran, S., Ramakrishnan, R., Reiffel, J. A., & Bloomfield, D. M. (2002). Autonomic nervous system influences on QT interval in normal subjects. *Journal of the American College of Cardiology, 39*(11), 1820-1826.

Malik, M., Cripps, T., Farrell, T., & Camm, A. J. (1989). Prognostic value of heart rate variability after myocardial infarction; a comparison of different data processing methods. *Medical and Biological Engineering and Computing, 27,* 603-611.

Malik, M., Farrell, T., Cripps, T., & Camm, A. J. (1989). Heart rate variability in relation to prognosis after myocardial infarction: Selection of optimal processing techniques. *European Heart Journal, 10,* 1060-1074.

Malik, M., Odemuyiwa, O., Poloniecki, J., Staunton, A., & Camm, A. J. (1991). Time-domain measurement of vagal components of heart rate variability in automatically analysed long term electrocardiograms: Prognostic power of different indices for identification of post-infarction patients at high risk of arrhythmic events. *Journal of Ambulatory Monitoring, 4,* 235-244.

Mallat, S. (1989). Multifrequency channel decompositions of images and wavelet models. *IEEE Transactions on Acoustics, Speech, and Signal Processing, 37,* 2091-2110.

Mallat, S. (1999). *A Wavelet tour of signal processing* (2nd ed.). Academic Press. San Diego.

Mallat, S., & Zhang, S. (1992). Characterization of signals from multiscale edge. *IEEE Transactions Pattern Analysis and Machine Intelligence, 14*(7), 710-732.

Manolio, T. P., Furberg, C. D., Rau Taharju, P. M. et al. (1984). Cardiac arrhythmias on 24-hour ambulatory electrocardiography in older women and men: The cardiovascular health study. *Journal of American College of Cardiology, 23,* 916-925.

Maron, B. L., Bonow, R. O., Cannon, R. O. et al. (1987). Hypertrophic cardiomyopathy: Interrelation of clinical manifestation, pathophysiology and therapy. *New England Journal of Medicine, 316,* 780-789, 844-852.

Marple, S. L. (1987). *Digital spectral analysis with applications.* Upper Saddle River, NJ: Prentice Hall.

Martínez, J. P., Almeida, R., Rocha, A. P., Laguna, P., & Olmos, S. (2006). Stability of QT measurements in the PTB database depending on the selected lead. *Computers in Cardiology, 33,* 341-344.

Martínez, J. P., Olmos, S., & Laguna, P. (2000). Evaluation of a wavelet-based ECG waveform detector on the QT database. *Computers in Cardiology, 27,* 81-84.

Mason, J. W. (1993). For the electrophysiologic study versus electrocardiographic monitoring investigators. A comparison of seven antiarrhythmic drugs in patients with ventricular tachycardias. *New England Journal of Medicine, 329,* 452-458.

Mateo, J., & Laguna, P. (2000). Improved heart rate variability signal analysis from the beat occurrence times according to the IPFM model heart timing signal. *IEEE Transactions on Biomedical Engineering, 47,* 985-996.

Mateo, J., & Laguna, P. (2003). Analysis of heart rate variability in the presence of ectopic beats using the heart timing signal. *IEEE Transactions on Biomedical Engineering, 50,* 334-342.

Merri, M., Alberti, M., & Moss, A. J. (1993). Dynamic analysis of ventricular repolarization duration from 24-hour Holter recordings. *IEEE Transactions on Biomedical Engineering, 40*(12), 1219-1225.

Merri, M., Benhorin, J., Alberti, M., & Locati, E., & Moss, A. J. (1989). Electrocardiographic quantitation of ventricular repolarization. *Circulation, 80,* 1301-1308.

Molnar, J., Weiss, J., Zhang, F., & Rosenthal, J. E. (1996). Evaluation of five QT correction formulas using a software-assisted method of continuous QT measurement from 24-hour Holter recordings. *American Journal of Cardiology, 78,* 920-926.

Moody, G. B., Koch, H., & Steinhoff, U. (2006). The physionet computers in cardiology challenge 2006: QT interval measurement. *Computers in Cardiology, 33,* 313-316.

Morillo, C. A., Klein, G. J., Thakur, R. K., Li, H., Zardini, M., & Yee, R. (1994). Mechanism of 'inappropriate' sinus tachycardia: Role of sympathovagal balance. *Circulation, 90,* 873-877.

Murphy, J., & Coleman, J. (1984). *The philosophy of law.* Totowa, NJ: Rowman and Allenheld.

Nademanee, K., Singh, B. N., Stevenson, W. G., & Weiss, J. N. (1993). Amiodarone and post-MI patients. *Circulation, 88,* 764-774.

Page, R. L., Wilkinson, W. E., Clair, W. K., McCarthy, E. A., & Pritchett, E. L. C. (1994). Asymptomatic arrhythmias in patients with symptomatic paroxysmal atrial fibrillation and paroxysmal supraventricular tachycardia. *Circulation, 89,* 224-227.

Pahlm, O., & Sörnmo, L. (1984). Software QRS detection in ambulatory monitoring—a review. *Medical and Biological Engineering and Computing, 22,* 289-297.

Parer, W. J., & Parer, J. T. (1985). Validity of mathematical methods of quantitating fetal heart rate variability. *American Journal of Obstetrics and Gynecology, 153,* 402-409.

Pinciroli, F., Pozzi, G., Rossi, P., Piovosi, M., Capo, A., Olivieri, R., & Della Torre, M. (1998). A respiration-related EKG database. *Computers in Cardiology, 15,* 477-480.

Porta, A., Baselli, G., Caiani, E., Malliani, A., Lombardi, F., & Cerutti, S. (1998). Quantifying electrocardiogram RT-RR variability interactions. *Medical and Biological Engineering and Computing, 36,* 27-34.

Prystowsky, E. N. (1994). Inpatient versus outpatient initiation of antiarrhythmic drug therapy for patients with Supraventricular tachycardia. *Cardiology Clinics, 17,* II.7-10.

Reiffel, J., Mann, D., Reiter, M. et al. (1994). A comparison of Holter suppression criteria for declaring drug efficacy in patients with sustained ventricular tachyarrhythmias in the ESVEM trial (abstract). *Journal of the American College of Cardiology, 23,* 279A.

Reiffel, J. A., Reiter, M., Freedman, R. et al. (1994). Did the number of premature stimuli used or the length of unsustained tachycardia induced affect the predictive accuracy of the electrophysiologic study used to guide therapy in the ESVEM trial (abstract). *PACE, 17,* 826.

Reiter, M., Mann, D., & Reiffel, J. (1994). Predictive value of combined Holter monitoring and electrophysiological testing in the ESVEM study (abstract). *Journal of the American College of Cardiology, 23,* 279A.

Sagie, A., Larson, M. G., Goldberg, R. J., Bengston, J. R., & Levy, D. (1992). An improved method for adjusting the QT interval for heart rate (the Framingham Heart Study). *American Journal of Cardiology, 70,* 791-801.

Sahambi, J. S., Tandon, S. N., & Bhatt, R. K. P. (1997). Using wavelet transform for ECG characterization. *IEEE Engineering in Medicine and Biology, 16*(1), 77-83.

Sahambi, J. S., Tandon, S. N., & Bhatt, R. K. P. (1998). Wavelet based ST-segment analysis. *Medical and Biological Engineering and Computing, 36*(9), 568-572.

Sarma, J. S. M., Sarma, R. J., Bilitch, M., Katz, D., & Song, S. L. (1984). An exponential formula for heart rate dependence of QT interval during exercise and cardiac pacing in humans: Reevaluation of Bazett's formula. *American Journal of Cardiology, 54,* 103-108.

Saumarez, R. C., Camm, A. J., Panagos, A. et al. (1992). Ventricular fibrillation in hypertrophic cardiomyopathy is associated with increased fractionation of paced right ventricular electrograms. *Circulation, 86,* 467-474.

Scherer, P., Ohier, J. P., Hirche, H., & Hopp, H.-W. (1993). Definition of a new beat-to-beat parameter of heart rate variability (abstract). *Pacing and Clinical Electrophysiology, 16,* 939.

Shusterman, V., Aysin, B., Shah, S. I., Flanigan, S., & Anderson, K. P. (1998). Autonomic nervous system effects on ventricular repolarization and RR interval variability during head-up tilt. *Computers in Cardiology, 15,* 717-720.

Shusterman, V., Beigel, A., Shah, S. I., Aysin, B., Weiss, R., Gottipaty, V. K., Schartzman, D., & Anderson, K. P. (1999). Changes in autonomic activity and ventricular repolarization. *Journal of Electrocardiology, 32*(suppl), 185-192.

Singh, J. N., Fletcher, R. O., Fisher, S. G. et al. (1994). Results of the congestive heart failure survival trial of antiarrhythmic therapy. *Circulation, 90,* 546(A).

Soderstrom, T. (1974). Convergence properties of the generalised least squares identification method. *Automatica, 10,* 617-626.

Speranza, G., Nollo, G., Ravelli, F., & Antolini, R. (1993). Beat-to-beat measurement and analysis of the R-T interval in 24 h ECG Holter recordings. *Medical and Biological Engineering and Computing, 31*(5), 487-494.

Stewart, J. T., & McKenna, W. J. (1994). Hypertrophic cardiomyopathy: Treatment of arrhythmias. *Cardiovascular Drug Therapy, 8,* 95-99.

Tarvainen, M. P., Niskanen, J., Karjalainen, P. A., Laitinen, T., & Lyyra-Laitinen, T. (2006). Noise sensitivity of a principal component regression bases RT interval variability estimation method. *Proceedings of the 28th Annual International Conference of the IEEE Engineering in Medicine and Biology Society* (pp. 1145-1147).

Tompkins, W. J. (1978). A portable microcomputer-based system for biomedical applications. *Biomedical Sciences Instrumentation, 14,* 61-66.

Tompkins, W. J. (1981b). Role of microprocessors in ambulatory monitoring. *Proceedings of AAMI* (p. 99).

Tompkins, W. J. (1982). Trends in ambulatory electrocardiography. *IEEE Frontiers of Engineering in Health Care, 4,* 201-204.

Tompkins, W. J. (1983). Arrhythmia detection and capture from ambulatory outpatients using microprocessors. *Proceedings of AAMI* (p. 122).

Tompkins, W. J. (198la). Portable microcomputer-based instrumentation. In M. S. Eden & M. Eden (Eds.), *Microcomputers in patient care* (pp. 174-181). Park Ridge, NJ: Noyes Medical.

Tompkins, W. J., & Abenstein, J. P. (1979). CORTES—a data reduction algorithm for electrocardiography. *Proceedings of AAMI* (p. 277).

Tompkins, W. J., Webster, J. G., Sahakian, A. V., Thakor, N. V., & Mueller, W. C. (1979). Long-term, portable ECG arrhythmia monitoring. *Proceedings of AAMI* (p. 278).

Van Huffel, S., & Vandewalle, J. (1991). The total least squares problem: Computational aspects and analysis. In J.M. Hyman (Ed.) *Frontiers in applied mathematics* (vol. 9, pp 1-300). Philadelphia: Society for Industrial and Applied Mathematics.

Vila, J. A., Gang, Y., Presedo, J. M., Fernandez-Delgado, M., & Malik, M. (2000). A new approach for TU complex characterization. *IEEE Transactions on Biomedical Engineering, 47*(6), 764-772.

Vullings, H. J. L. M., Verhaegen, M. H. G., & Verbruggen, H. B. (1998). Automated ECG segmentation with dynamic time warping. *Proceedings of the 20th Annual International Conference of the IEEE Engineering in Medicine and Biology Society* (pp. 163-166), Hong Kong.

Waele, S., & Broersen, P. M. T. (2003). Order selection for vector autoregressive models. *IEEE Transactions on Acoustics, Speech, and Signal Processing, 51*(2), 427-433.

Waspe, L. E., Chien, W. W., Merillat, J. C., & Stark, S. I. (1994). Sinus node modification using radiofrequency current in a patient with persistent inappropriate sinus tachycardia. *PACE, 17,* 1569-1576.

Webster, J. G. (1978). An intelligent monitor for ambulatory ECGs. *Biomedical Sciences Instrumentation, 14,* 55-60.

Webster, J. G., Tompkins, W. J., Thakor, N. V., Abenstein, J. P., & Mueller, W. C. (1978). A portable, microcomputer-based ECG arrhythmia monitor. *Proceedings of SIstACEMB* (p. 60).

Wolf, M. M., Varigos, G. A., Hunt, D., & Sloman, J. G. (1978). Sinus arrhythmia in acute myocardial infarction. *Medical Journal of Australia, 2,* 52-53.

Woo, M. A., Stevenson, W. G., Moser, D. K., & Middlekauff, H. R. (1994). Complex heart rate variability and serum norepinephrine levels in patients with advanced heart failure. *Journal of the American College of Cardiology, 23,* 565-569.

Wyse, D. G., Hallstrom, A., McBride, R. et al. (1991). Events in the cardiac arrhythmia suppression trial (CAST): Mortality in patients surviving open label titration but not randomized to double-blind therapy. *Journal of the American College of Cardiology, 18,* 20-28.

Zardini, M., Yee, R., Thakur, R. K., & Klein, G. J. (1994). Risk of sudden arrhythmic death in the Wolf-Parkinson-White syndrome: Current perspectives. *PACE, 17,* 966-975.

Zaręba, W., Maison-Blanche, P., & Locati, E. H. (2001). *Noninvasive electrocardiology in clinical practice.* Armonk, NY: Futura.

Ziv, J., & Lempel, A. (1977). A universal algorithm for sequential data compression. *IEEE Transactions on Information Theory, 23,* 337343.

Ziv, J., & Lempel, A. (1998). Compression of individual sequences via variablerate encoding. *IEEE Transactions on Information Theory, 24,* 530536.

Glossary of Terms

Abnormal Electrical Activity (Chapter II) is understood as unusual representation of particular elements of the heart cycle in time or amplitude. Such variations of electrical parameters are caused by too fast/slow or irregular rhythms and abnormal generation or conduction of the cardiac electrical impulses.

Adaptation Delay (Chapter IX) is defined as the time period from the patient status-domain transient occurrence to the moment when the diagnostic outcome altered by the interpreting software modification starts falling into a given tolerance margin ε around its final value.

Agile Software (Chapter V) is a sequence of calculation procedures having a possibility of limited changes in architecture and properties while in use. Agile software is controlled by itself (auto-adaptive) or by an external management procedure. In the case of the proposed system, the remote interpretation process is implemented as agile software and the central management process is implemented as rigid software.

Ambulatory Event Recorders (Chapter III) are portable devices smaller than Holter recorders, providing continuous buffered storage in digital memory of a specified period of the ECG. When the event button is pressed, not only electrocardiographic events from that point on are recorded, but also a period of the preceding ECG.

Ambulatory Recorders (continuous) (Chapter III) are portable devices providing between 6 and 72 hours of continuous ECG recording in 3 to 12 simultaneous channels. The raw signal is stored in digital solid state memory cards. The recorder does not contain interpretation software, and optional screening is used for signal control or messaging. Holter recordings are automatically analyzed in a workstation after the transfer of the collected data from storage media to a hard disk.

Arrhythmias (Chapter II) are specific patterns of abnormal heartbeat sequence. If ventricular beats are present, the arrhythmia is ventricular, otherwise it is supraventricular. The detection of an arrhythmia is essential to the assessment of stimulus generation and conductivity, while the frequency of an arrhythmia occurrence is the factor of conduction disease severity.

Aspects of Software Adaptation (Chapter IX) provide a qualitative description of the changes and the choice of procedures selected for modification in order to achieve overall improvement in the diagnostic quality of a given patient's status.

Asymptotic Accuracy (Chapter IX) is the absolute value of diagnostic error when the transient-evoked software adaptation is completed. Assuming no other transient is present in the subsequent signal, it may be expressed as a limit of the difference between the received value and the reference.

Atrioventricular (AV) Node (Chapter II) is a highly specialized cluster of neuromuscular cells at the lower portion of the right atrium leading to the interventricular septum; the AV node delays sinoatrial (SA) node-generated electrical impulses momentarily (allowing the atria to contract first) and then conducts the depolarization wave to the bundle of HIS and its bundle branches.

Attention Density (Chapter VI) represents the time the eye-globe spends over a time unit in the ECG plot (recorded typically at 25mm/s) and thus is expressed in seconds per second ([s/s]). It should be noted that although scan-path and ECG time are both temporal variables given in seconds, the eyesight and ECG record are not simultaneous processes.

Autonomic Nervous System (Chapter II) is the functional division of the nervous system that innervates most glands, the heart, and smooth muscle tissue in order to maintain the internal environment of the body.

Autonomy Time (Chapter IX) is the time of device operation without the necessity of battery replacement or use of external power sources. Because power source capacity in relation to physical volume ratio is limited by technology, autonomous operation time is a compromise between the size and the current drain. Therefore, a good design of electronic circuitry should be power-saving oriented and include intelligent methods of power dissipation reduction.

Auxiliary Information (Chapter XI) is the data about the device status that variability is very low (e.g., battery status). Therefore it makes no difference which data packet they are appended to, and such information may fill the spare bytes in data packet.

Baseline Estimation (Chapter II) stems from the fact that physiologic zero voltage does not coincide with the electrical zero of the digitized ECG since the baseline may wander. In many studies found in the literature, the isoelectric level is estimated from the voltage level of a single point, the fiducial point, identified in the PR segment. One way to obtain better estimates of the baseline is to interpolate between consecutive fiducial points.

Bedside ECG Recorders with Interpretation (Chapter III) are stand-alone devices with a embedded specialized computer, printer, presentation screen, and digital data link. The design of the software complies with the unique task of the interpretation of the acquired ECG. The device usually provides options for digital storage, transmission, and printing of the signal and calculated diagnostic parameters.

Cardiac Ejection Fraction (Chapter III) is the ratio of stroke volume (SV) measured as volume of blood expelled from the heart during each systolic interval and the end-diastolic-volume (EDV). Its nominal values range from 0.5 to 0.75; lower values are symptoms of disease.

Cardiac Functional Reporting (Chapter IV) is a multimodal record containing voltage time series, static images, motion images, displacement time, and magnetic fields measurement time series.

Cardiac Muscle (Chapter II) is the involuntary muscle possessing much of the anatomic attributes of skeletal voluntary muscle and some of the physiologic attributes of involuntary smooth muscle tissue. The SA node-induced contraction of its interconnected network of fibers allows the heart to expel blood during systole.

Cardiologists' Preferences (Chapter X) about the contents of the final diagnostic report in the context of the described disease were based on an investigation of the priority rules in the set parameters. The hidden poll method enabled the software to observe and record doctors' behavior of including or excluding a randomly preselected parameter from the final content of the report.

Cardiovascular System (Chapter III) fulfills the task of a general transportation network. It is purposely organized to make available thousands of miles of access pathways for the transport to and from a different neighborhood of any given cell and any material needed to sustain life. The cardiovascular system consists of blood vessels, the heart, the blood, and the control system.

Central Intelligence (Chapter IX) assumes that the ECG interpretation model assumes that the interpretation is performed by a central server connected to each remote recorder via communication channel. The remote device continuously reports raw signals, so it needs uninterrupted carrier availability, which makes the transmission cost very high.

Circular Memory Buffer (Chapter IX) is a signal buffer rewritten according to the pointer scanning perpetually all allocated memory. When new data arrives, the oldest value is first removed from the buffer and the new data is written in its place. This technique preserves the most recent signal strip for the calculation, and in the case of a multiple software update, the original signal is still available for calculation of the diagnostic results whose quality is being optimized.

Client Identification (Chapter VIII) procedures and access control serve as substantial tools for the service usage statistics. In the case of a payable subscription, access control may be considered as a first approach to the service's financial support.

Clinical Document Architecture (CDA) (Chapter IV) is an HL7 standard for the creation of clinical documents using XML (eXtensible Mark-up Language). XML uses non-printable characters within text documents to allow the computer system to process the text. The use of the bracket structure as <instruction> is the method of embedding instructions in the text.

Cognitive Process (Chapter V) is a sequence of logical reasoning and intuitive interpretation of perceived facts. The reasoning is usually alternated with the pursuit for additional data. The cognitive process cannot be objectively described by the subject itself, because the processes of tracking and verbalization are also cognitive processes concurrent with and influencing the process under investigation.

Commercial Tele-Diagnostic (Chapter IX) services in the United States and Europe offer the continuous monitoring of cardiac-risk patients. Such services typically use closed wireless networks of star topology. The interpretive intelligence aimed at the derivation of diagnostic features from recorded time series is implemented in the recorder or in the supervising server.

Communication Protocol (Chapter III) is a definition of data exchange rules between computers. Protocols are often subject to worldwide standards and must be implemented in a corresponding communication hardware.

Communication Standard is a collection of specific layers and implementations of corresponding protocols.

Compression Efficiency (Chapter VI) is measured as data volume ratio of the original signal and the compressed code. The denominator of this ratio should include all data necessary for a correct reconstruction of the original signal (look-up tables, etc.).

Computational Power (Chapter IX) is the measure of the microprocessor ability to perform computational (arythmetic, logic, etc.) operation in a given time unit. The computational power is usually expressed in number of instructions per second (Mips) or in number of floating point operations per second (Mflops) in the case of processors providing support for floating point arithmetics.

Control of Cardiovascular Function (Chapter III) is accomplished by two mechanisms: (1) inherent physicochemical attributes of the tissues and organs themselves (intrinsic control), and (2) attributes of the effects on cardiovascular tissues of other organ systems in the body—mainly the autonomic nervous system and the endocrine system (extrinsic control).

Controlling the Distortion (Chapter VI) is the approach to the lossy compression of the ECG that assumes the temporal variability of compression parameters allowing higher distortion in a medically less relevant part of a signal while preserving the most relevant sections undistorted.

Convergence (Chapter IX) represents the correctness of decisions made by the management procedure about the interpretation processing chain. If the software modification decisions are correct and the resulting outcome approaches the true value, the modification request signal is removed, thus decreasing error. Incorrect decisions lead to the growth of diagnostic outcome error and imply a stronger request for modification.

CSE Recommendations (Chapter II) on the precision of ECG waves delimitation may be found in the documents of the Common Standards for Quantitative Electrocardiography, a European organization that performed a 10-year worldwide project on the quality and repeatability of P, QRS, and T waves determination in the ECG by both cardiologists and computer software.

Custom Reporting Protocol (Chapter XI) is a proprietary open description of rules designed for non-uniform reporting between remote recorder and central server. This idea does not infringe on the interoperability issues, because the standard is flexible and designed for point-to-point communication between the elements of the network. The use of an existing standard of medical data interchange is restricted to regular reporting systems.

Data Bus (Chapter VII) is an inter-procedure information channel. Data busses are sorted by the value of expected throughput and by their priority level, meaning the degree of signal processing advancement. Each data flow was assigned a throughput level combining statistical parameters of the data: average datastream, frequency of usage, and probability of usage.

Datastream Reduction (Chapter VII) is a ratio of input datastream volume and output datastream volume estimated for each procedure. Most procedures have a significant data reduction ratio, therefore they are fed with a significant datastream and yield only sparse data. Putting the most reduction-effective procedures at the front of the processing chain reduces internal dataflow and resource requirements.

Decision Support Packages (Chapter IV) are elements of modern HIS implementations. They usually incorporate medical knowledge as rule sets to assist the care provider in the management of patients. A knowledge base system consists of a knowledge base and an inference engine. The knowledge base will contain the rules, frames, and statistics that are used by the inference applications to substantiate a decision.

Dependency Tree (Chapter IX) describes the dependency relation of each procedure and any other procedure in a form of aggregate variable (structure) built and updated each time the software is modified. The tree is specific for each procedure and may be generated automatically with the use of scanning the external calls in the source code. In the prototype system, the tree was fixed for each subroutine and written in the code description area.

Determination of Electrical Axes for Waves (Chapter II) is a process in which the electrical axis of a QRS vector helps estimate the correctness of stimulus conduction. If the conduction is affected by local necrosis of a heart wall tissue or by a bundle branch block, the heart axis has a permanently altered position, referred to as a right or left axis deviation.

Deterministic Sequential Machine (Chapter XI) is an automaton whose outputs being a partial description of its internal state are dependent uniquely of the inputs and the previous state. They assume that each change of the input could potentially influence the machine status and the output values.

Development in Computerized Cardiology (Chapter III) is currently made in three parallel and mutually dependent areas: medical methodology of the examination, recording electronic technology, and signal and data management and processing.

Diagnostic Data (Chapter VIII) are all the numerical values and string constants describing the final findings about patient status. Their form usually conform to human habits and standardization rules. Diagnostic data have the most concise form. The final decision is usually a binary choice.

Diagnostic Goal (Chapter V) is a set of diagnostic parameters confirming or contradicting a diagnostic hypothesis. The prevalence of diagnoses are hypothesis driven, and the particular information is expected to be provided by the diagnostic process.

Diastolic Phase (Chapter III) of the heart cycle is that the muscle is relaxed, the inlet valves of the two ventricles are open, and the outlet valves are closed. The heart ultimately expands to its end-diastolic-volume (EDV), which is on the order of 140 ml of blood for the left ventricle.

DICOM Services (Chapter IV) are embedded into a standard and involve transmission of data over a network; the file format is a later and relatively minor addition to the standard. Examples of DICOM services are: store, storage commitment, query/retrieve, modality worklist, modality performed procedure step, printing, and off-line media.

Digital Imaging and Communications in Medicine (DICOM) (Chapter IV) is a standard for handling, storing, printing, and transmitting information in medical imaging. It includes the definition of file format as well as the network communications protocol based on the TCP/IP standard. DICOM files can be exchanged between two entities that are capable of receiving image and patient data in DICOM format, also extensible to ECG signals.

Disease-Domain Sensitivity (Chapter XI) of an emergency detector is the ability to reliably detect patient status deterioration in a wide range of diagnostic states. In a perfect case the detector should provide an emergency alert with equal sensitivity and specificity for any signal change, representing patient status deterioration

Distributed Computing Design (Chapter X) assumes a process is initiated by one system and during the execution transferred to other system. The task sharing in the proposed network is always asymmetrical, therefore transfer of the process back to the remote recorder is inhibited.

Drug Dispenser (Chapter V) is a personal-use electronic device dispensing pharmaceuticals according to the prescription written as a program or controlled remotely. The use of drug dispensers is particularly beneficial in the case of elderly patients and provides better reliability than self-service by the patient.

Dynamically linked Libraries (Chapter V) are libraries of executable code that may be added (linked), removed, or commuted during the run of a calling procedure. Thanks to the uniform interface between the static and dynamic procedures, the commutation is as simple as redirection of the software area in the program memory.

ECG Interpretation Process (Chapter V) is a sequence of conditional computation steps aimed at deriving the quantitative diagnostic information from the digital signal representation. The composition of the interpretation process is dependent on the diagnostic goal. At several stages the interpretation process branches into data-dependent processing paths.

Electrocardiogram (Chapter II) is the paper or digital record of cardiac electrical activity. The ECG is recorded as a temporal representation of an electrical field resulting from the electrical activity of the heart muscle tissue at the cell level.

Electromagnetic Compatibility (EMC) (Chapter IX) describes the PED's ability to reduce the harm of other adjacent devices' functions and to be immune from environmental interference. Medical electronic devices should comply with the requirements of EMC since they may work in any unpredictable configuration; they should also guarantee the reliability of functionality and issued data.

Embedded Analysis (Chapter VIII) is the software providing the automated ECG interpretation programmed into a stand-alone ECG recorder by the manufacturer. The embedded analysis is usually tailored for an average client and consists of standard diagnostic procedures. The upgrade of embedded analysis is possible as a service procedure provided by the manufacturer or its representative.

Emergency Detector (Chapter XI) is a software procedure aimed at detection of patient status deterioration of any kind. The emergency detector must be computationally as simple as possible and provide a reliable trigger for a wide range of diagnostic states interpreted as patient status deterioration requiring detailed analysis.

Error Propagation (Chapter VII) is observed in any processing chain when subsequent procedures are using results of previous procedures as input data. These results are of limited reliability due to input signal uncertainty and the limited quality of computation algorithms. The value of expected error at the end of the processing chain cumulates the component errors along the processing chain.

Exercise Stress Test (Chapter II) is a 12-lead ECG + blood pressure rest phase (5 minutes) exercise protocol defining the applied workload during the stress phase recovery phase (up to 15 minutes).

Extended Connectivity (Chapter VIII) is the procedure enabling the cooperation of a stand-alone electrocardiograph with multiple method-specialized remote interpretation services, including data querying, process requests, and data exchange at various processing levels. Most current devices already have a basic network connectivity used only for electronic patient records.

Eyetracker (Chapter VI) or an eyetracking device is electronic equipment used to pursue and capture a sequence of eye globe positions. Eyetrackers use various physical principles: infrared light reflexes, electrical signal induced by the eye globe dipole, or video recording of the eye image.

FDA-Approved Device (Chapter II) is any medical device approved by U.S. Food and Drug Administration before being marketed. The FDA provides an Investigational Device Exemption (IDE) to allow interstate distribution of unapproved devices in order to conduct clinical research on human subjects.

Flags Area (Chapter IX) is the separate structure of binary variables representing the status of the interpretive library usage. The main flag is the "currently used" flag that reports the procedure is being used and stored in the system stack area. This inhibits the release or commutation of such procedure until the stack data are released and the program execution is returned from the procedure.

Flash Memory (Chapter V) is an electrically erasable and programmable memory providing fast access and high reprogrammation durability. Flash memory is constant memory in the sense that it does not have to be powered or refreshed to maintain the information. The flash memory is available as integrated circuits and also in a mobile standards like CompactFlash or Secure Digital Cards.

Functional-Growth Architecture (Chapter VII) is the most common diagram of internal procedures connection and dependencies within the ECG interpretation software originating from their version histories or the upgradeable modules concept. The advantage of such an approach is the usage of previously engineered modules, but the drawback lies in not considering the optimal dataflow and error propagation.

Half-Band Components (Chapter VI) are the output of an elementary step of binary tree-based signal decomposition. The components are the step-down signal approximation and the detail signal. Both have half the sample count and half the bandwidth of the original signal.

Heartbeat Clustering (Chapter II) is a single- or multipass procedure aimed at revealing the number and contribution of extra-sinus stimulators. The clusters are assumed to contain physiologically similar but not electrically identical heartbeats. The interest of the procedure consists of representation of the group of beats by a reference pattern on which the most time-consuming processing is done.

Heartbeat Detection Algorithm (Chapter II) is the mathematical method aimed at extraction of the heartbeats from the recorded ECG. Various techniques used to implement a QRS detector include: linear digital filters, nonlinear transformations, decision processes, and template matching.

Heart Rate Variability (Chapter II) is an RR-interval-based method of assessing physiologic and pathophysiologic mechanisms governing heart rate, and its oscillations are not only complex but also substantially irregular in their periodicity. The methods are divided into time domain and frequency domain. The time-domain methods are divided into statistical and graphical; the frequency-domain methods are divided into spectral (using FFT) and autoregressive (using ARMA models).

Heuristic Subroutine (Chapter VII) is a procedure engineered with regard to its output for input elements from the learning set of a known true value. Despite the application of very thorough testing procedures, no software engineer is able to foresee all possible signal recording conditions combined with all possible heart diseases. Heuristic procedures in the ECG interpretation chain show a non-zero probability of inappropriate processing and incorrect outcome.

High Variability (Chapter X) ECG parameters are diagnostic data showing the variability of order of the heart rate. Each parameter varying in a beat-to-beat interval belongs to this category. The exact limits of frequency range are hard to define since the physiological heart rate varies from 40 up to 210 beats per minute.

HL7 (Chapter IV), first created in 1987, is a protocol to create that common communication platform for healthcare computer systems that allows healthcare applications to share clinical data with each another. Its name refers to the application level of the OSI Basic Reference Model, since the protocol contains the definition of the data to be exchanged, the interchange timing, and the error messaging to the application.

Holter Monitoring (Chapter II) is an ambulatory 3- or 12-lead ECG using a portable recorder; typically 24-hour records are obtained, covering all sorts of daily routine activities including sleeping, waking up, and moderate exercise such as walking.

Hospital Information System (HIS) (Chapter VI) integrates patients and hospital information needs. Such systems must be able to provide global and departmental information on the state of the hospital. Current HISs support financial, administrative, and clinical data in order to provide specialized and task-oriented optimization tools, as well as materials for research in medical sciences.

Human Heart (Chapter III) is a muscular organ occupying a small region between the third and sixth ribs in the central portion of the thoracic cavity of the body. It is a unique organ propulsing the blood in the vascular system thanks to perpetual contraction. The heart is divided by a strong muscular wall—the interatrial-interventricular septum—into the right and left sides, each being a self-contained two-stage pumping device.

Human Relations (Chapter VIII) between cardiologists are all the applications of personal knowledge and interpersonal information exchange inspired by and resulting from the ECG interpretation process. Such relations may concern two humans of different skills or a team of coworkers (a consilium) aimed at collective interpretation of signal exchange or knowledge and education.

Hypothesis-Driven ECG Interpretation (Chapter XI) is usually performed by human experts and limits the diagnostic set to the most relevant results. A very general data analysis is a background for a hypothesis of the disease, and further diagnostic steps aim at confirming or denying this hypothesis.

Instantaneous Bandwidth Function (Chapter VI) is a time function describing local variability of the source in terms of expected bandwidth requirements for transmitting the signal undistorted. In the uniformly sampled ECG, the components using full bandwidth provided by the Shannon rule of sampling are relatively rare and the instantaneous bandwidth is significantly lower for the majority of signal.

International Organization for Standardization (ISO) (Chapter IV) is a worldwide federation of national standards organizations. It has 90 member countries. The purpose of ISO is to promote the development of standardization and related activities in the world. ANSI was one of the founding members of ISO and represents the United States.

International Standard IEC 60601-2-51 (Chapter II) specifies the testing range and conditions, as well as requirements for results provided by the automatic analysis embedded in the electrocardiographs or released as independent software packages. Requirements for amplitude measurements and for interval measurements are specified on analytical and biological signals. For the latter, the CSE database is indicated as a source of test signal.

Internet Reference Model (Chapter III) is a layered abstract description for communications and computer network protocol design. The five layers of TCP/IP are: the application layer (topmost), the transport layer, the network layer, the data link layer, and the physical layer.

Interoperability (Chapter IV) is the term describing the ability of a medical device to cooperate in a technical environment built of components from different manufacturers. Interoperability between medical devices and between host systems is a key requirement for the establishment of the electronic patient health record.

Interpretation Task Sharing (Chapter IX) is the set of software management rules describing the optimum assignment of the ECG interpretation tasks between two elements of the distributed system: the remote recorder which acquires the signal and starts the interpretation, and the central server which is responsible for issuing the diagnostic result.

Interpretation Trigger (Chapter XI) is an asynchronous event initiating the ECG interpretation process. The proposed system assumes two such events: patient status deterioration and expiry of validity period for diagnostic data.

Irregular Reporting (Chapter X) is the remote recorder operating mode characterized by irregular time intervals between consecutive reports. Irregular reporting may be a consequence of adaptive processing or may be programmed independently.

Knowledge Base Similarity Check (Chapter IX) is the method of automatic assessment of result reliability which uses diagnostic data and is performed for every received data packet. Each time a new packet arrives, the central server accesses the database for verifying the consistency of the received data by comparing it to the most similar database record and for estimating the trends of diagnostic parameters from changes observed in similar records.

Knowledge Space (KS) (Chapter VIII) is an information structure that integrates the signal with medical annotations as well as the information technology-based methods of data interpretation. KS is accessible to a wide range of medical researchers over the Internet. As a conventional database, the KS service contains downloadable reference ECG data, however its main advantage is to offer a choice of the most recent interpretation methods.

Lead Systems (Chapter II) relate to the electrical activity of the heart, which can be approximated by a time-variant electrical dipole, called the electrical heart vector (EHV). The voltage measured at a given lead is the projection of the EHV into the unitary vector defined by the lead axis. The lead set most widely used in clinical practice is the standard 12-lead system.

Levels of Software Adaptation (Chapter IX) quantitatively describe the interference of the management procedure into the ECG interpretation process. According to the adaptation level, various kinds of programming technology are used to achieve the adaptation aim.

Local Area Network (LAN) (Chapter III) topology is the layout of networking segments and their interconnections by devices such as repeaters, bridges, and routers. LANs, instead of the traditional point-to-point connections, have become the primary medium for computer communication at healthcare practice centers to the extent that all new computers are expected to be LAN compatible.

Local Conspicuity (Chapter VI) is the feature of the scene determining how attractive its particular fragment to the potential observer is. The values of local conspicuity measured for each point of the image forms the conspicuity layer over the visual content of the image. The correlation of the visual content and its conspicuity is considered by visual research.

Longitudinal Record (Chapter IV) may contain either a complete clinical record of the patient or only those variables that are most critical in subsequent admissions. In modern systems of high-capacity storage resources, the structure of the longitudinal file contained information regarding the encounter, admitting physician, and any other information that may be necessary to view the record from an encounter view or as a complete clinical history of the patient.

Lossy and Lossless (Chapter VI) methods concern data compression. Lossless methods guarantee the identity of digital representations for original signals and their reconstructed copy. Despite the common belief, lossless compression methods represent a continuous real signal when it results from the digitizing parameters. Lossless compression is featured at a cost of considerably lower compression efficiency and in many countries is the only legal way for storing medical data.

Low Variability (Chapter X) ECG parameters are diagnostic data showing the variability lower than a few consecutive heartbeats. The values are usually measured in epochs of the length ranging from 20 seconds up to 10 minutes.

Master Patient Index (MPI) (Chapter IV) contains the unique identifier for the patient and other entries necessary for the admitting staff to identify the patient (name, sex, birth date, social security number). This information is used by the program to select potential patient matches in the MPI from which the administration can link to the current admission.

Medical Waveform Format Encoding Rules (MFERs) (Chapter IV) are used for storage of any waveforms in temporal frames. Thus their major components are sampling information and frame information. The definitions of MFER are classified into three levels: level 1 is basic specification, level 2 is extended specification, and level 3 is auxiliary specification. MFER applies data encoding rules for maximum format flexibility.

Medium Variability (Chapter X) ECG parameters are diagnostic data showing the variability of order of several consecutive heartbeats. These parameters are usually measured in a beat-to-beat interval but then are averaged over a specified beat count or specified time interval.

Metadata (Chapter VIII) are all intermediate results yielded by interpretation procedures. Metadata are characterized by free data-forms, dependent only upon the requirements of the interfaced procedures, limited reliability, and average dataflow and volume. Metadata are usually not readable by humans.

Minnesota Code Classification System (Chapter IV) for Electrocardiographic Findings is a list of one- to three-digit codes attributed to the record as a diagnostic outcome according to a tree of finding relevance.

Modalities in Cardiology (Chapter IV) include various examination techniques based on different phenomena triggering the action, directly included in the action, resulting from the action, or accompanying the action of the heart.

Modulation of Remote Recorder Functionality (Chapter IX) is performed by the software and consists of deep modification of the external behavior (accessible via user interface) and the internal functionality (e.g., software architecture). The software modulation functionality is particularly interesting in a remote mode when the supervising server modifies the interpretive procedures on the run according to changes in patient status.

Modulation of Report Content (Chapter X) uses a flexible data report format, including raw signal strips, metadata, and diagnostic parameters. It may consist of inclusion or exclusion of automatically selected parameters, attributing the parameters with priority and validity period parameters, and/or continuous regular reporting.

Multimedia Communications (Chapter III) are technologies and standards ranging from application-specific digital signal processors and video chip sets to videophones and multimedia terminals, and relying on digital signal processing. Biomedical signals are integrated with other patient information and transmitted via networked multimedia.

Multithreading Operating System (Chapter V) is an operating system that allows the sharing of resources in a way to perform several independent tasks at the same time. The multithreading OS can also have multi-user access, and therefore an independent instance of the ECG interpretation process may run for each user, supporting cooperation with a corresponding remote recorder.

Non-Uniform Reporting (Chapter X) is the remote recorder operating mode characterized by irregular time intervals between consecutive reports and variable contents from one report to another. The non-uniform reporting best optimizes the use of a transmission channel if the processing is patient adaptive, but it also requires more computational power for the management of the contents of data packets.

OpenECG (Chapter IV) is a European-funded initiative with global reach, aiming to lower the barriers for seamless integration of ECG devices in e-health services and electronic health record systems. The means the consortium is achieving its goals of promoting ECG interoperability standards, providing input on global trends and developments, and ensuring conformance testing services addresses ECG records and electrocardiographs.

Optimal Patient Description (Chapter V) is a set of diagnostic parameters most wanted in the current patient state. In a technical implementation, for every possible patient state there is a list of mandatory, desirable, and optional diagnostic parameters with the attributes of priority, tolerance of value, and validity time.

OSI Basic Reference Model (Chapter III) is a layered, abstract description for communications and computer network protocol design. The seven OSI layers are, from top to bottom: application, presentation, session, transport, network, data link, and physical. A layer is referred to as a collection of related functions that provides services to the layer above it and receives service from the layer below it.

Pacemaker (Chapter VII) is an implantable electronic device generating pacing pulse for the heart. Pacemakers today have a wide adaptivity thanks to the embedded microprocessor programmed according to the patient's needs. Long-term recording is a valuable tool in assessing pacemaker malfunction due to electronic circuit failures or inappropriate programming.

Patient Health Record (Chapter IV) is a description of all parameters necessary to identify the patient and reveal his or her diagnostic data. PHRs are currently stored in digital databases and are printed in paper form when the patient is discharged. The electronic form of a PHR is the condition of applying automatic data management, storage, and retrieval systems.

Percent Root-Mean-Square Difference (PRD) (Chapter VI) is one of the most common distortion estimators, despite it is not reflecting the variability of signal importance in medical examinations. Such a technical parameter is therefore hardly interpretable in terms of medical diagnosis.

Perfect Reconstruction Property (Chapter VI) is the feature of a reversible signal transform (here referred to as a time-frequency transform) that yields a bit-accurate digital signal and originates from the combination of the forward and inverse transforms. The perfect reconstruction property is necessary in lossless data compression methods, but here is important to guarantee that all the changes in the output signal result from the manipulations in the time-frequency domain.

Personal Cardiac Prevention Program (Chapter V) is a preventive healthcare procedure ordered to healthy people individually in order to reduce their risk of cardiac diseases by change in diet, lifestyle, and medication.

Physiological Stimulation (Chapter II) is defined as when, in a physiological case, a heartbeat is electrically initialized by a group of cells located in the upper part of the right atrium, known as sinoatrial node (SA), having the ability of spontaneous discharge.

Raw Signal (Chapter VIII) is unprocessed digital representation of electrical measurements of the surface ECG and synchronous other phenomena (respiration, blood pressure, patient motion, oxygen saturation, acoustic, and many others). Various data-types follow their proper technical specification of measurement (sampling frequency, amplitude scale, etc.).

Read-Only Memory (ROM) (Chapter IX) is the section of the system memory for storage of the executable code. The name is justified because it is opposite the random access memory (or data memory); the software itself reads the code and does not use the program memory as storage space for variables. Nevertheless, using flash technology, the ROM may be rewritten multiple times by an external procedure.

Recipient Request (Chapter XI) is a data query present in a transfer mode initiated by a data recipient and not by a data source. The recipient request usually also triggers several calculation procedures in order to update the data whose validity expired.

Redundant Signal Re-Interpretation (Chapter IX) is the method of automatic assessment of result reliability that uses bi-directional transmission and begins with the raw signal request issued by the central server. The remote recorder does the interpretation independently, and besides the diagnostic result, returns the raw electrocardiogram as well.

Refractory Period (Chapter II) (approximately 200 ms) represents the biologically possible minimum interval between two heartbeats. After the depolarization the cells are not immediately able to receive or transmit new electrical stimuli. Consequently, the stimulation wavefront dies down after achieving the latter cell of the heart muscle tissue.

Relevance Coefficients (Chapter V) are numerical values determining the medical significance of the corresponding diagnostic parameter with reference to a given scale. The relevance sets the ordering relation translating the set of diagnostic parameters to a prioritized list. The list contains the most important parameters at its beginning and the least meaningful data at its end.

Report Content Optimization (Chapter XI) is a computational process of "reservation" space in the nearest report for irregularly appearing data. The optimization selects between two contradictory criteria: calculate each diagnostic parameter as late as possible and fill the data packet by the values within their validity periods.

Reporting Frequency (Chapter IX) is the frequency that data packets with particular content are sent by the remote recorder. This frequency can be set as constant and common for all the data, can be controlled by the server according to the patient status, and can be independently set for each diagnostic parameter. Continuous reporting is a real-time variant of constant reporting in which the remote recorder issues only basic diagnostic parameters and raw signal.

Resources Report (Chapter IX) is included in the remote device status word or independent record pooled by the server-issued request. The resources report contains a few variables representing battery use and status, ambient temperature, connection quality, processor usage, memory allocation, and codes of linked libraries. Receipt of this information is for the server a background for the estimation of available resources and software modification.

Rest ECG (Chapter II) is a 12-lead short-time recording of simultaneous ECG leads in a lying-down position.

Rigid Software (Chapter V) is the sequence of determined calculation procedures of the architecture and data flow defined uniformly for all data. The software is usually required to provide predictable results and thus the common definition of its behavior guarantees the unique dependence of the process state (partly manifested at its output) on the inputs and the previous state.

Scan-Path (Chapter VI) is the visual representation of the eyeglobe trajectory acquired during the investigated human-performed visual task. The superposition of the scan-path over a displayed scene reveals the zones of particular interest represented by the gaze time and the visual strategy of the observer represented by the order of gazing.

SCP Compliance Testing (Chapter IV) identifies the records resembling the SCP specifications; compliance testing is necessary. The compliance tests cover the following areas: the content of the record, the format and structure of the record, and the messaging mechanisms if records are communicated according to the SCP specifications.

Serial Communication Protocol ECG (Chapter IV) is a standard specifying the interchange format and a messaging procedure for ECG cart-to-host communication and for retrieval of SCP-ECG records from the host (to the ECG cart). In 1993 the Standard Communication Protocol was approved by CEN as a pre-standard ENV 1064. The SCP standard specifies that the information be structured in mandatory and optional sections.

Shannon Theorem (Chapter XI) is a basic theorem of the signal theory restricting the bandwidth of digital signal representation to a half of the sampling frequency.

Signal Decomposition (Chapter VI) is the representation of the digitized time series by the coefficients of the analytical function family. In the case of the Fourier Transform, such analytical function is a unitary spiral in the complex domain. In the case of wavelet transform, the role of analytical functions play wavelets of different scale and dilation values.

Signal Quality Assessment (Chapter VII) is an automated procedure working on the raw signal aiming at detecting the features of the desired signal and the features of the most probable interferences in order to compare them. The procedure issues a signal quality estimate, which is a background for optimization of channel information use in the ECG and for assessment of the reliability of diagnostic outcome.

Signal Quality Verification (Chapter VIII) is an initial step of the ECG signal processing by the subscriber service. Its purpose is to correct estimation of diagnostic outcome reliability, since in the case of weak amplitude, noisy signals, spikes, or baseline wander, the analysis may end with incorrect results. Suspicious input signals are identified, and a warning message is issued together with the diagnostic outcome.

Sinoatrial (SA) Node (Chapter II) is a neuromuscular tissue in the right atrium near where the superior vena cava joins the posterior right atrium (the sinus venarum); the SA node generates electrical impulses that initiate the heartbeat, hence its nickname the cardiac "pacemaker."

Social Impact of Cardiovascular Disease (Chapter III) manifests itself as the leader on the list of most frequent mortality causes. In other words, for many years in the United States and other developed countries, cardiovascular diseases have been the most frequent cause of death. This fact garners great attention from researchers and also considerable funds for the prevention, diagnosis, therapy, and prosthetic of cardiology.

Software Layers (Chapter IX) are defined in the remote recorder in order to distinguish the unalterable modules: data acquisition and wireless communication services as well as fundamental user interface procedures and the flexible overlay

include all interpretation and report formatting procedures programmed as diagnosis-oriented dynamic libraries, which may be charged and released upon request.

Specialized Interpretation Centers (Chapter VIII) are in a computer network the analogy to regional or national specialists and are realized as Unix-based multitask and multi-user servers scaled to the estimated demand for particular interpretation tasks. In particular, each heart disease may be supported by several physical interpretation nodes using independent interpretation methods and located in different parts of the world.

Spread Intelligence (Chapter IX) ECG interpretation model assumes that the recording device interprets the signal and issues an alert message in case of abnormalities. Although the *spread* interpretation *intelligence* reduces communication costs, the diagnostic quality is affected due to resource limitations typical to a wearable computer.

Standardization of Data (Chapter IX) is the process of preparing two sets of non-uniformly reported data for comparison. The standardization is also necessary when a non-uniform result of an adaptive interpretation system is to be compared to a uniform reference. As a data standardization tool, we used the cubic spline interpolation.

Standardized Interpretation Criteria (Chapter IX) are interpretation guidelines and parameter threshold values formulated by the professional organizations of medics. The criteria are uniform for all patients, regardless of diagnostic goals and patient status, and are believed optimal for the most expected patient.

ST Segment Analysis (Chapter II) is the analysis of the ST segment, which represents the period of the ECG just after depolarization, the QRS complex, and just before repolarization, the T wave. The possible abnormalities include displacements of the ST segment either above the isoelectric line (elevation) or below it (depression), and reflect metabolism and oxygenation disorders in the cells heart muscle tissue.

Subscriber Service (Chapter V) is a payable data processing task performed for a limited group of registered users by the remote center, and ordered and accounted for via the computer network. The subscription is based on a given period or given credit of a financial nature. The ECG interpretation processes may also be implemented as subscriber services of territorially unlimited range.

Subscriber Service Supervision (Chapter VIII) is provided to control the automated interpretation process in both medical and technical ways by the medical expert assistant and server administration. Help from a qualified cardiologist is crucial at the prototyping stage, because he or she not only resolves conflicts or misinterpretations, but also gathers and qualifies information on errors.

Support Compact (Chapter VI) is a support of the analytical function that is equal to zero except for a single compartment of a countable number of samples. The transformations using the support compact are designed similarly to digital filters and are able to represent the signal in a lossless way in a finite number of coefficients in the transformation domain.

Systolic Phase (Chapter III) of the heart cycle is the electrically induced vigorous contraction of cardiac muscle which drives the intraventricular pressure up, forcing the one-way inlet valves closed and the unidirectional outlet valves open as the heart contracts to its end-systolic-volume (ESV), which is typically on the order of 70 ml of blood for the left ventricle.

Temporal Distortions' Distribution (Chapter VI) is a time function of statistical difference measure between the original and the distorted signal. The distortion distribution is a much more elegant and meaningful way of compression quality estimation than a commonly used global coefficient like PRD.

Usability (Chapter IX) of a wearable recorder is understood as the influence of the device on the patient's comfort. Low usability, difficult maintenance, complicated operation, or continuous attention requirement will lower the acceptance of the recorder by the patient and leads to the failure of continuous surveillance.

Usage Probability (Chapter VII) is the estimator of frequency of calling of a particular procedure. Some procedures are mandatorily called, while others are called in very rare cases of specific diseases. Since the processing chain is switched conditionally on the metadata, the usage probability varies with the patient status. The usage probability is used for estimating the contribution of a procedure quality coefficient to a global quality coefficient of the software.

Validity Time (Chapter V) is for a diagnostic parameter the longest period in which the value should be updated in order to maintain continuity. The validity time is longer for diagnostic parameters of lower expected variability or bandwidth.

Vulnerability of Medical Data (Chapter VI) is the parameter referring to the change in manually derived or automatically calculated diagnostic outcomes as a response to the ECG signal distortion.

Wave Detection and Delimitation (Chapter II) relate to the three main waves in the heart evolution, whose temporal order is P, QRS, and T, following the consequent action of a single isolated stimulus propagating through the heart. Primary ECG diagnostic parameters are based on temporal dependencies between the waves, here representing the conduction of stimulus through a specified tissue or contraction of muscle.

Wearable ECG Recorders (Chapter IX) are electronic devices designed for digitally recording the ECG signal from the body surface that are small enough and lightweight enough to be worn continuously by the patient without affecting his or her usual behavior. The principal advantage of wearable recorders is that their seamless companionship in the everyday activity increases the probability of capturing the context of sudden events.

Wide Area Networks (WANs) (Chapter III) are applied by healthcare centers to connect networks at physically distant buildings, offices, clinics, or with different organizations. Recently data interconnections through WANs have exploded among care facilities, private physicians' offices, nursing homes, insurance agencies, health maintenance organizations, research institutions, and state and federal regulatory agencies.

Wireless Communication (Chapter IIII) uses different technologies depending on required bandwidth, range, and acceptable costs. These technologies include: WiFi, connecting a wireless local area network to the wide area network; WiMAX, providing wireless data over long distances in a variety of ways, from point-to-point links to full mobile cellular type access; and GPRS, a packet-switched GSM protocol allowing multiple users to share the same transmission channel.

About the Authors

Professor Ryszard Tadeusiewicz studied at the Electrical Engineering Department of the University of Mining and Metallurgy in Krakow (Poland) from which he graduated (with honors) in 1971. Additionally, after receiving his degree in Automatic Control Engineering, he studied at the Faculty of Medicine at the Medical Academy in Krakow, as well as undertook studies in the field of mathematical and computer methods in economics. He has written and published over 600 scientific papers, which were published in prestigious Polish and foreign scientific journals as well as numerous conference presentations - both national and international. Prof. Tadeusiewicz also wrote over 70 scientific monographs and books, among them are highly popular textbooks (which had many reprints). He was supervisor of 54 doctoral thesis and reviewer of more than 200 doctoral thesis. In 2003 Polish scientists elected him to be President of IEEE Computational Intelligence Society – Polish Chapter.

Piotr Augustyniak was born in Krakow, Poland in 1965. He graduated in 1989 in electronic engineering and received the PhD degree in electronics (1995, with honors) and DSc (habilitation) in automatics (2004) all from the Electrical Engineering Department AGH-University of Science and Technology, Krakow. Since 1989 he works at the Institute of Automatics AGH-UST, Krakow, as research engineer, since 1995 as assistant-professor and since 2007 as associate professor. He worked also at Aspel SA, the Poland-biggest manufacturer of ECG equipment as research engineer. His scientific interests include hardware and software problems of biosignal processing, currently he is working on perceptual model of electrocardiogram and data-dependent signal representation. He prototyped four acquisition and analysis systems for electrocardiography, electrooculography and electroencephalography. He published three books on electrodiagnostic signal processing, over 110 journal and conference papers and was a reviewer and program committee member of many international conferences. Prof. Augustyniak is a member of the *Institute of Electrical and Electronics Engineers*, *International Society of Electrocardiology* and of the *Computers in Cardiology Society*.

* * * * *

Prof Peter Macfarlane (DSc FRCP(Glasg) FESC FRSE, Professor of Electrocardiology) came to work in the Royal Infirmary over 35 years ago and was a founding member of the University of Glasgow Department of Medical Cardiology which was created shortly after he arrived. His major interest throughout has been the application of computer techniques to ECG interpretation. His work has been adopted commercially and applied world-wide. He has established an ECG Core Laboratory for handling ECGs recorded in national and international clinical trials and epidemiological studies. He is a Fellow of the British Computer Society, the Royal College of Physicians of Glasgow, the European Society of Cardiology and the Royal Society of Edinburgh. He is currently President of the International Society of Electrocardiology. He was awarded a D.Sc. on the basis of his contribution to research in his own field. He was also jointly awarded the 1998 Rijlant International Prize in Electrocardiology by the Belgian Royal Academy of Medicine. He currently directs an 8 strong group who work on various aspects of computer assisted reporting of ECGs (CARE) and Clinical Trials. His research interests are:

- Electrocardiography
  The ECG Group has pioneered many techniques related to computer analysis of electrocardiograms. Among these are the use of neural networks for ECG interpretation, automated methods of serial ECG comparison, extensive use of age, sex, clinical history and medical therapy in automated ECG reporting among other things. The Group has also established large databases of normal ECG measurements which are of immense value in the development of new electrocardiographic criteria. Developments are in hand to extend these normal limits to other ethnic groups.
  Recent work has included optimising age/sex based criteria for acute myocardial infarction. The new ESC/AHA/ACC universal defintion of myocardial infarction has included sex based ECG criteria for acute MI based on the work in Glasgow.

The Group has extensive commercial collaboration with Burdick, a Cardiac Science company,and PhysioControl, Heartlab (Agfa), Medcon (McKesson), Draeger Medical and Spacelabs Healthcare as well as a number of other companies (Epiphany Cardiology, Cardiolex, Schmidt GmbH).

- ECG Core Laboratory
  The Department has established an internationally recognised Core Lab for the management of ECGs recorded as part of national and international clinical trials as well as major epidemiological studies. A facility for undertaking Minnesota Coding and automated serial comparison is in routine use. Essentially this development arose from handling ECGs in the West of Scotland Coronary Prevention Study (WOSCOPS) from which many interesting electrocardiographic observations have arisen, particularly in relation to risk factors for ischaemic heart disease. The most recent WOSCOPS publication appeared in the New England Journal of Medicine in October 2007. Currently the Core Lab handles the ECGs from the following studies:
- Whitehall II (Phase 9)
- AIRWAVE
- MRC 1946 Study
- Scottish Family Health Study

Collaborative work continues with

- PROSPER
- British Regional Heart Study
- Graphic Study
- Newcastle over 85
- Leiden 85+

Index

A

B

C

D

E

F

G

K

L

O

P

Q

R

S

T

U

V

W

X

Z